MEDICAL ETHICS AT
NOTRE DAME

Library of Congress Control Number: 2007909576
BookSurge Publishing
North Charleston, South Carolina

ISBN/EAN: 9781419684463

MEDICAL ETHICS AT NOTRE DAME

THE J. PHILIP CLARKE FAMILY LECTURES

1988– 1999

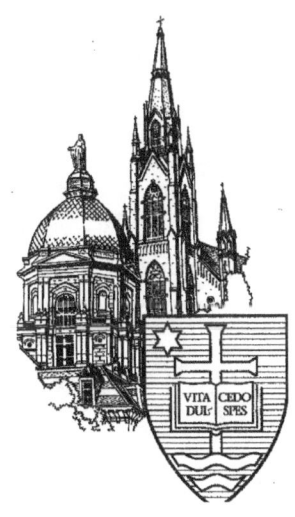

VITA DUL CEDO SPES

EDITED BY MARGARET MONAHAN HOGAN
AND DAVID SOLOMON

THE NOTRE DAME CENTER FOR ETHICS AND CULTURE

2008

CONTENTS

CONTRIBUTORS

REV. JAMES BRESNAHAN, S.J., J.D., LL.M., PH.D.
*Professor Emeritus of Medical Ethics and Humanities at
Northwestern University Medical School*

DANIEL CALLAHAN, PH.D.
Director of International Programs at the Hastings Center

CHARLES J. DOUGHERTY, PH.D.
President, Duquesne University

H. TRISTRAM ENGELHARDT, JR., M.D., PH.D.
*Professor in the Department of Medicine at Baylor College of
Medicine and Professor in the Department of Philosophy at Rice
University*

JORGE L.A. GARCIA, PH.D.
Professor of Philosophy at Boston College

STANLEY HAUERWAS, PH.D.
*The Gilbert T. Rowe Professor of Theological Ethics at the Divinity
School of Duke University*

REV. RICHARD A. MCCORMICK, S.J., PH.D.
*Late the John A. O'brien Professor of Christian Ethics at the
University of Notre Dame*

GILBERT MEILAENDER, PH.D.
*Richard & Phyllis Duesenberg Professor of Christian Ethics at
Valparaiso University*

THE HONORABLE JOHN T. NOONAN, JR., PH.D., J.D.
United States Court of Appeals for the Ninth Circuit

i

EDMUND D. PELLEGRINO, M.D., M.A.C.P.
*Chairman of the President's Council on Bioethics and
Professor Emeritus of Medicine and Medical Ethics and Adjunct
Professor of Philosophy at Georgetown University.*

MARK SIEGLER, M.D., F.A.C.P.
*The Lindy Bergman Professor of Medicine and Surgery and
Director of the Maclean Center for Clinical Medical Ethics at the
University of Chicago*

RESPONDENTS

MICHAEL J. BAXTER, PH.D.
Associate Visiting Professional Specialist in the Department of Theology at the University of Notre Dame

MARGARET MONAHAN HOGAN, PH.D.
Mcnerny-hanson Professor of Ethics and Executive Director of the Garaventa Center for Catholic Intellectual Life and American Culture at the University of Portland

JOSEPH M. INCANDELA, PH.D.
Joyce Mcmahon Hank Aquinas Chair in Cathoic Theology, Associate Dean, and Professor of Religious Studies at Saint Mary's College, Notre Dame

M. CATHLEEN KAVENY, PH.D., J.D.
John P. Murphy Professor of Law and Theology at the University of Notre Dame

KEVIN MCDONNELL, PH.D.
Edna and George Mcmahon Aquinas Professor in Philosophy at Saint Mary's College, Notre Dame

JOHN H. ROBINSON, J.D., PH.D.
Associate Professor of Law and Executive Associate Dean of the Law School at the University of Notre Dame

MAURA A. RYAN, PH.D.
The John Cardinal O'hara, C.s.c Associate Professor of Theology at the University of Notre Dame

DAVID SOLOMON, PH.D.
Associate Professor of Philosophy and W. P. and H. B. White
Director of the Notre Dame Center for Ethics and Culture

PAUL J. WEITHMAN, PH.D.
Professor of Philosophy at the University of Notre Dame

TODD D. WHITMORE, PH.D.
Associate Professor of Theology and Director of the Program in the
Catholic Social Tradition at the University of Notre Dame

PREFACE

Medical ethics is a very young field; just forty years ago, medical ethics as practiced and discussed today did not even exist. Now, however, issues in medical ethics dominate newspaper headlines and political campaigns. Despite the intense public focus on issues such as abortion and euthanasia, health care reform and stem cell research, Catholic and more broadly Christian teaching on these matters is often suppressed and overshadowed by the secular approaches of contemporary mainstream culture. The result is that many of those who seek advice and direction from the field of medical ethics and who hope for guidance that is more substantive and aligned with a broadly Christian ethical outlook are often at a loss. We at the Notre Dame Center for Ethics and Culture believe that the Catholic tradition in medical ethics provides splendid resources for articulating the new direction in which medical ethics should move. Indeed, we are confident that this rich Catholic tradition can provide guidance in confronting the most dramatic life and death issues, but also in dealing with the more hum-drum ethical challenges that confront the everyday medical practitioner.

The aim of the Notre Dame Medical Ethics Conference, which will celebrate its twenty fourth anniversary in March, 2009, has been from its inception to carry this message into the heart of medical ethics while engaging other traditions and views. Those who founded the conference also hoped to transform the field of medical ethics both as it is taught in colleges and universities and as it is practiced in health care institutions and serves to advise policy makers. Although the conference focuses on what the broad Catholic tradition offers to contemporary medical ethics, those who organize the conference have always welcomed diverse opinions at the conference and invited to the conference specialists in medical ethics from other religious traditions and viewpoints. Genuine dialogue and respectful and civil disagreement have always been the hallmarks of the conference.

While case discussion among physicians, theologians, and philosophers is the main activity at the conference, its centerpiece is the annual Clarke Family Lecture. In this volume you will find a collection of the Clarke lectures from the earliest years of the conference and commentaries on them. Both the lectures and the commentaries are authored by some of the most distinguished physicians, theologians, philosophers and jurists working in medical ethics today. Although some of these lectures were given twenty years ago or more, their message is as fresh as the day it was first presented to the audience. The underlying themes of respecting life and caring for the ill and the dying are permanent features of medicine and reflection on these themes never grows stale. The perspectives that these speakers and their commentators bring to the issues emerge from a long tradition of Christian reflection on these matters. Some of the lectures make reference to events contemporaneous with their delivery but which have now begun to recede into history. We have not edited out these references because we hope to retain the sense of occasion on which these lectures were given. For the same reason we have also left informal asides and locutions in the text of these lectures that might seem out of place in a more formal academic paper. These lectures always involved quite direct communication between distinguished scholars in medical ethics and practicing physicians and other health care workers in the audience. We have tried to preserve where possible the intimacy of that communication.

The Clarke Lecture Series and the Notre Dame Medical Ethics Conference that has housed that series both owe their existence to the creativity, generosity and commitment of a single individual, Dr. Philip J. Clarke, a distinguished physician and former Dean of the Medical School at the University of Colorado. Dr. Clarke was also a loyal and much honored alumnus of the University of Notre Dame as well as a dedicated and devout Catholic layman. Dr. Clarke's good friend and former patient, Father James Bresnahan, S.J., reflects on the special gifts of Dr. Clarke in the foreword to this volume. As he neared the end of his own very successful career in medicine, Dr. Clarke's deepest wish was that Notre Dame could found a conference where practicing Catholic physicians, Notre Dame undergraduates (especially pre-medical students), and distinguished scholars in medical ethics could meet and discuss in a cordial manner the deepest issues in contemporary medicine. Dr. Clarke saw clearly that modern medicine was both the conduit of many of the greatest benefits of modern scientific culture, but also of many of its greatest dangers. He saw that when medicine was practiced by virtuous and caring physicians in settings governed by genuine justice and charity, it contributed greatly to human well-being. When the powers of modern medicine were in thrall to money or to a Faustian desire for technological domination, however, they became a great threat to human decency. Dr. Clarke contributed financial support in his own name and in that of his family to initiate this lecture series and, while he was still alive, he participated actively in the selection of each of the Clarke Lecturers. It was a great honor for those of us who knew Phil Clarke to work with him and to be the beneficiary of his wisdom and kindness. This volume of essays should be seen as a token of our respect for him and for his memory.

There are many others, of course, to thank for their contributions to this volume, and the first of those must be the lecturers and commentators themselves. Their papers are truly wonderful. They stimulated much discussion throughout the conferences at which they were presented. Some have been privately circulated in the years since they were delivered and, in that form, have been widely influential. Now that they appear between the covers of a book, we hope their influence will only be increased and the number of their readers multiplied. The speakers were honored by applause at the conclusion of their presentations, and this volume will, I hope, awaken its echo in all who read their papers.

The single individual most responsible for bringing this volume to the press is Prof. Margaret Monahan Hogan, the McNerney-Hanson Chair in Ethics at the University of Portland and the Executive Director of the Garaventa Center for Catholic Intellectual Life and American Culture. Prof. Hogan transcribed the earliest talks, edited the later ones, arranged for and edited the commentaries, and worked tirelessly to see this volume through the editorial process. Her sanctity is surely assured by the patience with which she prodded her co-editor to complete his part of the job. In this volume she comments on Judge John Noonan's lecture and she later (2006) gave the Clarke Lecture herself , reminding her audience of some timeless truths about the respect due to life at its earliest stages. I am deeply indebted to Prof. Hogan for everything she did during her fellowship year spent at the Notre Dame Center for Ethics and Culture and in the following years working on this volume. Prof. Hogan was instrumental in bringing the Center for Ethics and Culture to its current prominence and has in more recent years brought her energy and insight to the University of Portland where she has made the Garaventa Center one of the most exciting and dynamic ethics centers in the country. This volume would not exist in its present form but for her diligent work.

The medical ethics conference that housed these lectures has been organized for many years jointly by the Center for Ethics and Culture and Notre Dame's Alumni Association. At the time of the lectures in this volume, Chuck Lennon directed the Alumni Association and Kathleen Sullivan, Ph.D. was the director of Alumni Continuing Education. Both, along with the Associate Director of Alumni Continuing Education, Judy Gibson, and her assistant, Jan Miller, worked tirelessly in support of the Conference and the Lecture Series. Dr. Clarke had great affection for the Notre Dame Alumni Association and was always extraordinarily grateful that it had been willing to take the organizational lead in making the medical ethics conference he envisioned a reality. A long succession of student assistants at the

Notre Dame Center for Ethics and Culture also played significant roles in making the Notre Dame Medical Ethics Conference and the Clarke Lecture Series possible. Megan Collins (now Megan Collins, M.D.) was for many years the organizational spark plug of the conference. She was succeeded by Margaret Watkins, Jennie Bradley, Cheryl Overmeyer, Mark Jensen, Katie Freddoso and, most recently, Karen Chan. The work of all of these student assistants was not only consistently of a very high quality, but they also lent a youthful quality and exuberance to the conference proceedings. I am extremely grateful for their dedication and hard work.

Finally, when the firm decision was made to bring this book to press, a long-time friend of the conference and great personal friend of mine, Prof. Kevin McDonnell, the Edna and George McMahon Chair of Philosophy at St. Mary's College, stepped forward to cut through a number of obstacles. He reformatted the texts, did re-editing were necessary, explored various publishing venues and encouraged others to do their best to bring this volume to completion. In pursuing all these tasks, he has earned the sincere gratitude of the many contributors to this volume. Kevin McDonnell is himself a distinguished and widely admired scholar of medical ethics, and he took valuable time away from his other scholarly endeavors to assist the two editors of this volume to complete this project. We thank him for that.

Dr. Clarke's firm desire was that the wisdom distilled in the Clarke Lectures would transform the medical practice of those students, physicians and other health care workers who were present in McKenna Hall at Notre Dame when they were presented. We are confident that he would have thoroughly approved of the project of making that wisdom more widely available through the publication of this volume.

David Solomon
January, 2009

DEDICATION

Dr. and Mrs. J. Philip Clarke

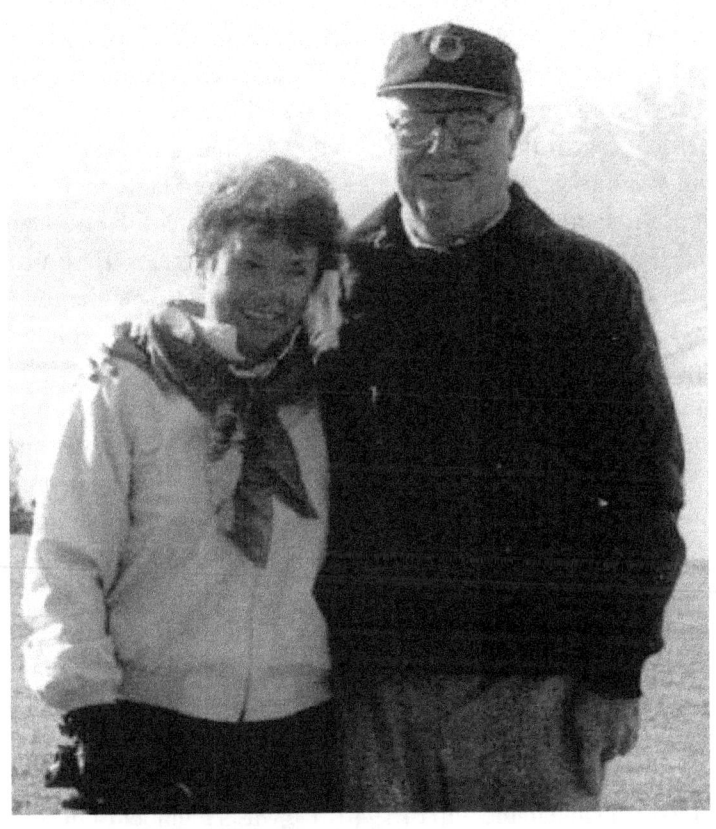

The J. Philip Clarke Family Lecture, an endowed lecture to be given at the annual medical ethics conference at Notre Dame, is the gift of Dr. and Mrs. J. Philip Clarke to the University.

Doris and Phil Clarke, a loving wife and husband, and parents of eleven children, shared a vision that there be a medical ethics conference at Notre Dame where physicians could bring the real problems that they encountered in their professional lives and discuss them with the best minds in the field of medical ethics. In 1987, when Phil received the Sorin Award, an award given to an alumnus who has rendered distinguished service to the University, he spoke of his vision. He said, "Now I share with you a dream – Father Sorin used to dream a great deal, according to Father Ted. As the greatest Catholic University in the world, I would like to see Notre Dame more fully involved in the entire field of ethics. In my judgment, Notre Dame should be providing a forum for addressing ethical issues from A to Z – advertising, business, government, journalism, law, medicine. . . . What we need is an Institute of Ethics on this campus in which the moral principles which we espouse can be discussed in relationship to the ethical issues of the day." In the year 2000, Doris offered this reflection on the conference which contributes to the continuation of that vision and in which the J. Philip Clarke Family lecture is presented: "Since Phil always presented me as 'the mother of the eleven children,' an identity I cherish, I recall thinking that the original medical ethics conference had some similarities to child birth – the conception of the idea, the planning, the anxious time of anticipation, the conferring with specialists, the nurturing, and, at last, the happy arrival. May this "offspring" continue in health and growth in its mission."

The public information about Phil's life begins when he entered Notre Dame in the Fall of 1940. He was a member of the class of 1944, however, World War II prevented his graduation with his class. After three years at Notre Dame, he entered medical school at the University of Colorado. He was awarded his Notre Dame degree after two years of medical school. After graduation from medical school, he served in the United States Navy at the U.S. Naval Hospital in San Diego and at the U.S. Amphibious Base on Coronado. His internship was completed at Saint Mary's Group Hospital at Saint

Louis University. He served residencies at the University of California Hospital in San Francisco and Saint Joseph Hospital in Denver. He was chief resident in medicine at the University of Colorado Medical Center in Denver.

Dr. Clarke was the quintessential professional. He served his profession, his church, and his community. He held hospital appointments at Saint Joseph Hospital, the Presbyterian Medical Center, Mercy Hospital, the University of Colorado Medical Center, and the Veterans Administration Hospital. At the University of Colorado Medical Center, he was clinical professor of medicine and associate dean for continuing medical education. He was a diplomate of the American Board of Internal Medicine and he served as president of the Catholic Physician's Guild. He was a member of the American College of Physicians and chairman of its Board of Governors from 1985-1986 and chairman of the Board of Regents in those same years. He was a delegate to the American Medical Association's Council on Internal Medicine.

He was awarded the A.H. Robins Award for Outstanding Community Service (1972), the Colorado Notre Dame Club Man of the Year Award (1974), the Outstanding Clinical Faculty Award at the University of Colorado Health Sciences Center (1983), the Distinguished Service Award of the American Diabetes Association (1984), and the Distinguished Service Award from the Denver Clinic (1984). His publications appeared in *Die Medizinische*, the *American Journal of OB & GYN*, *Linacre Quarterly*, the *Journal of the American Medical Association*, and the *Annals of Surgery*. His paper, "Carcinoid Syndrome: A New Clinical Entity" was awarded first prize by the Denver Medical Society.

Phil was a life long member of the Serra Club and served as its president in 1966. He was a life long member of the Ecumenical Commission of the Archdiocese of Denver and chaired that commission from 1971-1972. He was appointed by the Vatican as a lay observer at the World Methodist Congress in 1971. He was a participant in the Jewish-Roman Catholic Leaders dialogue from 1982 until his death.

My personal acquaintance with Phil began in late 1972. I had been assigned to the Religious Studies and Philosophy Departments of what was the Regis College – now Regis University – in Denver. Though I was not having any medical problems, I asked my friend and colleague at Regis, Fr. Ed Maginnis, S.J., if he knew a doctor I could consult. I felt I was of an age when I should have a regular physician. Ed replied that he knew just the person, Dr. Phil Clarke. Doris and Phil, along with other couples, belonged to a book club of which Ed was the mentor. An appointment was made for me with Phil at the Denver Clinic, a large group practice with physicians in all specialties. Phil was a partner practicing general internal medicine. I will never forget our first meeting. Phil took a history and did a physical, but for at least half of the considerable time he gave me, he inquired about my academic interests, my hobbies, and my life in general. He "examined" me to find out who I am, the person who sought to be his patient, so that he could care well for me should illness or injury develop. I was really impressed and liked him immensely from that first meeting. From our exchange that day, I had a sense of trust in his judgment.

This exemplifies the kind of doctor Phil was. His patients were persons whose personal uniqueness it was his privilege to come to know, and, should need arise, his awareness of this personal uniqueness would become, quite naturally, a central factor in the therapeutic alliance of doctor and patient in decision-making that would be required of them. This was clear to me when he spoke (carefully maintaining confidentiality) about situations that arose with patients, such as in the case he later submitted to the Notre Dame Conference for discussion – one he had spoken to me about years before and which is reproduced. This was a case of his compassionate support of a dying patient who had decided to forego further use of medication as that patient experienced great and increasing suffering in her treatment. Phil, unhesitatingly, took the truly Christian doctor's responsibility, which this patient asked of him. Phil made it possible for that patient to engage in a conversation with him about her dying, and he, then, took the responsibility, that too many physicians find hard or impossible, for discontinuing what had become for this dying patient "excessively burdensome treatment."

Well, as a result of our first meeting, Phil invited me to join him in discussing medical ethics issues on at least two occasions – the doctor and the ethician in dialog. One was a clinical conference on medical ethics issues at one of the hospitals in Denver, the other a memorable joint dinner meeting of the Denver Catholic Lawyers organization and the Denver Catholic Physicians organization. At this second occasion, the issue of being able to stop excessively burdensome treatments came up dramatically because one of the lawyers with a practice involving hospitals and doctors stood up to say that, after former President Harry Truman's recent death, he had received calls from several clients asking how they could prevent having done to them what was done to President Truman, that is, a prolonging of his dying by intensive treatment even though it was clear that it could not work to restore him to health. Shortly after that all of us would hear of Karen Ann Quinlan, "the girl in the coma" and litigation about her care would begin.

When I left Denver after only two years, in Spring 1974, to come to Chicago, one of my principal regrets was that I would no longer have Phil as my physician and close friend. Just before I left, Phil and I decided that I should undergo a relatively minor elective surgery before I left rather than wait longer, precisely because, in the future, we would not be able to decide together about a better time for it. Though I was still in general good health, this sense of confidence I had in Phil I knew was a special kind of grace in my life.

At that point, I simply did not expect to be able to have much contact again with Phil, but as he prepared for the first Notre Dame Conference, I received a call inviting me to participate as one of the ethics consultants from outside the University. This was, of course, at the suggestion of my old friend, Phil Clarke, who had persuaded the Alumni Association to bring physician alumni back to their *alma mater*. They would not return to suffer a barrage of lectures but to enter discussion with fellow alumni medical professionals at the place of their early formation in knowledge, wisdom, and affection, discussions about the kinds of ethical challenges they all experience in their practice. They would return to share experiences, and for some, to have a special kind of get together with their children now attending Notre Dame. And so, from the beginning, physician parents who were not themselves alumni were also invited.

While there would be one lecture, the rest of the time from Friday afternoon through Sunday morning would be devoted to discussion, first in small groups, then in plenary meetings to which the small groups would report and during which the ethics consultants, faculty of Notre Dame and invited faculty, would offer commentary and observations on the discussions. What an experience! Phil insisted that there be initiative from the physicians who would sign up – they would send in the cases ahead of time, and these would be distributed ahead of time to those who were coming. Then, when we arrived we were all prepared participants in the dialog. I must say that after taking part in all fifteen of these Conferences, I am utterly mystified by their uniqueness as always really stimulating experiences from which I depart, not exhausted but enlivened and energized and empowered.

Why isn't this the model for more, indeed for most professional meetings? At least for meetings where professional experience shared by all who attend is really the reason they are held? After all, most of us return from our professional meetings and say: "There were a few sessions I liked, but, really, the best thing about it was the individual contacts I was able to renew with old friends and the informal discussions I had with them." Yes, that's what we say, but we go on expecting and finding as the dominant model a plethora of one way lectures on various subjects, often valuable, but with a minimum of exchange afterwards.

What a genius Phil was in making these Conferences at Notre Dame what all of us long for and enjoy most about each other – a chance to talk, to talk back, to argue and to agree or disagree, but always to appreciate each year more that uniqueness of each of us that, years before in Denver, I came to know Phil valued above all in me and his other patients. Phil really deserved to be given the Sorin Award as an outstanding Alumnus of Notre Dame.

Yes, I loved Philip Clarke, and Doris – it was only at these conferences that I came to know Doris. We three shared some blessed private moments together each year until Phil died. He died at home, by the way, surrounded by Doris and his children and their families. Phil died of prostate cancer, which in his case was far from indolent in its progress! But, at the last Notre Dame conference he and Doris were able to attend together, though he was already weakened by the disease, he was still vibrant in his enthusiasm for discussion of ethical challenges faced by doctors, for the life together of fellow alumni that these conferences embody. Though he himself was entering his own dying, he was neither depressed nor unduly fearful. I sensed his loving trust in God's providence over him and his loved ones.

Knowing Phil Clarke and treasuring his having been my doctor and my friend, I must tell you that I pray to God that when my dying comes I may have a physician like Phil attending me. But, even if I am not so fortunate, I count on Phil Clarke's being near me in his nearness to Christ. I hope I have the courage and compassion both in my living and
my dying that Philip Clarke embodied so beautifully in his living and dying. Let us together be deeply grateful for God's precious gift to us of this wonderful Notre Dame man and truly good doctor.

James F. Bresnahan, S.J.
May, 2000

DOES BEING A CHRISTIAN PHYSICIAN REALLY MATTER?

Edmund D. Pellegrino

It is a genuine honor and a special privilege to launch this series of lectures in the name of the Clarke family. To do so in the presence of the family who have made the endowment adds to the honor of the invitation, but it also adds to my diffidence and anxiety lest I fail to do justice to that honor. This is, happily, the first lecture in the series. Subsequent speakers are certain to redeem my failings and make their lectures the notable occasions both Notre Dame and the Clarke family intend.

In deciding what I might talk about, Dr. Clarke's story about Father Kelly is very interesting. I want to tell you a little story in which I was, in fact, involved that had to do with the same kind of question. When I was President of Catholic University, I was having a discussion around the table with a number of my colleagues as we were awaiting the arrival of Archbishop Jadot who was then the Papal Nuncio to the United States. They were asking me a series of questions that had to do with reproductive biology and technology, and I said, "You know, I am so sick and tired of the school of pelvic theology." At that moment Archbishop Jadot walked in and said, "And what is this pelvic theology you're talking about . . . we've not heard about that in Rome." I am not going to talk about the pelvis either. Being an internist, it is foreign territory to me. What I want to do is try to respond to that question which Dr. Clarke gave you and which is my title today, namely: "Does being a Christian physician really matter?" My response is, yes! It really does matter. And I will devote this lecture to explaining why I respond in this way.

The most important realm of medical ethics today is the realm of professional ethics. All of the other issues we've been talking about are exquisitely important and I do not mean to deprecate them. But there is a kind of feeling that, when we are talking about Christian or Catholic medical ethics, we are concentrating on the challenges to sexuality, marriage, and procreation posed by recent biological knowledge. And while these challenges are certainly important, they do not comprise the whole of medical ethics from a Christian perspective. Indeed, they represent only one segment of the field of bioethics today. The oldest segment, twenty-five hundred years old, deals with the obligations of the physician *qua* physician. That segment of medical ethics is, at the moment, under very serious scrutiny. The Hippocratic ethic and tradition is really in a state of being deconstructed. Almost every one of the ten prescriptions in the Hippocratic Oath has been doubted, questioned, scrutinized, and, at present, it is very difficult to define what might be commonly held or commonly agreed to obligations by the profession of medicine. Our task, then, for the future, is to ask how do we reconstruct a medical morality. In what shall it consist? I will examine one exquisitely important part of it, the question of what difference does it make, as we look at this reconstruction, if one has, in addition to the findings of philosophical ethics--which is the dominant note and tone in medical ethics today, understandably in a pluralistic society--if one, in addition, has a commitment to being a Christian and, then, a Catholic Christian?

I want to pick up a challenge that I see in a quotation from Kierkegaard, a very brief one, and I would like you to have that in the background of your thinking, as I try to lay out what I think are the differences. The challenge is this, in Kierkegaard's words: "Without imitation of Christ, the fruit of Christian faith, Christianity becomes mere mythology or poetry or an abstract idea." What does it mean for a Catholic Christian physician to imitate Christ in Kierkegaard's sense? Lest you think you're going to have a sermon, let me disabuse you of that misconception. My response to Dr. Clarke's question will be in two parts. In the first, I shall examine the distinctive obligations that bind all physicians regardless of whether they hold religious beliefs. This is the moral minimum to which Christian physicians, or physicians of any religious persuasion, must adhere. In the second part of this lecture, I will examine the way in which a commitment to Catholic Christianity adds to, modifies, and enhances those obligations. I hope with that, I will have suggested at least some answers to the question: "What difference does it make?"

Let me start first with what I think is the fundamental and key question. I'm asked repeatedly, "Is it possible to be an ethical physician today given the climate of medical practice?" And the way the question is asked, predetermines the answer. People are referring to those many things that have caused depression, defection, and distress in conscientious physicians. Physicians who are not conscientious simply do not worry about these issues. The conscientious physician asking the question, "Is it possible?" typically, does not believe it is possible to be an ethical physician today. They are really agreeing with Machiavelli who said a long time ago, "The man who wishes to make a profession of goodness must necessarily come to grief in a world in which so many are not good." Many physicians are asking how they can be virtuous in a world in which others are not virtuous. Why are you asking more of me? Why am I different from the business man? Why am I different from the lawyer? Why am I different even from the minister? Everyone is lowering their standards and their objectives. Why are you asking more of me? Is there a place for altruism in the philosophical sense, and then for the Christian, is there a place for charity, in medicine? Some people have decided already that they will answer this question in the negative. Those are the ones who have decided that they will not treat the patient with AIDS. Those are the neurosurgeons who have decided they will not treat the patient in the emergency room for fear of malpractice litigation. Those are the ones who have decided to withdraw from the complicated obstetrical case. Those are the ones who will not see the Medicaid patient. Those are the ones who have enthusiastically gathered into themselves the idea of medical entrepreneurism or for-profit medicine. Those are the ones who have said, "Exigency . . . and survival . . . is the only answer. There is no place for virtue." They may not say this explicitly, but their actions reveal that to be their philosophical conception. They hold there is no place for altruism in medicine. While, they've all agreed to the principle of nonmaleficence (that is to say, not to harm the patient directly) beyond that, there is no obligation.

Now, the cynics among you will say that the history of medicine is filled with physicians who have behaved that way, and, unfortunately, that is the case. But our time is distinctive in that this view is being legitimated, being defended, and being put forth as the alternative to the traditional ethic of medicine. While the traditional ethic may have been violated in the past, those who violated it were considered social pariahs. They were no longer truly members of the profession. I need only to refer you to the first century A.D. to Scribonius Largus, a Pagan, who said that the physician who did not have compassion and altruism and the interest of the patient as his primary interest was not a physician. He said that it was intrinsic to what it was to be a physician that one had the interest of the patient primarily in heart, and suppressed his own self-interest. Now that view is being challenged. And it is that challenge that has caused distress and the moral desuetude. It is not that significant numbers of physicians have lost their idealism, but that their latent idealism needs to be reinforced and reexamined. We will not reinstate it by simply repeating the Hippocratic Oath since the Oath can hardly be sufficient for the problems of today.

In the face of the contemporary disarray of medical ethics, the inadequacies of the Hippocratic Oath, the cynicism, and the pervasive self-interest of some physicians, there remains universal human experiences on which medical ethics is based. These human experiences are the realities which provide the moral impetus for medical ethics and give medicine its special character among human activities.

First, the human experience of being ill requires altruism as an essential component of medicine. Are there any arguments that one can bring forth, philosophically, for altruism? There are certainly arguments to the contrary. There are those who hold, for example, that the sick have no moral claim whatever on us. According to this view, if we were born poor, if we were born sick, if we were born handicapped, we have no claim on society. This view doesn't deny that society might condescendingly help these folks, but it does deny the necessity for doing so. It does deny any moral claim that we offer ourselves to those persons as healers and helpers. In response to their claim, I would say that altruism is essential to the nature of medicine for the following reasons. First, being ill is not the same as being in need of a service or of commodities of other kinds. The sick person is in an altered existential state. A patient is someone who bears a burden. A patient is dependent, vulnerable, and, believe me, eminently exploitable. Anyone who has been a patient knows that it is not the same as being healthy--that you are in a position in which you are dependent upon the knowledge, the power, and the character of another person. The patient needs the physician's knowledge and the assurance that the knowledge will be used for the patient's benefit. The needs of the patient must be put ahead of the personal profit, power, or prestige of the physician. My first point is that we cannot treat health care as a commodity.

The second point is that medical knowledge is not proprietary. It does not belong to the physician. Why do I make that point? Reflect particularly on the process of becoming a physician. Many of us here today have gone through that process. In that process we invade and intrude upon the privacy of human beings. We dissect human bodies. We autopsy human bodies. We examine every orifice. We are allowed to do things which, if it were not in a medical school under the aegis of medical education, we would be jailed for – reducing a human body to an unidentifiable mass necessary to learn the anatomy of that body. We have access to all the knowledge of the medical world – knowledge gained from thousands of sick patients who have been the subjects of clinical investigations. We are allowed, in clinical years, to intrude into the process of healing in the care of a patient. Those of us involved in medical education know that treating patients in an educational settings sometimes involves discomfort for the patients and sometimes is dangerous for the patient. Surgeons, far more dramatically, but internists as well must learn their craft. We have been accorded an extraordinary privilege, but not primarily so that we will have a comfortable income. Even at the horrendous tuition that students pay at Georgetown, you cannot buy the privilege of a medical education. That knowledge is made accessible to us because society needs people trained with this knowledge. We hold that knowledge, therefore, in trust.

Finally, the physician also makes a public declaration of trust. I would suggest that we entered an implicit covenant when we accepted a medical education, so much so that I have suggested that we ought to take an oath on entering medical school as well as on exiting. It would say, "I understand that I have been given a privilege to intrude and invade, etc., etc., etc., and that this privilege is accorded me only because a, b, c." Certainly, when we graduate, the official entry into the profession is not the degree. (As a president of a university I have given out lots of those. That is mainly a certificate of exposure.) The entry into the profession is rather that symbolic oath. It is not the content of the oath that is crucial, because, as you've heard already, that the content is changing. It is rather that what we say is a promise to everyone present that (a) we have knowledge and competence, (b) we will use it in the interest of those who are sick, and (c) we can be trusted in the moment of truth (and those moments occur all too frequently in clinical medicine when there might be a conflict of interest between my interest and the patient's) to practice a certain degree of effacement of self-interest and to put my interest second to the patient's interest. We have, therefore, a covenant which we explicitly accept on graduation and which we repeat every time a patient enters the office and we say, "May I help you?" or "What can I do for you?"

I would submit, therefore, that altruism, understood first as taking into account the needs of others in medicine, is role-related. It is a role-specific obligation integral to the nature of medical activity and, therefore, on philosophical grounds alone, well-supported. That is not a new idea. The idea of role-related duties was brought forth very clearly a long time ago by the middle Stoics from Persodonius to Cicero. Trust lies at the foundation of the fiduciary or covenantal relationship between physician and patient. The patient must be able to trust the physician to use the knowledge entrusted to the profession. The good of the patient as the end of medicine requires certain traits of character or virtues from its practitioners. These virtues are defined by the degree to which they dispose the physician to act for the benefit of the sick person. Physicians, who are disposed habitually to act for the good of the patient, take on role related obligations which are exhibited in the virtues of competence, fidelity to trust, courage, benevolence, compassion, and altruism.

If those are the obligations that one would establish on philosophical grounds alone, what does a Christian perspective, a faith commitment add? What more is required? I would suggest that we might look at what a faith commitment might do to three dimensions of medicine and ethics. First, in what way does the Christian virtue of charity, which is the ordering principle of Christian ethics, alter the way we interpret the predominant principles of medical ethics which are arrived at philosophically? Second, what does it say about the nature of the physician-patient relationship? And third, what does it say about our moral obligations as a collectivity, as a profession united together in the common promise that we, all of us, are at the service of the sick?

Let us look at those primary principles of medical ethics first, and how the Christian perspective shapes those. Those principles are beneficence, justice, and respect for persons (which I prefer to autonomy). They enjoy widespread acceptance today, even in our morally pluralistic society. They are increasingly used as the template against which right and wrong, good and bad, judgments are made. Like the precepts of the Hippocratic ethic, they call for a high order of ethical sensitivity. What does Christian belief add, if anything, to this moral algorithm? How does charity inform each of them?

First, beneficence understood as acting for the good of the patient is the central principle of medical ethics. That principle is interpretable in several different ways and health professionals differ sharply today on precisely what degree of beneficence they consider binding. Some argue that simply not harming the patient is sufficient and they always quote that principle from the *Epidemics* of Hippocrates, "First do no harm." Is that sufficient when we look at the principle from the point of view of Christian charity? Christian beneficence is inspired by the ultimate beneficence of its founder, who suffered that all of us might be redeemed. Benevolent self-effacement is a minimum obligation consistent with the virtue of charity. Beneficence inspired by charity does good when it requires courage or sacrifice, when it costs something substantial in money, time, and hard work in the interest of the sick person. *Pro bono* work for the poor, courtesy, patience, and compassion even with the hostile, non-compliant, or self-abusing patient are obligations of those who profess a belief in Christ the healer. Clearly, patients have reciprocal obligations with respect to their physician. When patients fail, however, the physician is not justified in retaliating. Lesser degrees of beneficence would be inconsistent with the scripture exhortations with which we are all familiar – the story of the Good Samaritan, the Sermon on the Mount, and Jesus's own healing acts, day-in and day-out.

Further, a Christian perspective converts the profession into a vocation--a means of gaining our own salvation and the salvation of others and of witnessing the truths of the gospel in our own lives. Practicing medicine is inseparable from leading a life that is wholly Christian. There is a tremendously strong tendency to separate personal morality from professional morality. And we see that, unfortunately, in those who profess to be Christian physicians. The Christian physician is impelled to act in the interest of the sick, even when it means exposing himself to danger. I want to repeat that because I'm hearing over and over again, "I don't have to treat; it was not in my contract when I entered medical school."

The moral claim of the sick person exceeds any claim that we would find in a business relationship or in a commodity transaction. In business you may take advantage of the exploitability of your competitor, just not in a nasty way. But you don't survive in business unless you, in fact, take advantage of the weakness of the competitor. The used car salesman does not tell you about the shaky front end, the fact that the car was in a wreck. He kicks the tires and says, "Isn't she a beauty; take her out and ride her." And he's crossing his fingers hoping you'll bring it back in one piece and it won't fall apart . . . as he knows it will do eventually. Can the relationship with the physician be on that basis? Is *caveat emptor* to be the ordaining principle? Could it ever be consistent with the principle of charity?

Now we don't have an algebraic formula that's going to measure out precisely the degree of self-effacement a particular physician must practice in a particular situation and I'm not going to prescribe for you. This is going to depend upon how each physician balances the strength of his or her other obligations. Clearly, the Christian physician owes beneficence to his own family, friends, and himself. Even while being benevolent to his patients, these obligations must be met lovingly. Striking the right balance is a spiritual and temporal challenge which requires moral discernment. But what is clear is that there can be no easy justifications for interpreting beneficence as mere nonmaleficence or as beneficence which demands nothing of the physician or permits him to choose in his own interest against the patient's interest. The arguments that I am hearing over and over again for fiscal exigency, for survival, for adherence to the canons of competition of the marketplace are morally feeble, if not totally unacceptable, when viewed and weighed with a Christian Catholic perspective. The Christian physician is, and this is not a romantic notion, called to strive for perfection in charity, even though he or she must fall and fail given the exaltedness of the model which we, in our human weakness, want to emulate. That we do, in fact, fall short does not in any way excuse us from striving for the charitable interpretation of benevolence.

Let's take a look at justice, the second principle of the triad in medical ethics today. Justice is often portrayed symbolically as blindfolded and holding a balance to signify objectivity in judgment. When justice is interpreted in light of the Beatitudes, in which charity is the ordering principle, the blindfold is removed. A much richer and more compassionate weighing of what is due is entailed. Charitable justice has its origins in God, Who is just with us and to Whom we owe justice. Charitable justice goes beyond the strict rendering to others of what is due to them. It recognizes needs that go beyond duty. Its weighing includes taking into account the human context within which persons live. It seeks to redress the inequities of the natural lottery in which some are poor, some are sick, some are disabled, and some have great needs. It takes past injustices into account.

The Catholic response to injustice in health care distribution operates from the stance of charitable justice and solidarity. It speaks of a preferential option for the poor and of the provision of health care as a moral obligation of a good society to all its members. Those on the margins of society have a greater claim on us that those who are better off. This claim is not in terms of the kind of care we give them, but in terms of our information and knowledge. Some of the differences between a strict view of justice and a justice that might be charitable are revealed in the way we look at the whole question of health care delivery. In a strictly legal sense, it is difficult to justify any moral claim by the poor or the sick on us. Even more difficult to make convincing is the argument that the virtuous and the hardworking should sacrifice for the poor, the outcast, the sociopath. Yet again, it is precisely these groups that Christians, and specifically Catholic Christians, are expected to serve. The recent pastoral letter of the American bishops makes this clear. The social encyclicals of the popes since Leo XIII make this clear. And it is abundantly and exquisitely clear in Pope John Paul's beautiful apostolic letter on human suffering, *Salvifice doloris*. Charitable justice, therefore, fuses with beneficence in a way incomprehensible on a purely naturalistic interpretation of these virtues. It seeks out those who may not have deserved health care, those who are responsible for their ill health. It does so because the sick, the poor, the outcast are precisely those with whom our model spent His days. Where would Christ be if He were with us today? I'm certain He would be with the AIDS patients, among others, who are in that saddened kind of state.

Physicians are stewards, not sole proprietors, of the knowledge and skills needed by the sick. Health care is not a commodity whose cost, quality, and accessibility can be left solely to the invisible hand of the marketplace. Catholic physicians, therefore, cannot behave as if medicine were primarily a business and their skills proprietary possessions on which no one can have a moral claim. They cannot be primarily entrepreneurs driven only by the profit motive. They have special obligations to respond to the needs of those on the margins of society.

Finally, let's look at autonomy for a moment. Autonomy, that most strongly asserted principle of secular ethics and secular mores, must also be transformed by the ordering principle of charity. Kant grounded autonomy in an a priori respect for persons, but for the Christian that respect must be grounded in the worth the Creator has given to each life, the worth only God can judge. The antagonism some ethicists see between autonomy and beneficence is mitigated by a Christian ethic. This is not to justify medical paternalism, which is too often confused with beneficence, but to assert that respect for persons is in itself a requirement of beneficence. The two have fused. The possession of reason, foresight, and accountability for personal choices is elemental in human nature. To ignore, subvert, or override the capacity for self-determination is a maleficent act, especially in matters so personal as are encompassed in medical care. On the other hand, autonomy must be balanced against the maleficence of complicity with patients who make obviously detrimental choices. But what could be less beneficent than to violate the very humanity of the person you are treating? And what is more associated with being human than the capacity to make decisions for which you are accountable?

Viewed from a Christian perspective, however, autonomy is not absolute. A Christian is obliged to use his or her God-given freedom wisely and well. Autonomy is necessary to doing the right and the good, to fulfilling the stewardship we have of our own health. And this means, therefore, refraining from self-destructive lifestyles--suicide and other more subtle forms of self-killing. Patients are not free to make any choice they wish, such as a choice for euthanasia or assisted suicide or certain reproductive technologies or abortion. Here autonomy is held within the constraints of the morally permissible, as explicated in Magisterial teachings. Moreover,

Christian physicians cannot cooperate with patients wishing or willing to take unreasonable risks by choosing non-standard or alternative therapies which expose them to hazardous experiments whose effectiveness is non-existent or whose dangers are unknown.

In the same way, the patient or the family of the patient has an obligation in charity to respect the autonomy and the dignity of the health professional as well. Patient autonomy is limited when it violates the physician's autonomy or when the physician is asked to violate conscience. Today, some would extend the hegemony of autonomy so far as to demand the exclusion of Catholics from practice in certain specialties. Catholic beliefs, for example, are a constraint on procedures such as reproductive techniques, maternal-child medicine, and genetic manipulation, that physicians can offer their patients.

There is a move today to make the physician the willing instrument of whatever it is the patient might want. And that is a strong tendency, which I am encountering with greater and greater frequency. It says, "Well, if you talk about being the servant of the patient, then that means you must do everything the patient wants." And here again we have to respect the conscience of the physician as expressed by the physician's moral beliefs. You cannot ask the orthodox Jewish physician who believes, with Rabbi Jakobovits, that you cannot shorten life by a whit to do so. You cannot ask the Catholic physician to perform abortions. (And further issues will face us when euthanasia becomes legal.) We could never accept, on a charitable ground, the absolutization of patient autonomy and the absolute self-governance over life. If a physician cannot comply in good conscience with the patient's autonomous choice, the physician must, if possible, withdraw. Withdrawal should be done courteously, with an honest statement of reasons, and without vindictiveness.

Let us turn now to the manner in which a Catholic Christian perspective shapes the physician-patient relationship. The way Christian physicians perceive themselves and their patients is formed by the images of Christ's healing as they are given in the Gospels. In those Gospels, we see Jesus repeatedly healing the sick, showing them special solicitude, healing both body and soul, responding to appeals for help, and effecting His cures always in the name of His Heavenly Father. Next to preaching salvation, most of Jesus's time was spent with the sick, the suffering, and the outcast.

Christ, Himself, presents us with two images: Christ the Healer and Christ the Sufferer. He, Himself, is the physician of body and soul, but He is also the sufferer who experiences the pain, abandonment, and anguish of the sick person. Although He, Himself, is not ill, His death by crucifixion and His agony on the Cross prefigure all the sufferings of the sick. Jesus identified Himself with the person of the sufferer. He taught us that when we comfort the sick, clothe the naked, and feed the hungry, it is as if we were doing it to Him: "I assure you, as long as you did it to the least of my brothers, you did it to me" (Mt. 25: 35-40). For the Christian, the sick person is Christ seeking help from the doctor. The patient, therefore, can never be anything other than a *patient,* someone suffering. The authentic Christian physician can never see the sick person as a consumer, client, customer, plan member, insured life, contractee, or any of the other metaphors and euphemisms which are the standard talk of our present day commercialized, market driven, health care market place.

Today, the physician-patient relationship is dictated by forces beyond the physician's control. It demands too much to expect the individual physician to overturn the disastrous depersonalization of contemporary medicine. But every Christian physician must keep alive the image of Jesus as both healer and patient and, to the extent possible, preserve the idea of healing as a ministry in imitation of Christ's ministry. This means, at least, standing always for the patient, repudiating proprietary claims on medical knowledge, and countering the injustices of managed care as it exists today. The Christian physician cannot go on strike to advance the physician's own interests with the specious argument that a strike will help patients.

Medicine as ministry also means that many things now accepted as legitimate or at the moral margin in the secular world must be resisted. Among these practices are investment in for profit health care organizations, bonuses for restricting care, and high salaries garnered from profits arising from the buying, selling, or trading patients in mergers--that whole panoply of "deals" that characterize medicine as a business. Conflicts of interest must be avoided in fact, not just the "appearances" of conflict. Simply divulging information about conflicts does not validate their continuance as those infatuated with the operation of the unfettered marketplace seem to believe. Whenever the primacy of the welfare of the sick person is asserted against motives of power, prestige, pride, or prejudice, then the difference it makes to be a Christian is exemplified most clearly.

This is not a plea for physicians to practice monastic medicine or the heroic virtues in imitation of Mother Teresa, Fr. Damien, or St. Francis. Christian physicians are entitled to pursue legitimate self-interest and the interests of their families. But every time a choice or decision is made, the question should be asked, "How does my being a Christian shape this decision?" We are imperfect creatures, and we cannot possibly attain the level of Jesus's healing ministry. But we are obliged to strive in this direction and to examine our practices in the light of charity. We must learn to discern where we can work patiently for change within the system and where we have the obligation to object and dissent publicly. Silence in the face of injustice is complicity in that injustice.

We turn, finally, to the last area of practice to be touched by a faith commitment. The Catholic Christian physician has a special role to play in the community as members of a moral community with concern for the common good. I refer here to the teachings of the social encyclicals from Leo XIII to John Paul II. These encyclicals urge Catholics to work for justice in society. They exhort us to mount a sustained effort in the public arena to establish social institutions which will assure equitable access and distribution of health care and enable the Catholic health care ministry to flourish. They call for solidarity--the linking together of human beings in such a way that the good of the one and the good of the whole are simultaneously served. Catholic physicians are members of a professional community engaged in a Christian apostolate within a larger secular society. They have a collective obligation to do what is possible in democratic societies to make a whole society responsive to its sick members. It will be no surprise to anyone that in recent debates about health care policy, Catholic physicians have not made a concerted effort to foster a charitably just health care system. Yet, as believing Christians, they are bound together in a common ministry and share an obligation to evangelize, that is, to give witness to the kind of difference it does make in practice to be a Christian physician. Catholic Christians might have to begin their evangelization as a community by revitalizing the Christian virtue of charity in their own hospitals--Catholic as well as non-Catholic. Catholic hospitals have been too ready to accede to the demands of a commercialized, monetarized, market-driven health care system. This is an indictment of our commitment as Christians, which is not eradicated by arguing that survival excuses all. There is enormous power in collective action if it is motivated by moral concern. Even a glance at the Gospels is enough to tell us that care for the sick as Jesus did it would require all of us to feel responsible for a society and system that fails to meet the test of charitable justice.

The most significant thing for the care of patients, I believe, is how to reconstruct professional ethics and, in that reconstruction, how to understand the role of those who make a commitment to being Christians in addition. So the thrust of my message is for us to look first at ourselves rather than say we can't be ethical and moral in the climate in which we find ourselves. Let's start with looking at ourselves. There is a moral foundation on which the profession is built. That moral foundation has its source in the nature of medicine, the nature of illness, the nature of the acts of medicine. The obligations of medicine arise there. But, in order to be an ethical physician, we need help and we need reinforcement by our leaders. What would happen if we in the profession--all of the health care professions, five hundred thousand physicians, two or three million nurses, hospital administrators, all of whom should be dedicated to the good of the patient-- were to say, "We will not do a, b, and c. We cannot do a, b, and c." What would happen if we looked at health policies, as they come down the line, for their impact on the good of the patient? Our history has always been to say, "What is it doing to my privileges, to my prerogatives." The DRG (diagnosis related group), if it has a problem, is not because it limits the discretionary space of the physician. It is because limiting the discretionary space of the physician harms the patient. We have a moral obligation to demonstrate that, if it is true. However, if it is not true, we should not be saying it. Anecdotes will not do. If there are thirty-five million people not covered by medical insurance, and we know them and we see them, what are we going to say and do about it? Who is the advocate for all of the sick? Our profession has enormous power for moral good. I do not think we've exercised it fully or as effectively as we might. If we really want to recapture our moral integrity, the most important thing we could do would be to resist doing--to refuse to do--things that violate our promise to act in the patient's interest which is the very center, the moral center, and heart of physician-patient relationships.

Some years ago, Alasdair MacIntyre challenged theologians to demonstrate what theology might contribute to medical ethics. He suggested that theologians would have to show that it made a difference in three areas, namely, in morality in general, in a theological critique of morality and culture, and in the specific problems in modern medicine. What I have tried to do today is to show that being a Christian physician makes a difference: first, in fidelity to the moral precepts derivable by reason alone from the realities of medicine; second, in the way that Christian charity and the beatitudes reshape the principles of secular bioethics; third in the physicians view themselves and their relations with their patients; and, finally, in the way physicians conduct themselves as a community united in a common Christian apostolate of healing.

I hope I have answered Dr. Clarke's question with an unequivocal Yes! Being a Catholic Christian physician does make a difference, and a very great difference.

Response to
DOES BEING A CHRISTIAN PHYSICIAN REALLY MATTER?

John H. Robinson

In the inaugural Clarke Lecture, Doctor Pellegrino set out to prove both that physicians generally ought to think of themselves as professionals and that those physicians who are Christian have reasons for thinking of themselves in that way that go beyond those reasons that may be available to physicians who are not Christians. He thought it especially important to convince physicians to think of themselves as professionals at this point in history because, he thought, the shift from fee-for-service payment mechanisms to managed care poses uniquely harsh challenges to the integrity of the practice of medicine. In his lecture, Doctor Pellegrino was eloquent, even passionate, in his defense of the physician as professional, but it was inevitable that he would leave some important background considerations unexplored. When, furthermore, he sought to reinforce his secular arguments for physician professionalism with theological concerns, he left some serious theological questions unanswered. In my comment on Doctor Pellegrino's lecture I will attempt both to explore those background considerations and to address those theological questions.

The principal background consideration that I will focus on here is the very idea of a profession, with some attention to the normative questions raised by the existence of professions. As I understand them, professions are specialized occupational groups entry into which requires advanced education in the relevant field and proof that the applicant has acquired the knowledge and skills offered in that education. After an applicant has been admitted to a profession, the members of the profession socialize him or her to its particular mores and monitor him or her for continuous good-standing. In this way professions tend to monopolize the services that they provide and to become somewhat autonomous with respect to whom they admit and how they monitor the good-standing of those who have been admitted to practice. The state collaborates with the professions both with respect to their monopolistic tendencies and with respect to their autonomy, at least as far as the medical and legal professions are concerned. Certain evidentiary privileges, furthermore, significantly facilitate the communication of confidential information that lies at the core of professional practice. Independently of the state, civil society gives the professions a privileged position in the social scheme of things.

As Doctor Pellegrino would be the first to notice, my account of professions is, so far, bloodless and cold. The heart and soul of a profession – without which it becomes a morally and socially dubious entity – lies in the sort of relation that ordinarily subsists between professionals and the persons whom they serve. Professionals provide services that are vital to the physical, intellectual, spiritual, or social well-being of those whom they serve; they provide those services in ways that expose the deepest vulnerability of those whom they serve; and, finally, those whom they serve usually cannot rely on standard market mechanisms to choose or to assess their service-provider. Inherent in the professional relationship, therefore, are certain normative features, and it is those features that make professions morally interesting and morally controversial.

From the side of the recipient of professional services, the most outstanding moral feature of a professional relationship is trust. In the medical context, for example, a patient trusts that the doctor will not exploit the patient's vulnerability for the doctor's personal advantage, will not exploit the confidences that are ingredient to that relationship, will not put the patient to the doctor's own uses without the real consent of the patient, and will not abandon the patient in favor of another patient with a deeper pocket, a more winsome face, or a more interesting medical condition. The patient also trusts that the doctor will keep himself or herself current with respect to late-breaking medical developments, will bring an alert and unclouded mind to the provision of medical services, and will put the patient's well-being ahead of the doctor's self-interest if ever the two should conflict.

From the side of the physician, the most outstanding feature of the doctor-patient relationship is a commitment to respect that trust. Non-maleficence is the elemental form that this commitment must take; then comes beneficence, understood here as an abiding willingness to subordinate the doctor's self-interest to the perceived good of the patient. Much the same could be said of the moral structure of the priest-penitent relationship, of the teacher-student relationship, and of the lawyer-client relationship. In each case membership in the profession in question is thought both to require the professional to subordinate self-interest to the concerns of a vulnerable other in ways that might not obtain if the service-provider were not a professional, and to motivate the professional to honor that requirement. The Gospel message comes along at this point, Doctor Pellegrino suggests, both to reinforce the profession's demand for restraints on self-interested behavior on the part of the professional and to inspire the professional to observe those restraints. Similar work is done for Jewish and Islamic doctors by the sacred texts of their religions.

Doctor Pellegrino would admit, I suspect, that there is nothing particularly original in the account of the professions that forms the background for his lecture. He might even be pleased with the sheer orthodoxy of his professional ideal. Still it ought to give us pause. To see why, consider the neat fit between the moral dimension of professional relationships as this account presents them and the teaching of Jesus as Doctor Pellegrino describes them. It is true that both professional ethics and the Gospels subject our tendency to unwarranted self-preference to searching moral criticism, and to this extent all is well with the account just sketched. But there remains Jesus's unrelenting hostility to the professional elites of his day – the Scribes, the Pharisees, the priests, the lawyers – and his utter contempt for the moral smugness that they exuded. What are we to make of this, and of a similar hostility that Socrates exhibited towards the professional elites of fifth century Athens?

Could there be an underside to professional life that Doctor Pellegrino's account has missed? I think so. We find a hint of it in Doctor Pellegrino's suggestion that *outside* the privileged circle of professional relationships anything goes, morally speaking – as when used-car salesmen feel free to sell defective cars to gullible shoppers. But surely moral imperatives function in the marketplace, just as they do in a doctor's office, and surely our brothers and sisters who earn a living in the marketplace work out their salvation there just as professionals do in their more antiseptic settings. What kind of moral universe would professionals inhabit if they held themselves to high standards of self-denial and concern for others in their professional lives but felt free to deceive their neighbors in their extra-professional market behavior? In both settings the professional is required to deal honestly with the relevant other. That account of professional life must be flawed that presents extra-professional life as somehow exempted from the demands of morality and that does not see it as better – richer, fuller, more rewarding – for being lived morally.

It is one thing to see oneself (and one's peers) as called to a higher level of self-sacrifice than others are, and another thing to see others as less moral than oneself (and one's peers). Observing this distinction helps to rescue professionals from moral arrogance, and observing it makes it possible for us to imagine professionals respecting those whom they serve as moral agents capable of at least as much moral insight and of at least as much moral courage as professionals are. In that case beneficent physicians might well acknowledge the decisional autonomy of their patients without succumbing to any illusions about the real probability of autonomy under conditions of illness and ignorance. Lawyers, similarly, could serve as genuine and effective counselors precisely because they recognize their clients as moral agents seeking to preserve their integrity by means of the decisions that they make; priests could more easily discern the holiness of the penitents whose sins they shrive; and teachers could acknowledge the brilliance of the students whose papers they grade. In each case, if the professional observes the distinction between being called to an extraordinary level of self-sacrifice by virtue of the other's need and trust and being morally superior to the other by virtue of one's occupational affiliation, the professional might be able to recognize the other as at least his or her moral equal and therefore to deal with the other as capable of genuine (if limited) autonomy.

Observing the distinction between a call to extraordinary self-sacrifice and a claim to moral superiority could even help professionals to cleanse their professional organizations of their worst traits. As Doctor Pellegrino noted, the needs of those whom professionals serve ought to influence the positions that professionals take in public policy debates and in the functioning of their professional organizations. Too often, however, those organizations seem to be motivated more by a desire to protect the income flow of their members than by a desire to protect the public from quacks and scoundrels, and no profession in modern American life has done a good enough job of purging its ranks of unprofessional members, and none have been aggressive enough about pressing alcohol-abusers or drug-users into an effective therapeutic regime. Professionals should change their professional organizations so that this characterization no longer fits them, and perhaps they will once they develop a more adequate account of what it is to be a professional.

Perhaps. But when one considers how easy it is for those who enjoy wealth and social status to assume their own moral superiority, and when one considers how much the information revolution and biotechnology revolution will exacerbate the divide between the knowledge class and the under-class, it is hard to believe that our traditional professions will ever see themselves, and be seen by others, as the humble servants of people in need. If that is to happen, I suspect, it will be because some members of those professions have undergone a conversion experience thanks to which they identify more with the needy individuals whom they serve than with the powerful individuals who are their professional peers, and because those atypical professionals then lead their peers to embrace a new and better professional ideal than any that are now current. Perhaps Doctor Pellegrino's impassioned witness to the practice of medicine as a form of ministry will serve as a step towards that revolutionary change. In any case, he deserves to be praised for his years of witnessing to the ethical, even heroic, practice of medicine.

CLINICAL MEDICAL ETHICS: A REVIEW OF THE FIRST DECADE

Mark Siegler

It is a wonderful honor to be invited to deliver the second J. Philip Clarke Family Lecture. I want to thank Phil and Doris and I hope they'll extend my thanks to their family too. I also very much want to thank the University of Notre Dame for convening this conference. This is the fourth year of the Alumni Medical Ethics Conference and as far as I know, it's the only such gathering of alumni in the country. It was started, as I recall, with the inspiration of Father Ted Hesburgh. And Father Malloy has been a great supporter right from the beginning. So I do want to thank the Clarke family and the University.

I know that some of you are disappointed that Ed Pellegrino will not be delivering the second Clarke lecture. He did such a wonderful job in delivering the first, but for those of you who are disappointed you needn't worry very long. As I will quickly make clear, Ed is with me on the podium in spirit, but not just in spirit. He is with me as a co-author of the paper that I will be delivering – a paper, in fact, that was generated after Ed's talk here last year at this conference. We decided at that time that it would be useful for us to review the field of clinical medical ethics and to do it in a joint way. What I will be presenting this afternoon is the result of that year of collaborative work.

Sometimes people who hear the word medical ethics think of nothing but trouble and grim situations and I'd like to begin with a story that's reminiscent of some of their concerns. The story is told of a couple, John and Mary, who had been married for over fifty years, coming on to their sixtieth anniversary. John is lying on his deathbed and Mary is sitting beside the bed. John is reminiscing about their years together and he says, "Mary, you remember when we met over sixty years ago, the day we went to the county fair and I got kicked by the horse and you were right there to nurse me back to health?" And Mary said she remembered that very well. And John said, "Then I went off to war and I came back injured, but there you were right beside me to take care of me." Mary said, yes she was. John said, "Then we got married you remember and just a couple of years after that the stock market crashed and it took us eight or ten years to dig ourselves out of that financial hole but you were there to help me." Mary assured him that she was. And John says, "And now it's sixty years later and here I am dying and you're still right there beside me." Mary said, "Yes John, I'm right here." John stopped for a moment and then said, "You know Mary, I've been thinking, my God girl, you're bad luck."

Like poor Mary who really wasn't the cause of John's problems but always seemed to be around when those problems happened, ethicists seemed always to be around when the troubling and the tough and the grim situations occur, and perhaps we oughtn't to blame them for being there at the time. They don't bring on the situations. They merely respond to them.

What Ed and I talked about last year in planning this paper was that the health system and the medical education system reminded us of a great ocean liner that was going full speed ahead and was very difficult to slow down or divert from its course. I reminded Ed that in his effort to infuse humanities education back into medicine he had done an extraordinary job through the Institute of Medical Humanities in the 1970s to bring medical humanities and medical ethics into medical education. Ed's work was a substantial effort to slow down or modify the course of the ocean liner. He agreed that that was so, but then we thought that it was desirable to look at what happened in the last decade. That was the inspiration for this paper.

Thinking about the ocean liner though reminds me of just one more brief story before I turn to the paper. And that's the story of the sixth fleet's cruising in the Mediterranean. The admiral of the fleet happens to be wandering up on the bridge of his flag ship when he spots a blip on the radar screen and he turns to his ensign and he says, "Ensign, I want you to radio the other vessel and ask it to move out of the way." And the ensign gets on the radio and carries out the order and he says, "This is the S.S. Ticonderoga. You are squarely in the path of the American sixth fleet. Please alter your course." And after a few minutes he gets back a response from the offender saying, "I'm sorry. You'll have to alter your course." Well, the admiral gets angry and he tells the ensign to wire back immediately a stronger message. And so the ensign wires back, "This is the S.S. Ticonderoga. You are endangering the operations of the sixth fleet. You must change course." And a few minutes later a message comes back from the offender, "I'm sorry but you'll have to change course." Now the admiral gets extremely angry. He grabs the microphone, breaks silence, and gets onto the radio and says, "This is the most powerful fleet in the history of mankind. I am its admiral. And I command you to alter course." A few minutes pass and the message comes back which says, "Buddy, I don't care if you're John Paul Jones. If you don't change your course we're going to have a terrible problem because I'm a lighthouse."

I sometimes sense that American medicine and American medical education are rather like a lighthouse. You can't change their course. They're squarely in front of you and you have to somehow wander around them if you can. In any event, the rise of clinical medical ethics is one attempt to change the course, if ever so slightly, of American medical education.

To begin, let me tell you a little bit about clinical ethics. Clinical medical ethics is a relatively new field which explores ways to incorporate the new ethical insights that have emerged in the last thirty or forty years in response to the extraordinary developments in modern medicine into clinical practice, training, and research activities. In that respect, clinical ethics is a practical discipline whose central purpose is to improve the quality of patient care by improving the skill of health professionals to make good decisions for and with patients –

patients who come to them in a medical setting asking for care. Clinical ethics examines the important aspects of the doctor's central task which is the act of making a decision. The relationship between clinical practice and ethical practice is vitally important. Stated simply, skilled and excellent clinical practice is at the very center of the ethical practice of medicine. All the compassion and empathy and good nature in the world do not make up for an avoidable bad decision or an inadequate treatment plan. In coming decades it's likely that there will be increased concern about many ethical issues – end of life care, resource allocation, new technologies, the revolution in genetic engineering, and the like. And to this end it seems essential that we train a reasonable number of clinicians who can work alongside ethicists to teach and develop sound ethical policies for their hospitals, communities, and for the society in general.

Before I go on I would like to address the question of why I think it's important that clinicians be involved in medical ethics. There are a number of reasons. First of all, I think we need clinicians to identify the real clinical ethical dilemmas that can often go unrecognized by those who lack clinical experience. Second, clinicians can describe those dilemmas in language that's recognizable to patients and doctors and nurses in hospitals. Third, clinicians can work to resolve these problems in the context of clinical decisions using the expertise that comes to clinicians as a result of their training, experience and gradually accumulated practical wisdom. Fourth, I think clinicians are essential to teach clinical ethics to colleagues, to house staff, to students and, even very importantly, to the public. And in the public I'm including patients, judges, and legislators. And finally, I think the perspective of clinicians has to be part of the ethical dialogue because that perspective is very different from that of non-clinician theoreticians. The physician's role is to a certain extent unique. Once sought out by the patient the physician becomes involved in the patient's problem and never again is a mere observer. The obligations of involved professionals are different from those of mere theoreticians. The old Spanish proverb puts the point nicely when it says, "As one moves from the stands into the bullring the appearance of the bull changes."

With that as background let me then tell you what we did. Ten years ago Ed and I, I think, coined the term clinical medical ethics in a couple of papers that were published in "The Journal of the American Medical Association." At that time we suggested that ethics was central to clinical medicine for at least two reasons. First, ethical considerations can not be avoided when doctors and patients choose what ought to be done from among the many things that can be done for an individual patient in a particular circumstance. And second, the concept of good clinical medicine implies that both technical and ethical considerations are taken into account. We argued then that ethics informs the act of clinical decision – what Ed referred to as the moment of clinical truth. We proposed that clinical ethics must be taught at the bedside in the Oslerian tradition. And with a number of colleagues, including Al Jonsen, David Thomasma, and Bill Winslade, we introduced analytic systems for approaching clinical ethical problems. In the ensuing ten years, the field of clinical ethics has slowly developed programs in education, in clinical research, and patient care. Most medical schools offer preclinical courses in medical ethics. Some have rather vigorous teaching programs during the clinical years of medical school and a few have established post-graduate training programs. Medical journals increasingly publish reports both of empirical and theoretical research in medical ethics and many hospitals, as you know, now have ethics committees and some have ethics consultants.

What I hope to do in the time remaining is to assess the field of clinical ethics after this first decade and address some of the questions which have arisen about it. What is clinical ethics? How should clinical ethics be taught? What kind of research can be done in clinical ethics? What is the appropriate role of the ethics committees and ethics consultants? What are the future prospects of clinical ethics? Ed and I began by reaffirming the goal of clinical ethics that we had subscribed to initially – the goal was to improve the quality of patient care by emphasizing the importance of ethical considerations in patient-doctor decision making. Let me pick up on that point about the nature of clinical ethics and what is its relation to clinical decisions. Medicine is an inherently moral enterprise and the moral center lies in an act of the profession. Those of you who were here last year recognize that language. That language comes from Ed's thinking and reflection. Sick persons ask physicians to help them get better and physicians profess to be morally and technically competent to help the sick. This act of profession may lead to a physician-patient accommodation in which a joint decision is reached, first, that this patient will place his or her care in the hands of a particular physician and, second, that the physician affirms his or her ability to render care to the patient. This initial moral transaction between a patient and a doctor creates mutual responsibilities and establishes the context in which joint decision making can occur. Clinical ethics emphasizes patient-doctor decision making. Doctors make recommendations based on their knowledge, skill, experience, and personal values. Patients base their decisions on the medical information that is provided by the doctor. They interpret these medical facts through the filter of their own ambitions, preferences, values, and goals. Institutional, family, and societal pressures may constrain patients' decisions. The clinical ethicist then identifies, analyzes, and contributes to resolving the ethical problems that arise as patients and doctors make these decisions together.

I think clinical ethics has to be contrasted with biomedical ethics which is a broader concept. Biomedical ethics involves the application of ethical principles to the whole range of biological knowledge. Clinical ethics is a branch of biomedical ethics which focuses on the physician-patient interaction and concerns itself with individual decisions for individual patients. It uses ethical analysis to help resolve ethical issues and problems, but its primary aim is a right and good decision and action for a particular patient. Clinical ethics then is an urgent and concrete exercise that's filled with factual uncertainty. You remember Osler's comment about clinical medicine – that it is an art of probability and a science of uncertainty. Well, clinical ethics merely plays a role in that general atmosphere of clinical medicine. Clinical ethics is often conducted in an emotionally charged atmosphere. It requires a firm grasp of clinical language and clinical knowledge. And it has to conclude in an action for an identifiable patient. It confronts value conflicts among physicians, patients, families, and it deals with the law, social mores, and religious convictions. Many of these conflicts must in some way be resolved given the need to reach a clinical decision – and, of course, postponing a clinical decision is itself a decision.

Clinical ethics even relates to the standard of care in the following way. In earlier times when a paternalistic form of medicine was accepted, the standard of care referred to technical decisions that competent physicians would make for their patients. Increasingly, in the current era, the standard of care has come to represent decisions reached by competent adult patients after their physicians have provided them with the recommendations based on the best technical considerations. Thus, in the modern era, the standard of care involves decisions reached jointly by patients and physicians rather than physician decisions alone. Now, of course, ethical considerations operated in both eras, but the ethical considerations have changed. In former times the highest ethical value in medicine was physician competence and beneficence. In more recent times ethical concerns still take account of competence and beneficence, but they also have to take enormous account of patient values and self-determination. Clinical ethics then examines the process and outcome of medical decision making in an effort to foster excellent patient care. It is distinguished from clinical medicine primarily for pedagogic and heuristic reasons in much the same way that formal decision analytic models are distinguished from intuitive clinical judgment. But keep in mind that clinical ethics is intrinsic to the work of physicians and is inseparable from it.

I turn now to the question of teaching clinical ethics. In 1901, William Osler eloquently captured the need for clinical emphasis in medical education. This was in his great speech to the New York Academy of Medicine in December of 1901. Here is what Osler said, "In what may be called the natural method of teaching, the student begins with the patient, continues with the patient, and ends his study with the patient – using books and lectures as tools, as means to an end. For the student in medicine and surgery it is a safe rule to have no teaching without a patient for a text and the best teaching is that taught by the patient himself." Now that line of reasoning has been the mainstay of American medical education for the last eighty or ninety years. It was clearly picked up by the Flexner Report, written in Baltimore at Johns Hopkins by Abraham Flexner, which used that model of clinical education in which the patient was the best teacher of students.

Now over the past decade the teaching focus in medical ethics has moved gradually from the classroom to the bedside. Almost every U.S. medical school has incorporated medical ethics into its undergraduate curriculum and these courses increasingly have focused on clinical problems. A survey of physicians' perceptions – a survey done by Ed Pellegrino and colleagues – on the usefulness of medical ethics teaching concluded, "The most effective teaching was concentrated on specific cases and was taught in the clinical years by physician role models." An influential consensus statement, the DeCamp statement, proposed that ethics teaching "Should provide practicing physicians with conceptual moral reasoning and interactional abilities to deal successfully with most of the moral issues they confront in their daily practice." That DeCamp statement, published in January of 1985 in issue number four of "The New England Journal of Medicine," was very interesting. It identified seven or eight topics with which medical students and physicians should be familiar. But, more importantly, it agreed with the quote from the Flexner Report. It said that physicians and medical students ought to have cognitive knowledge about these seven or eight topics but also have to have behavioral skills in implementing that cognitive knowledge in the clinical arena.

Clinical ethicists have also begun to teach medical ethics to interns and residents. In a 1983 position paper, the American Board of Internal Medicine wrote, "A major responsibility of those training residents in internal medicine is to stress the importance of the humanistic qualities in the patient-physician relationship throughout the residency. The certification process must assure that this responsibility has been undertaken." A response to the American Board of Internal Medicine report echoed the view that ethics must be taught in a clinical setting, not as an academic discipline, but as a practical guide to action.

A few centers now offer specialized training in clinical ethics for professional ethicists and for physicians. Examples include the Hastings Center, the Kennedy Institute at Georgetown, and our own Center for Clinical Medical Ethics at Chicago. These centers and others engaged in similar work will train the next generation of clinical ethicists. Some people have asked me about our own fellowship program, that is our faculty development program, at the University of Chicago, and I think I will defer speaking about that right now but I will be happy to talk with people informally throughout this conference about it. Our group recently, however, was asked by a journal called "Academic Medicine," the successor to the journal formerly called "The Journal of Medical Education" published by the Association of American Medical Colleges, to do an issue this December on both the history and current educational practices in medical ethics throughout the country. And in fact on Monday we'll be distributing letters to the fifty major programs that we've identified requesting papers from them telling us about their work in the field of primarily undergraduate and house officer training in medical ethics.

A further question arises about the appropriate role for physicians and professional ethicists is in teaching clinical ethics. I've already said that the ethically sensitive physician is a superb role model. He or she can demonstrate that although the ethical and technical aspects of clinical decisions can be distinguished for pedagogical reasons they're ultimately inseparable in practice. It's a common observation that medical students respond better to demonstration than rhetoric. They do so in their clinical learning. It is likely that they'll do so also in their clinical ethics learning. It is essential that students see clinicians who are clinically competent and also able to engage in ethical analysis. In this way students will learn that almost all decisions involve moral choice and that most need not be referred for ethics consultation. The physician-ethicist is well equipped to demonstrate the conscientious exercise of moral responsibility in the clinical setting. The same would be true of the nurse, the dentist, and the social worker in their own clinical settings.

Now what might be the teaching role for the professional ethicist, the non-clinician ethicist? He or she would remain the resource to convey in the pre-clinical years of medical school, and perhaps even as importantly in the years before medical school during undergraduate school, the fundamental principles and theories of philosophical and theological ethics. Professional ethicists also serve as a vital resource in introducing medical students to the broader dimensions of medical ethics as they relate to public policy, social policy, and law. And finally, both in undergraduate medical school courses and in the clinical courses and hospital rounds, team-teaching between physicians and professional ethicists should continue to be encouraged.

Let me turn now to the question of research in clinical ethics. Research in clinical ethics focuses on ethical questions which arise in the practice of medicine and which may be susceptible either to data based or theoretical research. Examples of the kinds of questions I have in mind include the following. How should informed consent be applied in different clinical settings? Does informed consent accomplish its goals of increasing patient self-determination? How reliable are patient choices made in the midst of crisis and do patients change their minds frequently? What variables in a doctor-patient relationship modify patient choices and patient preferences? What is the effect of institutional constraints including economic considerations on modifying the choices patients make in reaching decisions? Now those four or five questions that I've just given you are questions for which there are no answers at the present time. The ideal approach to examining those questions would combine quantitative clinical research with ethical analysis. First, the investigator would collect data to describe the contours of the clinical ethical problem. Second, the data would be analyzed according to the methods of stochastic and scientific inference.   Third, one would analyze the inferential conclusions in the light of ethical guidelines, law, and public policy. And fourth, the investigator would evaluate these conclusions in the light of normative ethical theories based on virtue or duty or consequences.

Clinical research in medical ethics involves the collection and analysis of clinical data. It describes the way clinical decisions are in fact made, the values that are used, how they are used, by whom, and under what conditions. The methods of descriptive clinical ethics are those of quantitative social sciences – medical sociology and anthropology, health services research, decision analysis, and clinical epidemiology. Examples of clinical research in ethics include (1) the trade-offs patients make between length of survival and quality of life – work that McNeal, Pouker, Sox, and Weischelbaum did in Boston in the late seventies and (2) the prevalence of patients' withdrawal from dialysis – the work of Kjellstrand and colleagues in Minneapolis and (3) studies of the processes of obtaining informed consent – the work in which the Pittsburgh group of Appelbaum, Roth, and Meisel has been preeminent.

I appreciate that empirical studies in ethics are not going to resolve the normative ethical issues of what action is right or wrong in a particular circumstance. I want to suggest, however, that descriptive research of the sort I am talking about can help to structure ethical analyses and may ultimately contribute to a better understanding of the normative issues that lie at the heart of clinical ethics. Theoretical or analytic research in medical ethics builds, or should build, upon the conclusions of data based clinical research. Such theoretical research should attempt to identify conceptual issues and to structure coherent arguments for ethically acceptable practice.   This research should examine the clinical ethical problems from the perspective of fundamental normative principles of ethics. Examples of theoretical research in recent years include the distinction between killing or letting die, the moral implications of using placebos, the meaning of autonomy, the meaning of beneficence, and others.   Research in medical ethics examines the intersection of ethics and clinical medicine. And, if this is the case, interdisciplinary research is desirable and, perhaps, even mandatory. Quantitative clinical research would be carried out by clinical investigators trained in clinical epidemiology or the social sciences. Philosophical theoretical research would be the domain of the professional ethicist with strong foundations in theology, philosophy, or law. The physician-ethicist is analogous to the clinical researcher and the professional ethicist here could be seen as analogous to the basic scientist. Both are essential for developing a research base in medical ethics that can contribute to improving medical practice.

I turn now to the question of service, particularly that rendered to ethics committees and consultants. This is one of the service roles of clinical ethics. In addition to teaching and research, the clinical ethicist has service responsibilities. These are fulfilled in many ways including serving as a consultant or member of an ethics committee. Consultations and ethics committees can serve three functions: to educate staff, to help establish institutional policy, and to make patient care decisions. Committees and consultants improve clinical ethical decision making by educating hospital staff and by developing reasonable and sensitive institutional policies on ethics matters such as brain death, orders not to resuscitate, living wills, organ transplantation, to name just a few.

The critical question facing ethics committees and consultants is the following. Do they improve the process of clinical ethics decision making when they get involved directly or indirectly in individual patient care decision? The problem for committees and consultants is that by making patient care decisions they may diffuse or usurp the decision making responsibility that should be exercised by the patient and the attending physician. Regarding this difficult problem of patient care decisions it's useful to distinguish between the potential roles of ethics committees and ethics consultants. The difference between these two functions we, that is Ed and I, agreed is analogous to the difference between a court of appeals and a lower court. Ethics committees resemble the appeals court where all the evidence has been collected, not much further evidence can be entered into the record and the decision must be made on a careful review and analysis of the established clinical record. By contrast ethics consultations resemble the lower court where the record is being established and where all the relevant evidence is entered by the parties involved in the case. Ethics consultants will evaluate a patient on request and collect much of the primary data – the data upon which the clinical ethical decision will be based – in discussions with the patient, the family, the nurses, the physicians, the consultants, and the hospital administrators. The clinical ethicist who sees patients in consultation has to be able to do ethics under fire and in ambiguous situations. This requires balance, objectivity and compassion, a capacity to counsel and to psychologically support the participants without imposing the ethicist's own moral values upon them. The clinical ethics consultant must be available and accessible when the crucial decisions have to be made – day and night in the operating room, the clinic, the emergency room, or on the ward. The ethics consultant has to have an understanding not only of ethical theories and principles but also of relevant policy statements, legal cases, and published papers in the medical literature. The consultant should be knowledgeable in the clinical details of the situation and should be ready to apply clinical judgment to the difficult issues as they are encountered.

Now a physician who is competent as a clinician and trained in medical ethics can be particularly effective as a consultant. Physicians enjoy the advantages of a firm grasp of the factual material – diagnostics, prognostics, and therapeutics – upon which the ethical decision must rest. Physicians also have experience in making decisions which are urgent, complex, emotionally charged, and filled with uncertainty and they are accustomed to communicating with and counseling patients. The properly trained and clinically acculturated professional ethicist, the non-physician ethicist, should be able to meet many of these same requirements. This would, of course, mean that the professional ethicist must assimilate many elements of a medical education in order to approach the synthesis of technical and moral capability. The best professional ethicists today who are doing consultations have done just this.

Now the number of ethics committees and consultants in hospitals has increased rapidly in recent years. It is essential that these new health services be evaluated critically to determine their contribution to patient care. I'm going to depart for a moment from this paper to tell you that just ten days ago the American College of Physicians Ethics Committee put the final touches on the second edition of its ethics manual and approved it. Now this approval has to go to the College's Board of Regents for their approval in April but I'd like to read you at least what the American College of Physicians Ethics Committee said about ethics committees and ethics consultants. I am quoting now from our statement:

> Ethics committees and ethics consultants offer two different approaches to the same goal: improving the care of patients by attending to the ethical issues that frequently arise in clinical settings. Ethics committees and consultants contribute to achieving these patient care goals primarily by developing educational programs in the institution, by coordinating institutional resources, by providing a forum for discussion among medical and hospital professionals, and by assisting institutions to develop sound policies and practices. Although it is generally agreed that neither ethics committees nor consultants should have decision making authority it is less well established whether they should serve in an advisory capacity for physicians regarding difficult ethical matters about particular patients. Neither ethics committees nor ethics consultants have been adequately evaluated prospectively to know whether they can serve a useful advisory function. The legal status and potential legal liability of ethics committees remain unclear and physicians are strongly advised to seek legal counsel about the current state of local law in this unsettled area. When a conflict arises over a treatment decision and the conflict is thought to include ethical issues physicians have the discretion to seek consultation from clinical colleagues,

patient care review committees, ethics committees, ethics consultants, or legal advisors. Of course, final moral responsibility for the decision rests with the patient and the attending physician and not with a consultant or a committee.

In conclusion, then, let me look ahead to the future of clinical medical ethics. In this brief review of the teaching function, the research potential, and the service function of clinical ethics I hope that Ed and I have reaffirmed that the goal of clinical ethics is to improve the quality of patient care and that the focus of the discipline of clinical ethics is on the decision making process which occurs between physicians and patients. Ethics courses in medical school, research studies in ethics, and ethics committees and consultants should be seen as means to achieve this primary goal. Ultimately every physician and other health professional should feel comfortable with their ability to reach competent and humane clinical ethical decisions. Physician ethicists and professional ethicists will exist side-by-side for the future. One is not likely to replace the other completely nor would this be desirable because each brings a different perspective and different capabilities to the situation. Physician ethicists and professional ethicists must understand each other's potential role and contributions. Rather than competing, they must complement and supplement each other to advance the increasing quality of ethical decisions that are now being required, desired, and even demanded by patients and families. As far as manpower and womanpower needs are concerned, the field of clinical ethics is going to need a variety of trained personnel. First, all physicians will need to be better educated in making the day-to-day clinical ethical decisions which have become an intrinsic part of every branch and specialty of medicine. Second, to assist them with complicated cases physicians should have available some kinds of consultants. For the foreseeable future these consultants will be a mix of physicians trained in ethics and professional ethicists who are interested in the clinical application of their discipline. Third, professional ethicists and clinical investigators are both needed to pursue data based and theoretical research which should serve as the underpinning of clinical medical ethics.

When we come back ten years from now and review the field of clinical ethics my hope is that the focus will have shifted from ethics courses and ethics committees and ethics consultants to a more general understanding on the part of most physicians and medical students that ethics is an inherent and inseparable part of good clinical medicine. We hope that clinical ethics will then have been restored to its rightful place at the interstices of relations between patients who are sick and asking for help and the doctors who profess to be able to heal or comfort them.

Response to
CLINICAL MEDICAL ETHICS: A REVIEW OF THE FIRST DECADE

Maura Ryan

In a 1993 article entitled "Falling Off the Pedestal: What is Happening to the Traditional Doctor-Patient Relationship?" Mark Siegler observed, with some irony, that 1990 could be called the highpoint in the history of patient autonomy. (*Mayo Clinic Proceedings* 1993; 68: 461-467, 464. See also M. Siegler, "The Progression of Medicine: From Physician Paternalism to Patient Autonomy to Bureaucratic Parsimony," *Archives of Internal Medicine* 1982; 142:1899-1902.) With the Cruzan decision and the passage of the Patient Self-Determination Act, it was clear that the "age of the doctor" had given way to the "age of the patient." Growing recognition of the rights of patients, especially the dying, to determine the course of their treatment had, by 1990, dramatically shifted the traditional standard of care. No longer "doctor knows best," it had increasingly come to be taken for granted that good medicine should achieve more than just sound clinical outcomes; it should also serve the values and goals of the patient.

But even as the rhetoric of patient autonomy reached full flower, the "age of the patient" was already over. With the introduction of Diagnosis Related Groups in the 1980s we entered the "age of the payer" and the rapid rise of managed care would bring it fully upon us by the mid-1990s. We would continue to speak and act as though patient autonomy was the prevailing value in medical decision-making, but, as Siegler points out, even as the ink dried on the Patient Self -Determination Act, self-determination had already begun to be replaced by interests in profitability, efficiency, and broad resource management. Once comfortably insulated from institutional and social considerations, the physician-patient relationship in the present age of managed care has become an uncomfortable triad, with decision-making power often lying with a third party. It is neither the patient nor the physician calling the shots it seems but the case manager.

Dr. Siegler's Clarke Family Lecture surveys the birth of clinical medical ethics. His reflections on the importance of bringing medical ethics into clinical practice assume that medicine is inherently a moral enterprise, with the physician-patient relationship at its core. As Dr. Edmund Pellegrino has long argued, the sick person, in placing himself or herself in the hands of a physician, makes an act of trust in the profession which engenders mutual responsibilities. The challenge for clinical medical ethics in its first decade was to encourage recognition in clinical and educational settings of what is at stake in the medical encounter: a "right and good decision for a particular patient." It was also to break down the working dichotomy between ethics (a task for theorists) and medicine (the domain of clinicians). Teaching ethics at the bedside, as Siegler and others advocate, sought to make clinicians see that good clinical medicine *implies* that both technical and ethical considerations are taken into account.

What is the challenge for clinical medical ethics at the end of its second decade? With the exception of the genetic revolution, medical ethics in the 1990s has been most preoccupied with physician-assisted suicide and managed care. At first blush, these issues seem to be polar opposites. The movement to legalize physician-assisted suicide is a child of the age of the patient. It grew out of the broader movement to define and secure the rights of patients to refuse medical treatment. Legalized physician-assisted suicide is an extension of the philosophy that competent adults, especially when they are terminally ill, should be free to determine the time and manner of their death. For some, physician-assisted suicide symbolizes "autonomy run amok." Legalizing physician-assisted suicide in the United States, they suggest, is an ominous sign that medicine has lost its moral compass.

If the movement to legalize physician-assisted suicide is respect for autonomy at its extremes, managed care is institutional interests taken to their extremes. Touted as the great hope for our bloated health care system's economic woes, managed care reduces global expenditures by constraining both patient choice and provider discretion. Criticisms of managed care have centered on policies and practices which limit the physician's ability to pursue the best interests of a particular patient, e.g. fixed limits on the length of hospital stay, or which compromise the ideal, if not always real, intimacy of the physician-patient relationship. Even those who see some promise in managed care principles for addressing health care overspending in the United States find little to admire in the for-profit form of managed care that has proliferated since the failure of the Clinton Healthcare Plan. Given the intense resistance to government intervention that marked the debate over the Clinton Plan, it is no small irony that patients and providers alike are now looking to the legislatures to provide protection for patient rights within Managed Care Organizations.

One way to understand the challenges facing clinical medical ethics in the next decade, however, is to look at how the questions of assisted suicide and managed care overlap. M. Cathleen Kaveny and others have raised up the rapid transition to managed care as an overlooked danger in the debate about legalizing physician-assisted suicide. ("Assisted Suicide, Euthanasia and the Law," *Theological Studies* 58/1 (March 1997): 124-148.)   Under capitation arrangements, physicians are already placed in a position where there are financial incentives to undertreat. In addition, many of the resources that might be offered as alternatives to suicide, services such as aggressive palliative care and spiritual counseling, are low priority items when institutions begin cutting costs. Their concern, then, is two-fold. In a system where the bottom line is the prevailing value, will the terminally ill have access to the care needed to make a genuinely free choice *not* to commit suicide? Will physicians face subtle but powerful temptations to suggest suicide or to carry it out for economic reasons?

There is yet a deeper sense in which the problems of assisted suicide and managed care are joined. The movement to legalize physician-assisted suicide raises important questions about the meaning of privacy in a liberal democracy and about the limits of free choice. At stake in *Washington vs. Glucksburg*, at least in part, was whether the state's interests in protecting vulnerable parties against indifference or threat to the sanctity of life extends to preventing conscious, terminally ill patients from committing suicide. But the most profound questions raised by assisted suicide concern the nature of the physician-patient relationship and the meaning of care. The most persuasive proponents of legalizing physician-assisted suicide argue that it is the physician's duty to accompany the dying patient on a quest for a self-defined and self-controlled death with dignity. When, in the patient's view, death is the only escape from the physical and psychological burdens of terminal illness, the physician who refuses to act so as to bring death about violates the physician's commitment never to abandon the patient. From this point of view, physician-assisted suicide is merely a further step on the continuum from pursuing a cure to offering comfort when hoping for a cure is no longer realistic. Equally articulate opponents argue, to the contrary, that aiding in a suicide represents the very antithesis of the physician's role. To act so as to intentionally bring about a patient's death cannot fall within the physician's responsibility to seek the good of the patient.

Both positions assume that the medical encounter is a moral undertaking involving implicit and explicit commitments. They differ, of course, in their understanding of the nature of the moral commitments involved. If the physician is thought to be principally the servant of patient autonomy "a good and right decision for a particular patient" is ultimately whatever that particular patient wants, even if what the patient wants is to die. If, on the other hand, the physician's commitment is to the health and well-being of the patient, a good which can be known well only by knowing the patient's values and desires, but which is, nonetheless, not equivalent to the patient's wishes, it is legitimate to argue that a physician should refuse to act on a request to cause or assist in causing mortal harm.

The important issue raised here isn't whether physicians should have the freedom to refuse requests for assisted suicide. Even the most ardent supporters of the right to assisted suicide grant that an acceptable statute should protect the freedom to exercise conscientious objection. What is important is how we should understand the moral transaction at the heart of the medical encounter. To argue that assisting a patient to commit suicide violates the proper role of the physician begs the critical question of whether there is a proper role for the physician, a transcendent good or goal that medicine serves, that is subverted in the act of assisted suicide. The claim that assisted suicide is incompatible with the professional commitments of the physician assumes, as Pellegrino and Thomasma have argued, that there is an "internal" morality to medicine itself . . . derivable "from the nature of medicine as a particular kind of activity." (*The Christian Virtues in Medical Practice* (Washington: Georgetown University Press, 1996): 31.) In the same way, to argue either that assisted suicide can be considered as an extension of comfort care, or that it cannot be, assumes that it is possible to speak coherently about the purpose of medical care and its limits. But that is precisely what is now in question: What sort of activity is medicine? Which human needs and interests it should attempt to meet?

The advent of managed care also forces us to think about the ends or goals of medicine and the nature of those commitments taken to be central to the physician-patient relationship. One of the critical questions raised by managed care is whether medical services can and ought to be treated as any other commodity, dispensed and allocated according to the rules and practices of the market. For-profit managed care attempts to demystify the physician-patient relationship, turning medicine into a straightforward money making enterprise. Physicians and patients alike, however, have expressed repugnance, even outrage, at being treated as provider-consumer in a profit-oriented relationship. Indeed, in his 1996 Clarke Family Lecture, "The Crisis in Medicine: Professional Life in the Age of Managed Care," Pellegrino objected vehemently to the now commonly used term "provider." The physician practices the moral art of medicine; the physician does not simply provide a product. In the same way, our continued public discomfort at the disparities in access to care in this country, however lacking it may be in political will, suggests a deeper discomfort with the idea of treating health care like other consumer goods, available or not based on the ability to pay.

It may be, of course, that we will simply get over our discomfort as health care delivery moves increasingly to a for-profit corporate structure, just as we may get over our discomfort with the idea of a physician acting as the "angel of death." The resistance we now see assumes, however, that there is something at stake in the medical encounter that distinguishes it from other sorts of consumer transactions. At least in part, it seems to recognize what both Siegler and Pellegrino have identified as the moral core of medicine: there is a vulnerability in illness that makes the patient an unequal party to the physician-patient relationship and which necessitates an act of trust. The importance of the good involved (the restoration of health or the relief of pain and suffering) and the threat to the dignity of the person that comes with illness calls forth the act of profession, the promise to use one's skill for the good of the other. From this point of view, the problem with treating health care as a simple commodity is that it denies this vulnerability. The ill person in need of the surgeon's expertise is simply not in the same "purchasing position" as the person shopping for a color television. The particular risk of exploitation that results from the fact of illness and from differentials in power and knowledge makes medical care a dangerous sort of "product." Moreover, treating medical care as a simple commodity undermines the significance of the act of trust that forms the basis for the physician-patient relationship. Economic arrangements that create or permit the physician's economic interests to come into conflict with the interests of the patient fail to honor the sense in which the physician-patient relationship is inherently fiduciary.

Life in the age of the payer forces us to reflect on our expectations of medicine in another way as well. Two issues drove the debate over healthcare reform in the early 1990s: access to care for the then forty million under or uninsured Americans and rising health care costs. Whatever else we disagreed about, virtually everyone agreed that one problem could not be addressed without the other. At the end of the decade, we have a health care system that has been greatly restructured but hardly reformed. Access remains a popular platform issue. However, with the exception of some state initiatives to cover selected populations such as children, we have lost ground in the effort to secure universal coverage. Moreover, even if we set aside the ethical problems, managed care has not proven to be the great panacea for our staggering health care costs. Premiums continue to rise even with unpopular cost-containment measures and with the insured taking on an increasingly greater share of costs. After early promises, managed care plans are dropping Medicare patients across the country, citing high patient care costs and low rates of reimbursement.

Daniel Callahan and others have argued that we will not begin to address the global cost of healthcare or the problems of access until we are willing to question the demands we bring to medicine and the values that underlie health care delivery in this country. An unexamined focus on curing, coupled with a bias for the needs and interests of the individual patient, have brought us to the point where employers can no longer shoulder the costs of covering their employees and where overall costs are sustainable only at the expense of other important social goods. As Callahan observed in his provocative 1990 book, *What Kind of Life,* "nothing is more potent in driving up costs than the quest for unlimited improvement in quality combined with an unlimited desire to maximize choice, and then setting this combination in a system that is not a system" (p. 83).

"Revising our expectations of medicine" means, of course, that we accept the principle that medicine cannot or ought not do everything that could be done in every instance in which a patient might benefit. Callahan's work has been most controversial in its embrace of explicit, systemic rationing. But Callahan is not alone in arguing that eventually we will simply be forced to undertake explicitly and systemically the rationing of care that we now do implicitly (by failing to guarantee universal access) and on an *ad hoc* basis (by including some services under required emergency care and excluding others). Callahan is also not alone is questioning the bias in modern medicine on end-stage rescue care over preventative and palliative care. However, if we acknowledge the need for limits, either on medicine's aspirations or on the promises it makes to individuals, we return again to the questions posed by assisted suicide: What are the legitimate ends or goals of medicine? What human interests and needs should medicine address? If we face the fact that we cannot do everything for everyone, what values will motivate the choices we make concerning what we will do and for whom?

What does all this tell us about the future of clinical medical ethics? The goal of clinical ethics, Siegler argued, is "to improve the quality of patient care by emphasizing the importance of ethical considerations in patient-doctor decision making." Clinical ethics focuses "on the doctor-patient interaction and concerns itself with individual decisions for individual patients." It is an "urgent and concrete exercise." None of this is likely to change as we move into the next decade – nor should it. The physician's commitment to seek good of a particular patient through shared decision-making is at the heart of our understanding of medicine as a profession.

But even as clinical medical ethics continues to be a concrete and urgent exercise, oriented toward "good and right decisions" for individual patients, it will be increasingly important and necessary for ethical reflection to attend to these deeper questions of the goals and purposes of medicine. The framers of the Hastings Center's international project on the Goals of Medicine point to three reasons. The first is the practical matter raised by the movement to legalize physician-assisted suicide: we face serious and complex ethical questions today, the majority of which turn on "what is thought to be right or wrong, good or bad, for medicine to do for people in the name of preserving or improving their health" or relieving suffering. (*The Goals of Medicine: The Forgotten Issues in Health Care Reform*, Mark J. Hanson and Daniel Callahan, eds. (Washington, D.C.: Georgetown University Press, 1999.) And as the Human Genome Project opens up new possibilities for medical intervention, the assumptions we bring to the clinical setting concerning the meaning of "health" and the role of medicine in improving our lives will come even more sharply into question.

A second reason is that some of what we have taken for granted as the goals and purposes of medicine is now under attack. As we have seen, the modern bias toward curing individual patients is criticized for both for its role in driving up health care costs and its contribution to creating the conditions for the emergence of the movement to legalize physician-assisted suicide. But if we are in need of a reexamination of the priority given to some ends over others, e.g. to "curing" over "caring," it is important to look at what it is that we value in medicine, to "sense the ensemble of medical goals, and then ask how they should fit together" (*Ibid.*).

Still another reason is that, as we noted above, we have already entered the age of the payer; the drive for cost-containment is already underway and the need for systemic rationing of health care is probably inevitable. But we cannot usefully reform a health care system without knowing what we should be trying to do, what conditions are necessary to preserve the integrity of the healing relationship, and how we ought to establish priorities, e.g. how we ought to weigh the needs of individuals within a concern for the common good. At very least, attention to the fundamental goals or purposes of medicine helps us discern what we should be willing to fight for when up against the bottom line.   Obviously, the sort of philosophical and theological reflection called for here is the work of the theorist. Moreover, it is fraught with difficulty from the outset. Although we can identify certain "core" or "universal" values in the traditions of medicine, e.g. a commitment to the welfare of the patient, relief of suffering, and equity in access, we have nothing like a general consensus, within or across societies, on the nature of medicine as a profession or the ends medicine should seek. Medicine has always been shaped by the particular political, economic, and cultural forces of its setting. But I am suggesting that this sort of reflection cannot be *only* the work of the theorist. Clinical medical ethics and medical education cannot proceed immune from facing these fundamental questions. For all the reasons mentioned, the commitment to the individual that forms our understanding of medicine as a moral transaction, while of paramount importance, must be honored within and not in isolation from its inescapable social matrix. In the same way, reflection on the ends of medicine that is not informed by the practical experience and passion of the clinician risks neglecting matters essential for the good care of patients. And while aspiring to come to some working agreement on the ends and purposes of medicine in the twenty-first century may be hopelessly quixotic, it is nonetheless necessary if we hope to navigate safely the waters in which we now find ourselves. One thing is for certain: they are not likely to get any calmer.

WHO OR WHAT IS AN EMBRYO?

Richard A. McCormick

(This lecture later appeared in the *Kennedy Institute of Ethics Journal*, March, 1991, pp. 1-15.)

First a word about that title. It should read, "Who or What is the Preembryo?" Indeed, for the rest of this paper I'm going to refer to the preembryo. The word "preembryo" has raised some suspicion. It has been implied that such a usage has sinister motivations. I've heard that accusation often. For instance, Dr. Michael Jarmulowicz writing recently in the *London Tablet* asserts that this term was adopted by the American Fertility Society and the Voluntary Licensing Authority in Britain, "as an exercise of linguistic engineering to make human embryo research more palatable to the general public." I am afraid that Professor Jarmulowicz has a firm grasp on a preconceived idea that has led to a premature conclusion. I trust it was not premeditated.

Now, I can speak only for the American Fertility Society, not for the Voluntary Licensing Agency. I was a member of the Ethics Committee that discussed and adopted this term, "preembryo." Our discussion had nothing to do with embryo research or, even more generally, with embryo status. The term "preembryo" was used because the earliest stages of mammalian development do not primarily involve formation of the embryo and its parts, but the establishment of the non-embryonic trophoblast or feeding layer. As Clifford Grobstein, the distinguished basic scientist and a member of our American Fertility Society Ethics Committee, concludes, and I cite him, "The scientific rationale for the term 'preembryo,' accordingly, is its greater accuracy in characterizing the initial phase of mammalian and human development. The status implications of such a change in terminology were not at issue in the discussion." Now obviously, the status of the preembryo presents us with a set of questions with very practical implications. Some of these are the following. One, what may be done to preembryos before transfer into the uterus? Second, whether all preembryos must be transferred? Third, what may be done to preembryos that are not transferred? And then, of course, there is the extremely practical question of what is the acceptable treatment of rape victims.

Not all proposed clinical experiments directly affect the preembryo, for example, cytoplasmic transfusion. If eggs are harvested prior to peak maturity, they often fail to yield a pregnancy when they're transferred to the uterus. Assuming that this is due to the immaturity of ovum cytoplasm, researchers contemplate transfusing ova with the cytoplasm of mature ova. Other procedures are basically therapeutic. For example, this is the case with the removal of excess pronuclei. It can happen that more than one sperm enters an ovum. This results in the formation of three pronuclei. Such ova develop either not at all or abnormally as in a molar pregnancy.

Some actual or projected protocols, such as cryopreservation or freezing, directly affect the preembryo. Cryopreservation of extra preembryos decreases the number of stimulated egg recovery cycles for individual women and provides added flexibility in transfer protocols. However, significant numbers of preembryos die in the process of thawing. It is not a benign process. Moreover, cryo-injury cannot be altogether excluded, so it becomes an ethical issue. Down the road, a year or perhaps in ten years, lies pre-implantation genetic diagnosis. This would involve the removal of several cells from a preembryo developing in vitro. The DNA of these cells would be diagnosed, and then, only genetically normal preembryos would be transferred. With our growing knowledge of single gene defects and the rapid advance of amplification technology, it is not difficult to imagine scientists embarking on a variety of micro-manipulations of the preembryo in order to "learn something."

The status of the preembryo is, of course, not a new question or problem. Any number of advisory committees have addressed it. For instance, the Ethics Advisory Board, of which I am a member, agreed in 1979, that, "the human embryo," what I call the preembryo, "is entitled to profound respect, but this respect does not necessarily encompass the full legal and moral rights attributed to persons." The identical conclusion was drawn by the Warnock Committee in 1984 and by the Ontario Law Reform Commission in Canada in 1985, and by other bodies as well.

Catholic statements on the question differ in some measure. Prior to 1869, there was for centuries, as many of you know, a vigorous debate about the ensouled or the non-ensouled fetus. Most held for a theory of delayed ensoulment or animation, a position still defended by some contemporary authors such as Father Joseph Donceel at Fordham University. The distinction between the ensouled and the non-ensouled fetus was largely concerned with the canonical penalties for abortion, since all interruptions into the reproductive process were condemned as immoral. In 1869, Pius IX dropped reference to the ensouled fetus in the excommunication for abortion. Thus, excommunication was incurred for any abortion, even the earliest.

It is understandable, then, why recent Catholic literature would use the phrase "from the moment of conception" in its formulations of prohibited abortion. There are many examples, but one is sufficient. A very recent use of the "conception" terminology is that of John Paul II speaking to a group of scientists in 1982. He declared, "I condemn in the most explicit and formal way experimental manipulations of the human embryo, since the human being from conception to death cannot be exploited for any purpose whatsoever." Now, conception is understood as fertilization in these documents, though the two concepts are not necessarily coincidental or identical. By that I mean, that fertilization is strictly a biological term. Conception is not. It is still not absurd to ask when should a woman be said to conceive? In other words, conception is a movable term. In a 1990 letter to the Duke of Norfolk on the human fertilization and embryology bill, Cardinal Basil Hume seems implicitly to acknowledge this distinction. He writes, "I would assure you that there is no doubt that the church's official teaching is that human life is to be protected from the first moments of fertilization." You seldom find that phrase used. It is almost always "conception" you see.

The two most recent documents dealing with the status of the preembryo are the Declaration on Procured Abortion in 1974 and the 1987 document on reproductive technology, which I will call *Donum vitae*. (Its title, Instruction on Respect for Human Life in its Origins and on the Dignity of Procreation, is too long and therefore nobody quotes it anymore by its proper title. We all call it *Donum vitae* for short.) For the present, I want only to state the conclusions of these documents and, then, go into the argumentation. The Declaration on Procured Abortion is explicitly concerned with abortion and its legal regulation and, therefore, its chief concern is established pregnancy, not the preembryo. However, it does make all encompassing remarks about the protection of human life. Thus, it says, "In reality, respect for human life is called for from the time that the process of generation begins. From the time that the ovum is fertilized a life is begun, which is neither that of the father, nor of the mother. It is, rather, the life of a new human being with his own growth. He will never become human if he were not human already." (I apologize for the language in some of these ecclesiastical documents. Conversion is a word that is not too strong for what is needed now in the issuance of Vatican documents with regard to exclusive language.) Then, the Declaration goes on to make two points. First, it states that modern genetic science brings what it calls "valuable confirmation" to this perspective, since it shows that from the very beginning the genetic package is in place. I cite them: "Right from fertilization is begun the adventure of a human life." Second, the Declaration states that, "Its conclusion stands independently of the discussions on the moment of animation or ensoulment." Such discussions the Declaration expressly leaves aside. We shall see its argumentation for its conclusions just a moment or two later. What is clear, then, from the

Declaration is that human life must be protected from fertilization, even though the Declaration explicitly refrains from asserting that the person is present *ab initio*, from the beginning. For, if the soul is not present, the person is not present.

The next document, *Donum vitae*, is even more interesting. The Congregation for the Doctrine of the Faith asserts that it is "aware of the current debates concerning the beginning of human life, concerning the individuality of the human being, and concerning the identity of the human person." It immediately cites the Declaration on Procured Abortion, which I just cited, about the presence of genetic programming from the beginning. Then, it states, most interestingly, the following: "The conclusions of science regarding the human embryo provide a valuable indication for discerning by the use of reason a personal presence at the moment of this first appearance of a human life. How could a human individual not be a human person?" It then notes that the Magisterium has "not expressly committed itself to an affirmation of a philosophical nature" about the presence of personhood or not, as to whether personhood coincides, therefore, with fertilization. In summary, then, the Congregation for the Doctrine of the Faith looks at genetic uniqueness and, on the basis of genetic uniqueness, the Congregation is strongly inclined to see a personal presence from fertilization. From this basis, it makes two remarkably different statements. First, it is a person . . . how could a human individual not be a human person? The second statement is that it must be treated as a person. Now, those are different statements. What is called a "preembryo" here has rights in this document, and, indeed, a right to the same respect that is due to the child already born and to every human person. Harmful, nontherapeutic experimentation is a crime against their dignity and destruction of preembryos is abortion. So much for some of the literature by way of introduction. Let me now turn to embryological science to see what help it can possibly offer in these deliberations. I think two things ought to be kept in mind and, in a sense, in tension. First, as the Declaration on Procured Abortion notes, it is not the competence of science to decide the question of ensoulment or personhood. This is a philosophical problem. On the other hand, as *Donum vitae* notes, the conclusions of science provide, "a valuable indication for reason's deliberations about personhood." We might say then, putting these two together, that if science cannot decide the question of personhood, neither can the question be decided without science. What, then, does science tell us? Now, here I am relying unblushingly on three sources: the work of Clifford Grobstein, one of the most distinguished embryologists in the country; the work of the American Fertility Society and its embryologists – its basic scientists; and the work of the Catholic Health Association and its basic scientists, some of whom overlap with scientists in the American Fertility Society. The union of sperm and ovum at fertilization yields a new hereditary constitution, a genome, a unique genetic individual. This single fusion cell, called the zygote, has the theoretic potential to become an adult, a potential that is theoretic and statistical because relatively few actually achieve this in the natural process. It is to be noted that the genetic individual is not yet developmentally single, or a source of only one individual until a single body axis has begun to form near the end of the second post-fertilization week when implantation is underway. After fusion of egg and sperm, the zygote, that single initial cell, undergoes successive equal divisions or cleavage with little intervening growth. The product cells, or blastomeres, become successively smaller, but the size of the aggregate remains about the same. After three divisions, the aggregate contains eight very loosely associated cells.

Several things should be noted here. At this stage, as we know from other mammals, each cell or blastomere has the same potential as the zygote. If separated from the others, it can produce a complete adult. Furthermore, if two eight-cell stages of different parentage are fused, a single adult is still produced. As the American Fertility Society's Committee put it, "Current scientific interpretation of these and other results from animal experiments is that first cleavage divisions in mammals produce a packet of cells, each of which still has the full developmental potential of the zygote, that is, to produce a complete adult." Stated another way, at the eight-cell stage the developmental singleness of one person has not yet been established. The second thing to be noticed is that beyond the eight-cell stage the individual blastomeres begin to lose their zygote-like properties. As the American Fertility Society report notes, "The impression now conveyed is of a multicellular entity, rather than a loose packet of identical cells." This multicellular entity, the blastocyst, has an outer cellular wall, a central fluid-filled cavity, and a small gathering of cells at one end, known as the inner cell mass. Developmental studies show that the cells of the outer wall become the trophoblast, or the feeding layer, and are precursors to the later placenta. All of these cells are discarded at birth.

Now, notice, most of the development up to this point has taken place at precisely that point with those cells that will be discarded. As the blastocyst is attaching to the uterine wall, the inner cell mass becomes more adherent and organizes into two layers that make up the embryonic disk or the primitive body axis. The indication that this is happening is the appearance of the primitive streak. It is at this point that developmental individuality or singleness is established.   Two conclusions ought to be underlined here. First, these facts indicate that early events in mammalian development concern, above all, the formation of the extra-embryonic, rather than embryonic structures. "This means," according to Clifford Grobstein, "that the zygote cleavage and early blastocyst stages should be regarded as preembryonic rather than embryonic." Not much embryo development is taking place yet. As Dr. Howard Jones of the Jones Clinic in Norfolk puts it, "While the embryoblast segregates and is recognizable toward the end of this stage, pre-implantation, it consists of only a few cells which are the rudiment of the subsequent embryo." The second conclusion is that, as the scientist, Grobstein, has noted,

Genetic individuality and developmental individuality do not coincide. At fertilization uniqueness in the genetic sense has been realized and nobody questions that anymore, but, for example, unity or singleness has not.

The zygote with its unique genome may give rise in either natural or induced twinning to two or more individuals with identical heredity. In some species this occurs naturally and regularly – the armadillo, for example. Moreover, in mice – and probably in most, if not all, mammals including humans – cells of two or more different genotypes can be combined to form one embryo, which develops into an adult that is a mosaic of more than one genotype.

Dr. Andre Hellegers, when I knew him before he died, used to argue that he knew of six cases where this was only the plausible explanation. Dr. Jones tells me that at the present time there are well over twenty cases of such recombination. Before leaving this scientific overview, several other points should be mentioned. First, the product of fertilization may end up as a tumor, a hydatidiform mole, or worse, a chorioepithelioma. Quite aside from such anomalies, there is enormous loss of fertilized ova prior to implantation – conservative estimates hovering around the two-thirds figure. This was mentioned by Father Hesburgh at lunch today. I was hoping he wouldn't say too much more, because he was stealing everything I had to say.

What is to be made of these facts? I will proceed in three steps corresponding to the three sources of moral reflection. I will turn, first of all, to the Declaration on Procured Abortion and then, secondly, to *Donum vitae*. Finally, I will add my own theological reflection and conclusions. First, then, the Declaration on Procured Abortion. As noted, the Declaration sees in science valuable confirmation for protection of germinating life from fertilization. By "valuable confirmation" it refers to genetic individuality. It has nothing to say about developmental individuality. I doubt if the authors knew about that in the year 1974. But, since the crunch issue is not ultimately scientific, but moral or philosophical, the Congregation states its principle: "From a moral point of view this is certain. Even if a doubt existed concerning whether the fruit of conception is already a human person, it is objectively a grave sin to dare to risk murder." You can't act in the face of such a doubt. The Congregation is admitting, then, the presence of doubt about personhood, but asserting the immorality of acting in the face of such a doubt. The age-old chestnut is this: when the hunter doubts about what moves in the underbrush, whether animal or human person, there is a certain obligation not to shoot. I shall return to this below.

The second document is *Donum vitae*. As I noted above, *Donum vitae* makes two different statements. First, the preembryo is a person. Secondly, it must be treated as a person. Again, I insist they are different statements. Now, these are different statements because, even if one conceded that the preembryo is not yet a person, there might be powerful and persuasive reasons for holding that it ought to be treated as a person, <u>at least most of the time</u>. I underline "at least most of the time" because I'm going to return to that, and it represents my own position. Let me say first off then, that *Donum vitae* makes absolutely no use whatsoever of the distinction between genetic individualization and developmental individualization. For the Congregation of the Doctrine of the Faith, if the preembryo is genetically individualized, it is individualized in the most radical sense. For it asks, "How could a human individual not be a human person?" A possible and, in my judgment, sufficient response to this question is this – by not yet being a human individual, that is, developmentally single. Yet *Donum vitae* shows no awareness that in its early stages neighboring cells are loosely associated – that the cells of the inner cell mass of the early blastocyst are little different in developmental capability from the zygote. Each can contribute to any part of the embryo and separation of the mass into two parts can still yield two or more embryos. *Donum vitae* shows no awareness that only with implantation do we have primary embryonic organization, the embryonic disk. That a biologically stable subject is not present from the beginning seems factually established as long as twinning and recombination are possible. That it should be present as a minimal, by that I mean necessary, but not necessarily sufficient, biological substrate for personhood should appeal strongly to those in the Catholic tradition. This tradition originally defined person as *naturae rationalis individua substantia*, the individual substance of a rational nature, or, in Thomas's phrase, an incommunicable substance. The heart of these definitions originally concerned with the Trinity and the incarnation has come down to modern times so that "person" still refers to the actual unique reality of a spiritual being, an indivisible whole existing independently and not interchangeable with any others. The second assertion of *Donum vitae* is that the preembryo must be treated as a person. It does not develop this extensively, except to say that it must be treated as a person because it is a person. Well, that's clear. How could a human individual not be a human person? It is a person because it is genetically unique. Yet, it explicitly acknowledges that the Magisterium has not expressly committed itself to an affirmation of a philosophical nature, which of course is precisely what the assertion of personhood is.

Now to my third point. After examining those two documents, I turn to a bit of theological reflection which will, of course, as in all moral matters, be controversial and will invite your enlightened disagreement. Obviously, the question of personhood – and its constitution – is both critical and controversial. It is critical because it may determine what is morally acceptable or appropriate to do with preembryos. If they are persons, then they have rights and, presumably, that most fundamental right – the right to life. If they are not persons, then we must investigate further the claims they make on us as those *en route* to personhood. Now, that the matter is controversial is obvious. The strongest case for personhood from the beginning, *ab initio*, that I have heard argues from the fact that there is no stage of nascent development that is so significant that it points to a major qualitative change – not implantation, not quickening, not viability, not birth. In the simplest terms, no one in this world exists who did not exist as a preembryo. As Bishop Mario Conti, the Bishop of Aberdeen in England, put it about a month ago, "Human beings commence their lives at fertilization." This he sees as simply the common sense view.

In contrast to this is the view that demands a certain biological stability in the organism before personhood is possible. This stability is not present prior to the stage of primary embryonic organization. As Clifford Grobstein puts it, "The first sign that primary organization is underway is the appearance of what is called the primitive streak. Prior to this time twinning and recombination can occur." In other words primary embryonic organization is the time when singleness is being established. *Donum vitae* demurs. It states, "The conclusions of science regarding the human embryo provide a valuable indication for discerning, by the use of reason, a personal presence at the moment of this first appearance of human life." With all due respect, this is not what the conclusions of science provide, if beyond genetic uniqueness, there is also required developmental uniqueness. Bishop Conti, whom I just cited, has attempted to undermine this conclusion by locating developmental individuality earlier. Let me cite him from a recent issue of the *London Tablet*. He says,

> However, long before the formation of the primitive streak, there is already differentiation of cell function so that the inner cell mass present at the fifth day represents a distinct center of organization within the embryo playing a role analogous to that associated with the later primitive streak. In the case of identical twins there are two distinct inner cell masses at this stage. If the individual is already established at the fourteenth day with the primitive streak, the same individual is already established at the fifth day.

It would be immodest of me to try to referee this scientific point. Let me rather cite Professor R. V. Short of the Department of Anatomy and Physiology at Monash University in Melbourne, Australia responding directly to the Bishop. Professor Short says in this straightforward statement, "It is untrue to state that in the case of identical twins, there are two distinct inner cell masses at the fifth day. When spontaneous cleavage of the embryo is delayed until eight or more days after fertilization, the two resulting embryos have come from a single inner cell mass and share one common set of all placental membranes."

Where does this leave us? Norman Ford's book, *When Did I Begin?* lays out the facts of embryological development with admirable precision and objectivity. He knows the difference between genetic individualization and developmental individualization. Yet, interestingly, and, I think strangely, he agrees with the conclusions of *Donum vitae* that a preembryo must be treated as personal even though it is not a person. He puts it as follows: "Wherever there are reasonable doubts about the personal status of the early embryo, moral principles, without prejudice for the search for truth, require that the human embryo, from conception, be treated as a person." There are two statements there, two elements in that statement – moral principles and reasonable doubts.

A word about each. First the principles. It's been accepted teaching in Catholic theology for many decades that one is free to act on the basis of a doubtful obligation, based on a doubt of fact, provided that one does not thereby risk harm to a third party. For example, if you don't know whether it is Sunday or not, you are not obliged to go to Sunday mass. All right. The doubt of fact, in this case, concerns the personhood of the embryo. In the case we're discussing, the specific doubt is whether it is a person or not. Because the doubt cannot be resolved, the risk to the third party remains. And a doubtful fact does not convert to a doubtful obligation. The traditional illustration that I mentioned is the hunter who doubts whether the object moving in the underbrush is a nonhuman animal or a person. It was said that he had a certain obligation not to shoot and the axiom used for many decades was the following: it is one and the same thing in moral matters to do something and to expose oneself to the risk of doing it. *Idem est in moralibus facere et exponere se periculo faciendi.* Thus, the preembryo must be treated as a person.

The principle here, of tutiorism, appealed to by Ford, fails to mention, I think, several things in my opinion. First, it does not

mention the circumstances of the hunter. Is the hunter perhaps a
starving hunter or one on whom others depend for their lives? Would
such circumstances not purge the risk of imprudent recklessness? It
is precisely, in other words, the freedom not to shoot that renders
shooting a morally imprudent risk and brings into play the axiom I
just quoted, that is it is one and the same thing in moral matters to do
something and to expose oneself to the danger of doing. Second,
Ford does not discuss the degree of doubt. When he refers to
reasonable doubts about his own position concerning the personhood
of the fetus, he says, "Unless my thesis is shown to be certainly true
I hold in accord with the Congregation for the Doctrine of the Faith
that morality requires the human embryo be treated as a person from
conception." I think that's too sweeping. "Certainly true" is the type
of certainty we rarely have and more importantly rarely require for
human action. I agree with the Jesuit moral theologian, John
Mahoney of London, when he states that "the most one can regularly
hope for, as Aristotle and Aquinas realized, is certainty sufficient to
justify a choice of action. Such certainly is constituted by the
presence of very strong reasons for maintaining a particular view."
Are there very strong reasons then for maintaining that the preembryo
is not yet a person? I believe so. In this, I agree entirely with
Mahoney. He sees the probability that the preembryo is a person as
a possibility, at most.   There are two arguments officially adduced
to defend personhood from the beginning. The negative one, the
absence of any subsequent development so significant as to indicate
a qualitative change, he regards, and I agree with him, as upon further
examination to carry little if any force. The possibility of twinning
and recombination are key here. The positive argument, the one from
genetic uniqueness, is an argument used by the Declaration on
Procured Abortion and *Donum vitae.* It shows only genetic, but not
developmental uniqueness. Mahoney's conclusion, then, that the
opinion holding the move toward personhood to be a process is a
quite impressively strong one. Similarly, he argues that the risk of
destroying a person at this stage is correspondingly slight. I would
conclude, therefore, that Ford's moral assertion that the preembryo

must be treated as a person, because there are reasonable doubts about whether it is a person, is not a defensible conclusion in the light of most recent scientific data. And, if the preembryo is not yet a person, it cannot be the subject of human rights.

This does not mean, however, that preembryonic human life is simply disposable tissue. Not at all. I want to raise two considerations here that must be carefully weighed as we try to discern our obligations toward germinating life in this pre-implantation period. The first is the issue of potentiality. Under favorable circumstances, the fertilized ovum will move through developmental individuality, then, processively through functional, behavioral, psychic, and social individuality. In viewing the first stage, one cannot afford to blot out subsequent stages. Granted the statistical potential for survival of any given preembryo is significantly reduced. Yet, it remains potential for personhood and, as such, deserves profound respect. This is *a fortiori* weighty for the believer who sees the human person as a member of God's family and the temple of the Holy Spirit. Interference with such a potential future cannot be a light undertaking. The second consideration concerns our own human condition. I want to gather the subsequent reflections under the general word uncertainty. There is uncertainty about the controllability of human research enthusiasms. That is, if we concluded that preembryos need not be treated in all circumstances as persons, would we, little by little, extend this to embryos and then to established pregnancies? And then, perhaps, to some of our weaker fellow citizens? Would we gradually trivialize the reasons justifying preembryo manipulation? These are not abstract worries, I assure you. I have experienced their realization on the Ethics Committee of the American Fertility Society. Furthermore, there is uncertainty about the effect of preembryo manipulation on personal and societal attitudes toward nascent human life in general. Will there be further erosion of our respect? I say "further" because of the widespread acceptance and practice of abortion. There is grave uncertainty about our ability to say "No" and backtrack when we detect abuses, especially if they have produced valuable scientific and therapeutic data. Medical technology has a way of establishing an irreversible dynamic.

Let me conclude my paper with two proposals: one a moral statement, the other a practical policy. I hope my moral statement builds upon what I have laid before you. In view of the fact that the preembryo is not yet a person and that its statistical potential for becoming such is greatly reduced, it is not clear that nontherapeutic experiments can be excluded in principle. However, because the preembryo does have intrinsic potential, and is, in a sense, a person in the process of becoming, and because of the many uncertainties I just mentioned, I would conclude that there are good grounds for concluding that the preembryo should be treated as a person. But, that this "should" is a *prima facie* obligation only, albeit a strong one. This conclusion is virtually identical in substance with that reached by John Mahoney. After noting that depriving a preembryo of its future cannot strictly be called homicide, Mahoney says of actions that terminate its existence, "Even in the very earliest days, moreover, such an action could not responsibly be undertaken for any but the most serious reasons going far beyond considerations of convenience or scientific curiosity and affecting either that being's own prospects for the future, as in cases of genetic abnormality, or the life and welfare of others, as in cases of rape and incapacity in a woman to carry a child to term without risk to herself."

My second proposal is procedural. This matter, I think, is so important and controversial. It is important because, if we go the wrong way, we are for the first time sanctioning the use of living human beings (I didn't say persons) for the purposes of other people. Any exceptions, therefore, I judge from this *prima facie* duty to treat the preembryo as a person, should be based on criteria established at the national level. For this reason, I dissented from the report of the Ethics Committee of the American Fertility Society. That committee had demanded approval of an institutional review board for experimentation on preembryos – an experimentation which would lead to their demise, their death. My dissent read as follows: "The matter is of such grave public importance that approval of preembryo research should depend on conformity with guidelines established at the national level."

One final note by way of conclusion and protection of you, not me. Does this analysis, the one in this paper, correspond with current official Catholic formulations? No, not in every respect. I have indicated that the two key Catholic documents, the Declaration on Procured Abortion and *Donum vitae,* do not consider developmental individuation, a point key to my paper. I must point out, however, that John Mahoney's analysis, in his book *Bioethics and Belief* which I have cited, is practically identical with mine. Mahoney's book, containing an *imprimatur*, was published in 1984. In 1986, the *imprimatur* was removed. In a joint statement, John Mahoney and Right Reverend Ralph Brown, vicar general of the archdiocese of Westminster, explained why the imprimatur was withdrawn. At one point, they state that the imprimatur is no more than a declaration that a book or a pamphlet is considered to be free from doctrinal or moral error. This does not totally disperse one's anxiety . . . specifically, mine. But, then, they state, very interestingly, the following: "However, the question can arise, particularly in light of the passages of the second Vatican Council, as to whether a work which contains passages which are at variance with the church's current official teaching on a particular moral matter is to be considered by that fact as containing moral error." The claim here seems to be that the mere fact of divergence is not necessarily indicative of error.

If history is our guide, the answer to this question is a clear and, I would say, a rather thudding "No." Being at variance with the Church's current official formulation of her teaching is not tantamount to being wrong. If it were, the above reflections would be an exercise in intellectual folly and unquiet conscience.

Response to
WHO OR WHAT IS AN
EMBRYO?

Margaret Monahan Hogan

In the1990 J. Philip Clarke Family Lecture, Fr. Richard McCormick addressed the issue of the status of the preembryo. (The name preembryo or preimplantation embryo is the designation being applied, in the current literature, to the entity which or who exists after the union of the gametes and before either the appearance of the primitive streak or before the beginning of implantation. In this paper, as in Fr. McCormick's lecture, the term preembryo will be used. It characterizes a stage of human development similar to the way the term preteen characterizes another specific stage of human development.) In the lecture Fr. McCormick claims that the moral determination of status of the preembryo, within a medical-technological horizon in which *in vitro* fertilization and embryo transfer is an actuality and preimplantation genetic diagnosis a real possibility, is a matter of considerable importance. He maintains that the moral status of the preembryo exercises a governing function on the medical/technical interventions permitted on the being in question. He says, "at stake are such issues as: (1) what may be done to preembryos before transfer; (2) whether all preembryos must be transferred; and (3) what may be done to preembryos that are not transferred ... [and] ... what is acceptable treatment of rape victims."
To this list may be added the use of the abortifacients such as the chemical RU-486. McCormick's thesis is that the moral status of the preembryo – and specifically the controversial issue of personhood – is related to the attainment of developmental individuality not

genetic individuality. He offers several conclusions, one theoretical and two practical, in regard to his thesis. The theoretical conclusion is that the preembryo differs in moral status from the embryo. The difference in moral status, he claims, follows from the attainment of developmental individuality, that is, being the source of one individual, on the part of the embryo. The preembryo, he claims, has not yet developed to the stage of developmental individuality. The practical conclusions are contained in the concluding two proposals. The first of these, which McCormick characterizes as a moral statement, is the proposal that there is a strong *prima facie* obligation to treat the preembryo as a person. Here, the controlling notion of person seems to be the juridical fiction whereby one has standing in the law. The second practical proposal is a procedural one, that is, how the determination should be made as to which obligations may intervene to dispense from the prior obligation to treat the preembryo as a person. McCormick's proposed policy is found in the following statement: "any exceptions from the *prima facie* duty to treat the preembryo as a person should be based on criteria established at the national level."

McCormick's thesis is that the determination of the moral status of the preembryo is important (although a strange claim for an alleged proportionalist). However, his theoretical conclusion, that the preembryo differs in moral status from the embryo because the preembryo has not yet attained developmental individuality, is problematic. Moreover, his first practical conclusion regarding the *prima facie* obligations to the preembryo is not consistent with his denial of personhood to the preembryo. Furthermore, his second practical conclusion, the manner of specification of appropriate exceptions to the *prima facie* obligation to treat the preembryo as a person, is otiose if his theoretical conclusion is correct and elitist (the powerful confer value on the vulnerable) if his theoretical conclusion is incorrect. Since, however, the theoretic conclusion should exercise a governing influence over the practical, this response will focus on the theoretic conclusion. For if the doubts regarding the differentiation of the moral status of the pre-implantation embryo from the embryo are sustained and if the being in question is not a living developing human individual, then the conclusion that it is not a person, a bearer of rights in the law, seems correct. If the being in question is not a person, then the ethical injunctions that apply to persons and the laws protective of the interests of persons do not apply to this being.

This response to Fr. McCormick's lecture will examine his theoretic conclusion. It proceeds with (1) the examination of the development of his arguments, (2) the presentation of responses to the major arguments that advance his position, and (3) the delineation of an appropriate metaphysics, developing the rich notion of potentiality, to describe human life at this earliest stage of development.

In the establishment of the empirical foundation of his thesis, McCormick first examines the relevant scientific information, that is, the empirical data describing the ontogenesis of individual human life. He then gathers representative statements from various secular and religious sources regarding the status of the preembryo. He next takes up the controversial and critical question of personhood as that notion applies to the preembryo.

Prior to the exposition of this embryological data, he repeats two important observations found in contemporary Vatican documents. The first, from the *Declaration on Procured Abortion*, is "it is not the competence of science to decide the question of personhood or ensoulment." The second, from *Donum vitae*, is that "the conclusions of science provide a 'valuable indication' for reason's deliberations about personhood." These observations direct his own assessment of the role of science *vis à vis* the question of personhood. He says, "if science cannot decide the question of personhood, neither can the question be decided without science." His claim, here, that the sciences furnish information describing the empirical substratum which information directs and limits the ascription of status to the object of inquiry, seems correct.

In the presentation of the embryological data, McCormick notes that event, normally referred to as fertilization, which is the significant event for the emergence of a unique genetic individual. More precisely the event is syngamy, which is process in which the chromosomes borne by each pronucleus conjugate along a mitotic spindle supplied by the sperm and pair to reestablish the full species complement of chromosomes. This fusion of the chromosomal material of the pronuclei that results in the emergence of a new individual has been designated as the ontogenetic zero point in the development of the individual (Carmichael, ch.6. [Sources are referenced at the end of this essay.]). One standard embryology text describes the power of this moment in the following: "Within the fertilized ovum lies the capability to form an entire organism." (Carmichael, Leonard. "Onset and Early Development of Behavior." *Carmichael's Manual of Child Psychology*. Vol. I, 3rd Edition. Edited by Paul H. Mussen. New York: John Wiley and Sons, Inc., 1970, Ch. 6.) While McCormick concedes that this event may mark the emergence of genetic uniqueness and individuality, he claims that it does not mark the occurrence of developmental individuality. And, he maintains, that it is developmental individuality, the condition in which the entity is the source of one and only one individual, that is the significant occurrence for determining the moral status of the preembryo. McCormick adduces several arguments of varying strength to support his contention that, rather than a developmental continuum, there is an ontological shift in human development, after which there is one and only one human being present. Among his arguments, which appear to have their source in Clifford Grobstein's *Science and the Unborn* are the following: (1) vulnerability, (2) organization, and (3) purpose. In regard to vulnerability, he reports that only a small minority of the unique genetic individuals which come into existence survive to become adults. He says, "prior to achieving implantation – conservative estimates suggest at least two-thirds of them are lost."

In regard to organization, he reports that the preembryo is more accurately described as an aggregate of loosely associated cells. It does not appear, at this early stage, to be an integrated whole. It is not until about eight days, with the appearance of the blastocyst, that it becomes a multicellular unity. He says, "As the blastocyst is attaching to the uterine wall, the inner cell mass becomes more adherent and organizes into two layers that make up the embryonic disc or primitive body axis. The process is reflected in the appearance of the primitive streak. It is at this point that developmental individuality or singleness can be said to be established." In support of the claim of lack of singularity in the organization of the preembryo, McCormick alludes to several issues of biological fact in regard to the entity at this early stage of its development. They are the totipotentiality of each blastomere, the possibility of monozygous twinning, and the possibility of mosaic formation.

In regard to purpose, he says among the main tasks of the preembryo is work of the formation of the extraembryonic structures rather than the formation of embryo itself. He quotes the conclusion of the Ethics Committee of the American Fertility Society in support of his contention that because the purpose of the entity at this time is not specifically directed to embryo formation, the entity is not yet the embryo. That assessment in the words of the Committee is, "This means that the zygote, cleavage and early blastocyst stages should be regarded as preembryonic rather than embryonic."

In the assessment of the preembryo, this paper responds first to the specific arguments of McCormick and then to his major contention, that is, discontinuity of development. The three issues at hand, vulnerability, organization, and purpose, are matters of fact. It is their assessment that is at question. An alternative interpretation is as follows.

The fact of the vulnerability of the being at this stage, McCormick's claim that only one third of preembryos survive to become adults, even if true, does not sustain the claim of lack of individuality any more than the vulnerability of any member of the group of living human beings who have reached the stage of octogenarian would suggest loss of individuality. McCormick confuses predictions of the future with descriptions of present states of existence. He fails to distinguish between classical laws and statistical laws. Classical laws describe regularities – "a one to one causal relationship . . . other things being equal." (Lonergan, Bernard J. *INSIGHT: A Study of Human Understanding*. Edited by Frederick E. Crowe and Robert M. Doran. Toronto: University of Toronto Press, 1992, p. 88.)

An example of a classical law in operation is syngamy – the union of the human sperm and the human ovum with the restoration of the diploid number of chromosomes along the mitotic spindle which marks the beginning of a new human life. Here there is anticipation of invariance, the mark of a classical law. Statistical laws relate to probabilities, that is, assessments based on relative actual frequencies. The statement that only one third of preembryos survive to be born may be used to formulate a probability statement, that is, a statistical assessment of the likelihood that a preembryo will survive to be born. It says nothing of the nature of the surviving being. What might be concluded from this probability statement is that existence is precarious at this period in one's life. At the other end of the life continuum, it may be the case that only thirty-five percent of those who reach the age of seventy-five live to be eighty. This does not make those who are now seventy-five only thirty-five percent persons. It simply means that those who have reached the age of seventy-five are now vulnerable in a statistical sense.

The claim of lack of unity of organization as evidenced by general appearance and as evidenced by the specific time-limited capacities of totipotentiality, monozygous twinning and mosaic formation, does not seem to sustain the claim of lack of individuality. In regard to the unity of organization, this so called "aggregate of loosely associated cells" has an immediately apparent unity as an individual organism in its containment within the zona pellucida and within the corona radiata. In addition, the individual cells, the blastomeres, even at this earliest stage, while giving a superficial appearance of loose association, are in constant and intense interaction as the organism, through its genetically determined internal dynamism, continues its self-development. As early as the eight cell stage the process of compaction takes place. This process has been described in the following:

> During compaction the blastomeres flatten and become tightly joined so that they cannot become distinguished from one another with the light microscope. The intercellular connections, which are the dominant feature of compaction, serve two purposes. Tight junctions prevent the free exchange of fluid between the inside and the outside of the embryo, allowing the accumulation of a fluid with special properties inside the embryo. Gap junctions couple all the blastomeres of the compacted embryo and permit the exchange of ions and small molecules from one cell to the next. (Carlson, Bruce M. *Patten's Foundations of Embryology.* New York: McGraw-Hill Publishing Company, 1988, pp. 167-68.)

Totipotentiality, rather than a suggestion of lack of individuality, might be considered a particular strength of the human being at this particularly vulnerable stage of development. Because this stage of human development is particularly vulnerable, each of the blastomeres has the capacity to repair, by means of a biological process designated regulation, damage to the developing individual human being. The individual cells at this early stage of development have a prospective potency, that is, the capacity to form many types of cells, which is greater than its prospective fate, that is, the capacity to form the types of cells it normally does if its course of development is not disturbed (Patten/Carlson, p. 173). After this stage in human development, there is a subsequent decline in the human potentialities. This is true of human development in general. As certain potentialities are actualized, others are lost.

As to the lack of unity as evidenced by the occasional occurrence of monozygous twinning or mosaic formation, it is appropriate to indicate that very little is known in regard to the etiology of either process. It may be environmentally caused and, hence, accidental or circumstantial. And what occurs accidentally is not a determinate of the norm. Furthermore, monozygous twinning, understood as a type of regulation process, may simply be a particular kind of totipotentiality called into operation on the occasion of significant circumstantial damage to the developing entity. Or the unfolding of the phenomenon of monozygous twinning may be in the program present in the particular zygote. Neither assessment of the phenomenon of twinning precludes individuality as the norm for the preembryo. Mosaic formation may be another way of compensating for a different set of developmental defects or environmental circumstances.

In regard to the specification of purpose, McCormick indicates that the focus of development at the blastula-blastocyst stage is directed to the formation of the extraembryonic membranes. Since this purpose is preembryonic rather than embryonic, the entity at this stage must be a preembryo rather than an embryo. Inasmuch as the extraembryonic membranes are the source of the early support system for the entity in development, which support system is necessary for the continuation in existence of the entity, the appropriate conclusion seems to be that this is the specific function of the being in question at this stage of its continuous development. That is, the preembryo directs the development of its support system which is necessary if the next stage in its development, the generation of a body of a special sort for having a conscious life, is to be accomplished.

Obviously, this alternative set of assessments does not prove the individuality of the pre-implantation embryo. It is simply a set of biologically respectable alternative assessments. The function of the alternatives is to cast doubt on the doubts put forward by McCormick. It would seem more precise to say that the phenomenon of developmental individuality probably has its source in genetic individuality. Moreover, because the preembryo appears to be but a particular stage in the unfolding of an individual human life, it should be accorded the same moral status that it enjoys at later stages of development. That is, the ethical injunctions that apply to persons and the laws protective of the interests of persons apply to this being.

This description of the unfolding of individual human life from its genetic constitution at syngamy requires a metaphysics adequate to the task. That metaphysics requires attendance to the rich and ancient notion of potentiality (an explication which is painfully absent from the current debates regarding reproductive rights). Neither the zygote stage nor the preembryo stage can be regarded as a pure potentiality, for both are stages of a being in act. Each stage, as a series of events in the life of an individual human, possesses potentialities as determinate capacities which are actualized over time. A nuanced explication of potentiality requires attendance to the distinctions of potentialities as active/passive, as natural/specific, and as remote/proximate. In passive potency, a being has the capacity to receive modification, but the agency of the modification is an external agent. In active potency, a being goes from not acting to acting, and is, also, itself the agent of the acting. The zygote, and, *a fortiori*, the pre-implantation embryo possesses active potentiality in regard to whatever human perfection, physical or psychological, is in question. There are two distinctive features that make up the notion of active potency. One of these is constitution; the other is tendency. Constitution determines the kind of acting and tendency determines acting. These two determinants of action have been described in the following: "(1) the prefixation of the agent's nature or constitution which describes the 'sort' of action it will do; (2) the prefixation of the agent by tendency which prescribes action rather than not." (Wade, Francis C., S.J. "Potentiality in the Abortion Discussion." *Review of Metaphysics.* (1975) 29: p. 243.) Neither constitution nor tendency are sufficient of themselves to explain the act of an agent when the agent does or becomes something. Tendency is the intrinsic dynamism of the being towards the realization of the constitution. Constitution is the underlying manifold that determines the direction of the tendency. The constitution is that which the tendency, by its dispositive thrust, urges to completion. The notion of active potency is that of the capacity of a being for a particular perfection because of its constitution, and the action of a being towards the perfection rather than not acting because of its dispositive thrust toward completion. The preembryo is, by its constitution, determined to lay down the inner cell mass and the primitive body axis as well as the support system and, by its tendency – its inner dynamism – to bring about that development, without the direction of any external agency.

Furthermore, tendencies are differentiated as natural and specific tendencies with a subsequent differentiation of active potencies into active natural potencies and active specific potencies. In regard to the active specific potencies, the agent has a degree of freedom. The agent may specify the manner in which to actualize the potency. However, the active natural potencies take place in a completely determined manner, as determined by the constitution. The agent is not free to choose whether or not to actualize the potency. In regard to the actualization of the active specific potency, something is needed beyond the constitution of the agent to fulfill the potency. For the actualization of the active natural potency nothing further is needed on the side of the agent beyond its constitution. Factors external to the agent, such as the destruction of the normal environment, can inhibit the actualization, but the agent itself cannot inhibit the action.

A final distinction is to be made between those potentialities which may be designated remote and those which may be designated proximate. This distinction is a function of time and development. The presence of the proximate potentiality allows the possibility of immediate realization. The presence of the remote potentiality allows the possibility of future activity and future realization. However, the remote precedes the proximate and is the necessary condition for the existence of the proximate in terms of both constitution and tendency. The proximate is nothing more than the further specification of the remote. "The remote tendency is the source of the drive and the determiner of any of its specifications; and a proximate potentiality is only a modification of its ever-present and active remote, fundamental potentiality" (Wade, p. 249).

A more detailed consideration of the zygote, and *a fortiori* the preembryo, the earliest stages of development of the human individual, in terms of the metaphysical notions described above seems appropriate. The existential reality of the zygote is that of a human being in act. It expresses that being as a unified whole, unified in itself and distinguished from others, including the mother. It is living as indicated by its growth, its development, and its ability to utilize materials from its environment to sustain its existence. Its individuality – unless proved otherwise – and uniqueness derive from its genetic constitution. It is human and in it reside not only the biological potentialities but all the potentialities – creativity, spontaneity, truth seeking, loving – that are distinctive of individual human existence.

The present reality of the zygote in relation to the adult human being is not that of passive potentiality which requires extrinsic agency for actualization. In the act that is the zygote, there resides the active natural potentiality to become a more fully developed human being. The zygote is, by its constitution, determined as an individual human being and is, by its tendency, determined to become – in a fashion prefixed by its constitution – rather than not. Since the tendency of the zygote in regard to fuller human development proceeds in a completely determined manner and since it cannot become something other than what the constitution determines it to be, and since it cannot of itself not become, it may be said that the potentiality of the zygote for more fully developed human life is an active natural potency. In regard to specific functions characteristic of more developed stages there exists in the zygote the remote potentialities which specify the proximate potentialities which proximate potentialities are necessary for action. For example, in the chromosomal material there exists all that is necessary, in a relatively unachieved state of affairs, for the becoming of the primitive body axis or the becoming of the neocortex or the becoming of any system that is to serve as the material basis for a higher process.

In terms of the metaphysical notions developed above, a minimal notion of the life of a human person emerges. A human being is an open, unfinished being who begins existence at syngamy – its ontogenetic zero point of development – and who becomes what it is by developing its potentialities. The becoming which is described in various stages is a time-conditioned unfolding of the possibilities given at fertilization. The essential reality at each stage of development is different only in degree of actualization. What exists in the more fully developed human being, as a relatively achieved state of affairs, existed in the zygote and preimplantation embryo as a relatively unachieved state of affairs. If there is to be intellectual development, there must be prior psychic development. If there is to be psychic development, there must be prior organic development. Each prior stage is the necessary condition for the emergence of each successive stage, and each prior stage anticipates in its development the specification of the next higher stage. It is the same human being who begins in existence, who develops, matures, declines, and dies. The adult human being cannot be more than the reality contained in the zygote. The existential reality of the adult is that of a being who is in action the fulfillment of the existential reality of the zygote in whose act the sum of the potentialities of the being reside. The zygote is a living individual human being at a particular stage of its development. It is what the human being should be at that stage. The preembryo is a living human individual at a particular stage of its development. It is what a human being should be at that age. And so on ... It is the same individual who develops organically, psychically, morally, and intellectually.

If the position developed above – that (1) the arguments presented by McCormick are not sufficient to sustain doubts regarding the moral status of the preembryo and that (2) individual human life is better understood as a continuum from syngamy until death – is found to be more adequate, then the prembryo is to be considered a specific developmental stage in the life of the individual human being. While it is distinguished from the stage before it and the stage after it by structure and purpose, it is the same individual human being, in act. Hence, the ethical injunctions that apply to persons and the laws protective of the interests of persons apply similarly to the human being at this early, particularly vulnerable, yet internally powerful, moment. At a minimum these injunctions would include proscriptions against killing and non therapeutic experimentation. Moreover, "for the believer who sees the human person as a member of God's family and a temple of the Holy Spirit," this individual human life is sacred.

EUTHANASIA: WHERE IS THE DEBATE GOING?

Daniel Callahan

It is a great pleasure to be here. First, I am honored to be giving the J. Philip Clarke Family lecture. I never knew him, but he sounds to me like everything a physician ought to be. Secondly, I'm pleased to be here because my wife, Sidney, preceded me. She took part in this program three or four years ago, and I remember at the time feeling distinctly jealous, thinking, "Why didn't they invite me . . . after all, I'm the one in the family who writes on medical ethics." But they invited Sidney, and it is a pleasure finally to make it. And I will tell her it was a pleasure, and say that she led the way very nicely.

I'm here today to talk about the euthanasia issue. I chose this topic some months ago thinking it was topical then, but it has, of course, become even more topical. What we can see simply by turning on the television set or reading the newspaper is that we are in the middle of some fundamental changes in public opinion and medical attitudes toward the subject of euthanasia and assisted suicide. Public opinion polls indicate a striking increase in the last ten to twelve years in the number of people favorable toward active euthanasia and assisted suicide. The growth has been very striking. The leading medical journals – *The Journal of the American Medical Association*, *The New England Journal of Medicine*, *The Archives of Internal Medicine*, and others – have all run articles or editorials over the past few years favorable to a change.

This represents, then, not simply a quirky Dr. Kevorkian kind of phenomenon, but, it seems to me, something much more central to the highest reaches of the medical establishment. We saw, most recently, a report in *The New England Journal* of a physician,

Dr. Timothy Quill, who helped a patient commit suicide. And I was struck some months ago with the Dr. Kevorkian case. My initial reaction to it was, "Well, my gosh, those who are in favor of assisted suicide and active euthanasia are surely going to be embarrassed by Dr. Kevorkian. He is going to really set that cause back." I don't think it happened that way at all. In fact, my wife Sidney said, "Now watch out; be careful; he will probably help it." And I think in general he did indeed help it – people tended to overlook the strange circumstances and to praise him for his courage. And most recently, Dr. Quill has been even more roundly praised. Last Sunday an editorial appeared in the *New York Times* which said that what he had done was courageous and that the woman he helped was "very plucky." The state of Washington has passed a ballot initiative to legalize euthanasia and assisted suicide. It is rather complicated, so I won't go into details. It still has to go before the legislature. If the legislature does not act, it will go back to a ballot initiative, but it's very possible that the state of Washington will see the first law legalizing euthanasia and assisted suicide. The Hemlock Society, once a kind of a joke, has risen in prominence and is well thought of by many people I know in my New York circles. They see the Hemlock Society as a bold organization dealing with a problem that has been hushed up for too long. Finally, I would mention the legalization of euthanasia in Holland. Holland is a country very much like ours, in that Holland has very powerful traditions of civil liberties, of freedom, and of choice. The fact that they now make euthanasia available says, I think, a great deal about a shift that is felt first there, but is beginning to be powerfully felt here as well.

Now, the question I want to pose in a fundamental way right off is: What is going on here? Why are we seeing this kind of shift? After all, the issue of euthanasia has been around for well over a hundred years. England, as a society, has had euthanasia advocates going back well over a century. In this country one can find scattered attempts in the thirties and forties to pass laws legalizing euthanasia, but for some reason the drive to legalize euthanasia has really taken off of late. The first question I want to ask is: Why is this? Well, I believe we have a fundamental and extraordinarily difficult dilemma before us. First of all, the effort to improve the conditions under which people die – what I will call allowing to die, which is important and represents a valuable movement – has been much too slow and much too ineffective. In effect, we are beginning to see more and more people terrorized about their dying. Or, if they are not terrorized about their dying, they are terrorized about their old age and particularly terrorized about the possibility that they will end up spending years as demented people. It is that failure of the movement to allow dying more easily which is fueling the interest in euthanasia.

I believe that the interest in euthanasia represents a move in a very dangerous direction. So what I want to put before you right off is that we have a very tough dilemma on our hands. If it is indeed the case that we are doing poorly in allowing to die – and I want to suggest it is going to get harder not easier – and if that is in fact fueling an interest in active euthanasia and assisted suicide, and if it is the case that to go in that direction is dangerous, then we are caught in a terrible bind indeed. I want to present arguments to suggest, that we are not going to get out of this bind very readily.

What I'd like to do in talking about this subject is three things. First of all, I'd like to say a bit about the rise and the fate of what I will call the allowing to die movement and what seem to me to be some of the problems it faces. Secondly, I want to take a look at the euthanasia movement itself – looking at the arguments in favor of euthanasia and the arguments against. And, finally, I want to come back to the initial dilemma I set for you and see if we can get out of the dilemma in some way other than legalizing active euthanasia.

First, let me say something about the allowing to die movement. I became interested in biomedical ethics in the mid-1960s and even then one was beginning to hear discussion about the conditions under which people were dying. By the 1960s, a large majority of people began to die in institutions and more and more people were dying in the company of the high technology medicine which blossomed after the end of the Second World War. So that even by the end of the sixties, and certainly by the early seventies, there were any number of calls for reform. Elizabeth Kubler-Ross, among others, popularized the fact that many people were dying high technology, impersonal, deaths. A movement rapidly developed to do something about that.

Those of us who were initially concerned with the problem quickly came up with three general reforms which we thought would do the job. The first reform was that of the advance directive movement. Here the emphasis was initially on living wills and then later on the appointment of a surrogate. If everyone would sign a document specifying the conditions under which they wanted to be treated and, in particular, the conditions under which they did not want to be treated, patients would thereby be empowered to make their own decisions and be able to avoid these unpleasant deaths. Secondly, if we could start a hospice movement, that is to say, if we could provide an alternative way for people to die other than in the company of high technology medicine and other than in the modern hospital and if we could find a way of dying where the emphasis was primarily on care, comfort, and palliation rather than treatment, we would then have an alternative to the high technology deaths which were increasing. The third assumption was that if we could simply point out to physicians, particularly during their medical education, that an excessive emphasis on high technology medicine, particularly the technological prolongation of life, was likely to harm – not benefit – patients, then we could add still one more powerful move – a counter move – against the pressures toward high technology dying which seems to be so prominent and increasing. In short, there were three assumptions: (1) give people power, (2) create an alternative in an hospice movement, and (3) train physicians better. We believed that, if those three reforms were put into place, the problem would go away.

What I'm struck by is that here we are over twenty years later and the problem has not gone away. Many physicians report to me they think things are worse than they were twenty years ago. We see a steady stream of court cases and, while one may think that we may have run out of the possibilities of taking issues to court, it turns out that the possibilities are endless. I would expect that we will see a continuing stream of court cases in the years ahead. Despite some twenty years of effort, it is estimated that less than fifteen percent of the population have signed advance directives. And even if we have a massive educational effort, it would be amazing, at least to me, if we got that up to twenty-five or thirty percent. That would be a great change, but it may never happen. We have not, of course, managed very successfully to change the training of physicians. When I talk with people in medical schools these days, I find that, in fact, they don't give much time to the care of the dying. It's a topic that arises sporadically, say in medical ethics segments, but they are usually short. Frequently, the subject is still not much dealt with in the clinical years or in a systematic fashion. The hospice movement is here. Medicare supports it. But from all reports the hospice movement has reached a plateau. And I think it has become pretty clear that the hospice movement is really most appropriate for cancer patients and less helpful with other kinds of patients.

What I want to suggest here is that these are valuable reforms and there is still a long way we can go with some of the reforms. But I am beginning to suspect that, even if we could put most of them in place, we would still have a very tough problem on our hands. The reason for that is that as fast as we have found ways to give patients more power – to provide alternatives – new problems emerge. We are seeing a society in which, on one hand, there is an aging population in which there is an increase in chronic and degenerative diseases and, on the other hand, constant technological progress. The fact that the chronic and degenerative diseases are now most common and that they are the main killers, means one thing of great importance, namely, we are dealing with diseases which generally show a rather slow decline over a long period of time. They don't show the rapid deaths that marked earlier death by infectious disease. This means that it becomes harder and harder to know where the line between living and dying is, and that the problem is further complicated by constant technological developments which, increasingly, make it possible for physicians to do something for patients, even if not everything. The possibilities of extending the vitality of an organ another week, another month, of keeping a body going, of keeping organ systems going, constantly increases.

There is in our society a fundamental ambivalence toward death. Despite all the easy talk about death with dignity and natural death, the truth of the matter is that we don't like death in our society and we are not easily going to be persuaded that death can be natural or good. I suppose the most striking manifestation of this attitude is the paradox, which I take to be pretty obvious, that even if we recognize that death is inevitable, that it comes to us all, it is not clear that scientific medicine is prepared to accept that fact. The National Institutes of Health has campaigns against every known cause of death – cancer, heart disease, stroke, Alzheimer's. You name it; they don't like it. What I really would try to suggest to you here is that even if, at the clinical level, physicians understand that patients die and patients understand that they must die, the enterprise of medicine – as a modern scientific enterprise – does not, in its heart of hearts, buy that at all. At least it is prepared to make a very sharp distinction between being dead and what brings about death. It is very hard for me to see how the enterprise of medicine can ever accept death as a human reality, if it is unwilling to accept anything that causes death. I don't think we can easily have it both ways. We want the best of both worlds – which is somehow a recognition of the inevitability and indeed acceptability of death as a part of the human biological cycle – and yet, on the other hand, we don't like anything that brings it about.

In short, our reforms have not fully succeeded and, even if they could succeed much more than they have so far, I believe the very nature of scientific technological medicine is going to make it increasingly hard to find ways to allow people to die in the future. And I believe the public has caught on to this. There is a loss of public confidence that medicine can manage our dying well, a loss of public confidence that it can manage our decline well. Furthermore, there is a kind of tacit belief even within the medical profession that medicine cannot manage our dying well. That, to me, explains, in part, why many leading medical journals and many prominent figures in medicine have now become more sympathetic to active euthanasia and assisted suicide. They do not believe that medicine can well manage our dying. Now, the consequence of this has been an increased fear on the part of people and a fear tacitly supported by some segments of the medical profession who say "You are absolutely right, we can't manage this all that well." Hence, we see a very strong movement toward euthanasia. Let me, before I go any further, quickly make some distinctions, just to avoid any semantic confusion here. When I use the term euthanasia, what I really mean is active killing. There was an earlier tradition that sometimes distinguished passive and active euthanasia. I do not want to use that language. What I will mean by euthanasia is active killing. I will mean by assisted suicide, that circumstance where a physician helps a patient to kill himself or herself, where the physician does not act directly but makes it possible for a patient to so act. Finally, by allowing to die I will mean that circumstance in which treatment is terminated and the patient is allowed to die of underlying biological causes.

Now, what are the attractions of euthanasia and assisted suicide in our society? The most obvious attraction is that they build upon two widely accepted, deeply ingrained values – the value of self-determination, that is to say, the right to control our destinies and our body and the right to be relieved of our suffering. Along with our right to be relieved of suffering, if it is possible to do so, there is a correlative perceived duty on the part of physicians to help us be relieved of our suffering. In short, the main attraction of active euthanasia, philosophically, is that it starts off with very familiar common American values. The embracing of active euthanasia and assisted suicide does not involve a fundamental change of values. It involves taking values that are already out there, widely shared and widely respected, and moving them simply one step further. If I were a betting person, I would bet that active euthanasia and assisted suicide will become legal in this country simply because they draw upon such popular values. I think that would be a great mistake. And I want to suggest ways we can cope with it. But precisely because, with some exceptions, the movement toward active euthanasia and assisted suicide is not proposing to do something radically deviant from values now held in our culture, it is going to have a very powerful appeal.

The main arguments in favor of euthanasia come down to a relatively few and they are familiar. Some of the arguments build upon culture and some, at least one, do not. The right to control one's body is an argument which is a very strong one in our society and has been backed up by the courts over a long period of time. The medical duty to relieve suffering, the moral value of beneficence being called upon here, is deeply ingrained. There are many philosophers, and a few physicians, who argue that, morally speaking, there is no real difference between allowing to die and direct killing simply because in both cases the net result is a dead person. You can turn off a machine and somebody is dead, or you can give that person an injection and that person is dead. What is the difference then? Many would argue that there is no significant moral difference. Many would argue that there is a lack of social consensus on the matter and, therefore, in a pluralistic society we should leave the choice up to individuals. No one should be forced into euthanasia or assisted suicide, but given our diverse moral traditions, it should be available as a choice for all of us. Finally, the most sophisticated defenders of euthanasia and assisted suicide are well prepared to admit that there could be dangers and hazards. They will say, "Sure there could be a slippery slope here." However, they have two arguments in response. First of all, if the problem is serious enough, it is worth running the risk of a slippery slope. And secondly, it is possible to control slippery slopes by means of careful regulation, oversight, and monitoring. Those in brief are the arguments in favor of euthanasia and assisted suicide. They are the arguments that in each case have a great deal of persuasiveness behind them. They persuade people who are otherwise decent people, who, I think, are aiming to do the right thing. They are persuasive precisely because of their familiarity.

What are some of the objections? The one objection I don't want to invoke here because I think it is not helpful is the Nazi analogy, although it is used by many. The argument is simple: if we legalize euthanasia in this country, the next thing you know we'll have death camps. First of all, that argument is not likely to win much support. I know enough people, many of them Jews, who were horrified by the Holocaust and by what the Nazis did, and who are simply not swayed by that argument. I think it is as a rhetorical move, not a strong one, and it ought not to be used. Moreover, having been the victim of it myself on occasion on other issues, I think it is more often an *ad hominem* argument rather than a serious argument. So I would suggest that we forget the Nazi experience and look at some other issues.

To begin, a turn to euthanasia would represent a corruption of the role of the physician. The tradition of medicine has been one of healing, of comforting, and not of killing. As far one can go back in the history of medicine, there has been a powerful aversion to the physician as killer. But beyond that, there is another consideration of a rather different kind. I'm concerned about giving too much power to the physician. To put the physician in the role of someone who makes euthanasia possible means the physician has to diagnose the condition of somebody and then determine if that condition merits euthanasia. A patient reports, "I'm suffering unbearably. I can't stand it." The physician will have to make a moral judgment on the validity of that kind of comment. In the nature of the case I believe that suffering is an undiagnosable condition. People we know suffer. We know that individuals suffer, but there are no medical means of diagnosing suffering. And certainly one thing that every physician can tell you is that you can have three patients with similar conditions, similarly manifested physically, in which one patient can find that circumstance unbearable and the two others perfectly bearable. So the very problem of diagnosing the problem and deciding when to act seems to me to pose some insuperable problems.

Even more importantly, it is a great mistake to give any individual absolute power over the life of another. It is an intrinsically wrong relationship. A physician ought not ever to be in a position of being able to kill somebody, even if that patient wants to be killed, precisely because that is too much power to cede to any individual – physician or not. This is a kind of intrinsic argument about the intrinsic wrongness of euthanasia. That is to say, it is only possible if we allow one person to have absolute power over the life of another. Here I say absolute power, even if it is done on the virtue of a request – even if it is a free consent. It is still to give somebody absolute power.

Here, I will move one step further. When we think about the conditions under which we allow people to kill in our society we already have enough problems. We allow killing under three circumstances: capital punishment, self defense, and in the case of a just war. We surely know historically that we've had trouble with all of those categories. We surely know in the case of our country, at any rate, that in the name of self defense, in the name of the right to bear arms, and particularly to have handguns or semiautomatic weapons, we create an awful lot of carnage. We have not been able successfully, certainly in our country, to manage self defense well. We surely have not been able to manage capital punishment well. We may differ on that issue, but I think most people would recognize it as extraordinarily difficult to carry out capital punishment in a fair and equitable way in our society. And, of course, it is striking that most other western civilized societies no longer have capital punishment because they do not think that it can be fairly carried out. Finally, in the case of just war, one can run through most of the wars of humankind and find that it is extraordinarily difficult to have just wars. Furthermore, it is even more difficult to carry out just wars in just ways. Abuses and atrocities seem to be common to all wars.

The proposal to add euthanasia to the list of reasons for acceptable killing has to take into account the precedence for the three conditions for killing that are already present. Our experience in these three areas should not to give us confidence that we're going to manage this one any better. We have to ask, "Do we want to add a whole new condition of killing?" A kind of killing that I would call consenting adult killing? Killing that involves the demand, "You, doctor, kill me because I want you to kill me. I give you this absolute power over my life." We should not ever give anybody that power. When you give people that kind of power, abuse is to be expected.

A third set of reasons I would bring forward turn on the inherent instability of some of the arguments themselves. The two primary reasons given for acceptance of euthanasia – the ones I've mentioned, self determination, and mercy – bear some careful analysis. If self determination is a requirement, that is to say, if one of the reasons I have a right to euthanasia is that I want to be able to control my body and my destiny, then the question, of course, is why should I have to be dying in order to exercise self determination? Why should I have to be in any terminal condition at all? If it is merely self determination, and if that is a powerful right, why can't I ask to be put out of my misery for anything that comes along that I find bothersome? Why must I have the arbitrary condition of being in a terminal condition to call upon this?

The argument for mercy, similarly, has some problems. If we believe that it is merciful for physicians to help competent patients be relieved of suffering, then how can we deny it to the mentally retarded and others who are suffering but unable to ask for it, unable to give consent? Are we to restrict this privilege only to middle class, educated people who are competent, informed, and can read the literature, and make up their mind – and deny it to people who are suffering, but can't ask? In short, it is not clear why mercy requires that there be self determination. Now, what I would note, of course, is that most people put these two together. They say there has to be both self determination – competent patients asking for euthanasia – and mercy as a motive. But the joining of mercy and self determination is arbitrary. There is no logical reason why those two have to be brought together, and, in fact, it seems an arbitrary stipulation. So I've come to believe that if we embrace mercy and self determination, we will have to be on a slippery slope because the very concepts, those two concepts, only accidentally joined, each when taken separately, lead inevitably to a breaking of the boundaries that we would now specify. That is to say, there is no reason why people should have to set any conditions for euthanasia. We see, of course, how things have gone in the abortion debate. Once a woman is given the choice, it is her business – that's the nature of the choice. She doesn't have to have a reason. And I believe the same thing would inevitably happen once we accepted euthanasia. Moreover, if we believe mercy is necessary, we set ourselves up to provide mercy for those who can not give consent.

Finally, although I won't go into this in much detail, in the Dutch experience we already see those abuses. I spent some time recently in Holland and I am persuaded that they are not in danger of the slippery slope. They are already on it. Only ten percent of the actual cases in Holland are reported. It is estimated there are four to six thousand cases of euthanasia, but only some three hundred were actually reported to the authorities. Physicians I've talked to admit that it is just about impossible to diagnose unbearable suffering which is one of the stipulations of the Dutch courts. I have also talked with a few physicians who will candidly admit that they are interested in nonvoluntary euthanasia. They are interested in euthanasia of the incompetent and the retarded on the grounds of mercy. They now embrace a voluntary approach as a first step, as one said, as a tactic to move on to that other class of people. Furthermore, I've found many physicians who will admit there have been cases already of nonvoluntary euthanasia. In short, Holland, far from being a model of how well things might go, is, at least in my judgment, providing a wonderful model of how things can go wrong.

Let me come back to my starting dilemma. I hope I might at least have given you some reasons to think that a move toward active euthanasia and assisted suicide would be dangerous, but remember I began by saying that I believe that the whole movement of allowing to die is in deep trouble as well. So if that is the case, we have a very tough problem on our hands. We have a genuine dilemma. If the one doesn't work well, and its failure is precisely what's helping to generate the move toward euthanasia, and if euthanasia is dangerous, what in the world are we to do? I will give you no definitive answer, but I want to suggest a kind of strategy to deal with this. We have to try to return to some very fundamental values that underlie our ideas of medicine, our ideas of the self, and our ideas of the management of technology. I want to argue, in short, that it is precisely some of the values that we embrace in the name of the sanctity of life and in the name of medical progress, that are setting up this dilemma and that if not better managed will almost inevitably lead us to euthanasia.

There are three areas that we are going to have to think about in the future. First of all, there is one very fundamental issue, namely, the question of the control of our lives. Here is a value which is deeply ingrained in America. We believe we have a right to control our life. We believe we have a right to control our death. We also believe that modern medicine has as one of its primary values that it allows us to control life and death. We've given up fatalism. We have embraced the Enlightenment, which said that with the power of science and medicine we are no longer hostage to the fickle hand of nature. This is something we can manage. The very nature of the modern medical enterprise is an enterprise bent on control. Hence, the campaign is against the causes of death. Hence, the effort is to enable us to be rehabilitated, to function again, to be psychoanalyzed in order that we can feel well. The effort is to cure us, our physical ailments, in order that we won't die. The ideology behind modern medicine is an ideology of control. The difficulty here, of course, is that once you buy that ideology it is very easy then to want to take that next very short step to say, that if we fail in the control of our life and death through medicine, why not give us the control or put the control in our own hands so that we can make up for the deficiency of control that medicine itself generates? In other words, I see a kind of phrase used somewhat differently in this auditorium, a kind of seamless garment here if you will. You buy into control of life and death with medicine and once you've done so it is very easy to then buy into euthanasia.

I believe, then, that we must change our thinking about control. We've got to get medicine to think differently about the ideal of control. We have to demythologize control. We have to find ways to make control seem less attractive, less humanly valuable, less humanly viable. And this doesn't mean changing our views by just rejecting euthanasia. It means changing some of the ways we think about medicine and health care. We're going to have to recognize the obvious – that aging, disease, and death are inevitable. However much medical progress we get, however much control, aging, disease, and death are still going to be here. We can push things around, we can change the circumstances a bit and the timing, but we can't overcome any of those human realities. Somehow or other we have come also to think that we can not be happy as individuals unless we have full control of our destiny – that, somehow, the very meaning of being human is the power to have choice. Well, one can see the attraction of that, particularly the attraction in the face of a history which shows people so often overwhelmed by forces beyond their control. It is easy to understand why we want control. Nonetheless we're really going to have to ask the question whether the ego ideal, so to speak, of control, which is part of our bourgeois society, part of our middle class values, is not itself potentially dangerous if pushed too far.

Can we get a new image of the self though? This to me is the tricky question. Can we come up with a new image of the self – one better prepared to live with reality, better prepared to accept limits rather than feel that control is the name of the human game? This, I think, can only come about by asking some fundamental questions about what we want the control for, asking some fundamental questions about what kind of a person an obsession for control makes of us, asking the question of whether one can have really good control over one's life without having some understanding of the purposes of human nature and the contribution of control toward that. I can't develop this in detail since it is a whole subject in itself, but I want to suggest that the first thing we've got to work on is our self image as people and part of that self image is how we are to better situate the control. Unless we find a better way to limit control, we are not going to deal well with the euthanasia problem.

Secondly, we're going to have to understand nature and reality better. Those philosophers who believe there is no difference between killing and allowing to die are wrong. Death is still out there, nature is still out there. The premise that killing and allowing to die are identical comes from a mistaken view that somehow nature has been erased, that all is human agency, that we now are as gods, that whatever we do is what really counts, that omission and commission are the same. This seems to me a wrong metaphysic, a wrong way of looking at nature. You can pull the plug on me, turn off the machine, and I will stay alive because there is no underlying terminal condition. The fundamental philosophical reason there is a difference between killing and allowing to die is that, if you turn off the machine, people will only die if there is some underlying disease that brings about death. The crucial question to ask is not whether we can stop nature. We cannot stop nature. We will all die. The question is, what ought to be appropriate circumstances and timing of death? When ought we to allow nature to have its say? The mistake is to think we now control nature, that if a doctor stops treatment the doctor has killed. Families often experience this. Families feel that, unless they want treatment to continue, they then will be responsible for death. That is philosophically mistaken in a very fundamental way. But I think we are stimulated by the notion that somehow human agency and natural causes have become identical.

Our question ought to be, if we die simply because we are biological creatures all of whom die, what of the timing and the circumstances of our death? When is the wrong time to die? What are improper circumstances of death? Death *per se,* whether we consider it a good or evil, is nonetheless an inevitability.

When is death wrong? To summarize very briefly some of my thinking here, death is wrong if it is markedly premature. Death is wrong if there is significant human potentiality left – by which I mean the potentiality to think, to feel, to relate – and if the motives for death are wrong. I would propose to you two sorts of acts of historical imagination as one tries to think about these issues. When I try to think about questions of whether it's proper to turn off a machine, whether it's proper to pull a feeding tube, whether it would be proper to deny an antibiotic to a severely demented person, I ask two questions. First of all, if that person had died a century ago would it have been considered a tragic death? Would it, a century ago, have been considered a tragic death if somebody in a persistent vegetative state had simply died because there was no artificial feeding available? My guess is no, they would not have considered that a tragic death. They would probably have considered that a benefit. Secondly, a century ago, would one have invented a technology precisely to keep somebody alive in that state? Would one have sat down and said, "I wish we had tubes to keep people in persistent vegetative state alive indefinitely?" Would one have pined for such a technology? Would one have pined for an antibiotic, a century ago, in order to combat infection in someone severely demented in order to give them more years?

What I want to suggest by asking questions of that kind is really to see if we can pull ourselves a little bit back into an earlier set of circumstances when people did die natural deaths, that is to say, deaths brought on by disease. Can we recognize that very often in earlier times we were prepared to say that those deaths were not tragic, they were not wrong. Indeed they were often accepted, not simply because there was nothing to do about them, but because there was a recognition that life in those conditions was not a genuinely full and human life.

Well, there's a lot more to be said about nature, but let me turn to my third category, technology. Here we are going to have to rethink things, that is say, we are going to have to find some way much better than we've done to the present to domesticate our technology. We've engaged in a kind of technological gamble in modern medicine. What we've tried to do, in effect, is to say, "Look, it is our obligation and it is within medical possibility to keep people alive as long as possible." That is to say, we should use all of our medical ingenuity to maximize the length of life, and ideally, at the same time, to maximize the quality of life. So we've engaged in a kind of technological gamble. We've taken ourselves to the technological edge. We've tried to see how close we can get to the edge without regretting what we've done. The evidence is pretty good that this gamble is not paying off. We have, by trying to push things too far, ended up by creating some terrible dilemmas for ourselves. And indeed, even worse, we have created an enormous anxiety on the part of people – the fear that once we get ourselves within the health care system, that gamble will be taken.

We will be pushed as far as we can go, and, as often as not, it's likely that the gamble is not going to turn out well. As to why we take the gamble, two things have come together. There is our belief in the sanctity of life – a very powerful, important value. That makes us want to go right to the technological edge. Then, there is also the power of technology whose very dynamic is to push as far as it can go. If you look at the issue of sanctity of life on the one hand, and issues of how far to press technology on the other, in each case you could find ways to set some limits. But when you put the two together, and they work in tandem, it pushes us very very far. We're stuck precisely because we believe by virtue of our respect for life, by virtue of our belief that we ought somehow to conquer disease and death, that to stop too soon would be morally wrong somehow. So we try to push things as far as they will go.

How can we do something about that? How can we change the nature of the enterprise? Well, I would suggest we have to go back to a very fundamental old question, "What is a good death?" I want to suggest that a good death is a death that takes place when one is still conscious and takes place over a relatively short period of time. This is what death used to be for the most part. Interestingly, studies done one hundred fifty years ago indicated that the average course of a fatal illness was something in the vicinity of eight weeks. Records seem to indicate also that often the death was more painful, at least prior to good analgesics and the like, but it was shorter. I want to raise the question, "Can we begin, really, to think how to recapture some of that kind of a death?" Can we find a way to move back from that technological edge, back from taking that technological gamble? We might begin by simply asking of any technology if we use it, whether it will diminish the likelihood of our having a good death, instead of asking the question, whether it will prolong life? We can add a third question, and maybe make it even the first question, "What will the technology do about my dying? What is its likelihood of giving me a good or a bad form of dying?" We're going to have to find ways to stop sooner. We're going to have to find physicians who will find ways to help people who don't want to get into the system. We already see people who want to die at home, but what about the people who don't want to have to be tested for potentially fatal diseases? What about people who, when their physician says, "Well, I'd like to check that out," say, "I don't want it checked out; forget it; stop right now." This is very hard to do in our culture, very hard to do in our medical society, and very hard to do with our physicians. What if somebody says that he or she wants to be treated only if there's a certainty of a very good outcome, not a marginal outcome, but a terrific outcome? In short, I believe that there are many ways of thinking about the stopping of treatment, the moving away from this technological edge, of reducing the gamble, but that's going to take some rethinking of the way we practice medicine.

We can surely also work on, spend a lot more money on, research and technology to relieve the burden of chronic and degenerative disease. Twenty years ago the greatest fear of dying was the fear of pain. Now among the greatest fears are the fear of Alzheimer's disease, of ending up as a demented person. It is now much more common for people to talk about the fear that they will end up as demented, not themselves, or that they will become a burden upon themselves and a burden upon everyone else. People fear that they will simply linger on and on as something less than a human being. Well, we can in part respond to that by investing much more money in a science aiming to relieve that condition. We still spend most of our research money on diseases that bring about death

– diseases that cause mortality. We need to shift the balance more toward those conditions that reduce the quality of life even if they don't necessarily shorten life.

Finally, and maybe most crucially and most delicately, I think we're going to have to begin shifting the burden of death. Right now I think it would be part of medical practice in this country, part of our values, to say, "When in doubt, treat." I've told my wife, "When in doubt, don't treat." What if we begin shifting the burden? What if we say, "I am more fearful of getting too close to that edge. I'm too fearful of being kept alive too long. I'm too fearful of being demented. I'm too fearful of dying an excessively technological death. I would prefer to gamble in the other direction. I would prefer to have as much possibility of dying well, even if that means that I lose some productive life, conscious life, valuable life. And I want to die conscious. I want to die over a relatively short period of time. I don't want to push things as far as they'll go."

There is a lot more to be said here, but what I really want to leave with you is the following idea. The euthanasia debate is one that is powerful in our society because it does invoke values that are so central and so deep. Its power is precisely that it feeds off of those values. Those values themselves have to be rethought and, if one is going to make way against what I see almost as a tidal wave of euthanasia, it is not going to be good enough to talk about slippery slopes. It is not going to be good enough to invoke the Nazi situation. One must have some very different images of a human life, a different notion of what it means to have control of one's self, of how much control, and a different philosophy. That different philosophy should included a better understanding of our relationship to nature and particularly to our own mortality and toward the efforts of medicine to cure all the causes of death. And finally there needs to be a wiser perspective on technology – a greater reluctance about using technology and a greater recognition that our commitment to technology can do us harm. Those changes are not just changes in medicine, but they are changes that are necessary in American culture. They're not going to be easy to bring them about, but I leave you with that task, if you want to take it on.

POSTSCRIPT

I gave this lecture more than ten years ago. The arguments for and against euthanasia and physician assisted suicide have not changed during that decade, but there has been a shift in the politics. Proponents now press for physician assisted suicide rather than euthanasia, and it was that shift which, apparently, was important in the passage of the ballot in Oregon that legalized physician assisted suicide for the first time in the United States. The public, it was judged, would more readily accept a physician's helping a patient to commit suicide than tolerate direct killing by physicians, a shrewd and probably correct assessment. There has also since then been a Supreme Court decision declaring that there is no constitutional right to physician assisted suicide but that states are free to legislate it if they choose to do so. Public opinion polls have remained favorable to physician assisted suicide, as they have been for over two decades.

What has not happened is the "deluge" of euthanasia that I predicted. Ten years ago that seemed likely because of the public opinion polls and the fact that ballot initiatives in California and the state of Washington had come so close to passing. Dr. Kevorkian, meanwhile, was able for a while to avoid prosecution because juries refused to convict him. Why, then, has there been no deluge despite all the signs pointing in that direction? I am not sure about that, but the fact of the matter is that no state has followed the example of Oregon, no other ballot initiatives have been introduced, and no proposed state bill to legalize physician assisted suicide has even made it out of committee. Politicians favorable to physician assisted suicide, I would guess, have decided that the issue is either too controversial to take on, not likely to help a political career, or too likely to fail in a final legislative vote, and thus not worth the effort. At least on the surface, then, it appears that the apparent tidal wave in favor of physician assisted suicide has abated and that, at least for now, it is a movement that is not going anywhere.

What we don't know, however, is the extent to which it is actually taking place underground. I would surmise that few prosecutors are going out of their way to catch physicians taking part in physician assisted suicide and, in any event, there is no easy way for them to know about, or catch, such physicians. While I have long felt that there would be no viable way to monitor laws permitting physician assisted suicide – the confidentiality of the doctor-patient relationship works directly against effective monitoring – that same reality no less works against effective monitoring of the present prohibition of physician assisted suicide. The unanswerable question is whether physicians favorable to physician assisted suicide feel less threat in carrying it out illegally than was earlier the case? My guess is that they might.

One additional reason why physician assisted suicide has not gone as far as I might have expected a decade ago is that the movement to improve palliative care has gained enormous momentum, no doubt fueled by the worry about a turn to physician assisted suicide. The hospice movement – which now encompasses 500,000 patients a year – has also done better than I expected, with efforts now underway to extend its scope beyond cancer patients. While it is still easy to find cases of physicians who over-treat, who insensitively refuse to stop aggressively treating a clearly dying patient, their number seems to be declining. A younger generation of physicians appears to be emerging with greater sensitivity to the dying and a greater willingness to turn to palliative care.

Will there be a resurgence of legislative activity in favor of euthanasia and physician assisted suicide? Not for the moment I believe. The real test will come in another decade or so, when the baby boom generation begins to age and die in large numbers. It is a generation raised in a culture of choice and control. Furthermore, the public opinion surveys have always showed younger people to be more favorable to physician assisted suicide than older people. If those younger people retain their present leanings as they get older, a new push for euthanasia and physician assisted suicide could be expected – which could, of course, be counterbalanced by even more effective palliative care programs in the future. Together with the financial crisis expected in the Medicare program as the baby boomers retire, that may well be a fateful struggle.

Response to
EUTHANASIA: WHERE IS THE DEBATE GOING?

Paul J. Weithman

(At various points in this commentary I have drawn on my "Of Assisted Suicide and the 'Philosophers' Brief,'" *Ethics* 109 (1999): 548-78.)

In the decade since Daniel Callahan delivered his J. Philip Clarke Family lecture, public debate about euthanasia and physician-assisted suicide (PAS) has indeed continued. Since 1991 there have been popular movements in several states to legalize PAS either by enacting legislation, as in Oregon, or by challenging existing laws which prohibited physician assisted suicide, as in California and New York. These two challenges to the existing legislation made their way through the federal courts. Eventually, they reached the docket of the United States Supreme Court in 1997. In *Washington v. Glucksberg* and *Vacco v. Quill,* the Supreme Court famously refused to find a right to physician assisted suicide in the Constitution but also refused to invalidate the Oregon statute.

Though neither side would say that it lost the cases, neither can claim that its arguments prevailed. This is especially noteworthy because of the moral authorities who threw their weight behind arguments for the competing positions. "The Philosophers' Brief," filed with the Supreme Court and published under that title before the Court reached its decision, urged the justices to find a constitutional right to PAS. (Ronald Dworkin, et al., "Assisted Suicide: The Philosophers' Brief," *New York Review of Books* 44 (March 27,

1997): 41-47; pp. 41-42 are an introduction authored solely by Dworkin. The signatories were Dworkin, Timothy Scanlon, Judith Jarvis Thompson, Thomas Nagel, Robert Nozick and John Rawls.) It was signed by six prominent moral thinkers one of whom, John Rawls, is unarguably the greatest political philosopher of the century and arguably the greatest of the last two. The authors of the "Brief" contended that terminally ill people should be left free to decide for themselves what meaning to attach to their deaths and how they ought to face them. Society should not enforce one conception of a good death by making physician-assisted dying illegal. Joseph Cardinal Bernardin of Chicago took the opposite view. In an open letter to the Supreme Court, he urged the justices to strike down statutes legalizing PAS. (The letter was published in Joseph Bernardin, *A Moral Vision for America* (Georgetown University Press, 1998) ed. Langan, pp. 129-30.) The letter was backed by the Cardinal's ecclesiastical authority and by the moral authority he earned as a loving conciliator in the American Catholic Church. It had additional force and poignancy because he wrote it at a time when his every action testified that he thought death can be welcomed when it comes on its own.

In the end, of course, neither the philosophers nor the Cardinal carried the day. The medical profession, which enjoys a moral authority of its own, can learn important lessons from the facts that they didn't and that neither side conceded defeat. (For the philosophers, see Ronald Dworkin, Assisted Suicide: What the Court Really Said, *New York Review of Books* 44 (September 25, 1997): pp. 40-44.) To draw those lessons, I want to look at the social and intellectual forces that pose the dilemma Callahan identified in 1991. Though I think he has correctly identified most of them, (I say "most of them" because I do not think Callahan is right about the reasons "many philosophers . . . argue that, morally speaking, there is no real difference between allowing to die and direct killing." Of course whether or not he is right could only be settled by looking at the work of the philosophers to whom he alludes. Callahan does not name any in his Clarke lecture. Were he giving the lecture now, he would no doubt mention the authors of "The Philosophers' Brief" since both Dworkin's introduction to the "Brief" and the "Brief" itself contain just the line of thought Callahan is trying to explain.) I think they bear a closer look. A somewhat more searching examination brings to light ways the medical profession might intervene in debates about PAS and euthanasia. The examination requires a certain amount of armchair sociology, for which I hereby offer a warning but no apology.

Callahan is surely correct that the movement for PAS and euthanasia draws energy from values that are commonly held, prominently including the value we attach to control over our own lives. The need for control is felt most urgently in the face of natural, technological, and social forces that threaten to overwhelm us. The value of control is at its most politically potent in the presence of these threats. And so the political movements it galvanizes are most often defensive maneuvers. The movement for PAS is a movement of this kind. It is best seen, I believe, as attempting to allow people control of life in the face of infirmity, dependency, and terminal illnesses which end in death only after protracted and meaningless decline.

Once we see the movement for legalizing PAS and euthanasia as defensive, it is natural to ask from what point of view the life of a dying patient lacks meaning and from what point of view infirmity and dependence are threats. The answer, I suspect, is that these are most threatening in prospect to those in the so-called "the prime of life." This is the stretch of maturity during which adults are at the height of their intellectual and physical powers and at the peak of their earning capacity. This is also the stretch during which at least the most privileged of them have the greatest control of their lives. It is from their point of view that old age and dying are perceived as threats grave enough to inspire a movement for reasserting control by legalizing PAS.

A great deal of our reasoning about social policy and the good life begins with the way things look from this point of view. As a consequence, a great deal of policy is enacted or rejected as it advances or hinders the interests of those who inhabit it. One of the pathologies of our politics is that we – the electorate and those we put in office – have so little ability or incentive to think about issues from other viewpoints. We do not think about child welfare policy in ways that adequately take account of the interests of children or about hate crime statutes from the perspective of victims or about plant-closing legislation from the point of view of workers, or about PAS from the point of view of those elderly and terminally ill people who may feel pressured to avail themselves of it when they fear others regard them as burdensome or useless. This is not, of course, to deny the existence of unions, child-advocacy groups, or the AARP. But the existence of these groups and the way they are typically described confirm rather than refute my conjecture. The AARP, for example, is often called a powerful "special-interest group." What makes its interests "special" is precisely that they deviate from the interests that we reflexively take as the benchmark when we debate social policy.

If all of this is correct, then it is small wonder that the prospect of dependency and infirmity are threatening enough to make the legalization of PAS attractive. Cultural, intellectual, and political forces that push us to reason from the benchmark point of view are deep and powerful. One thing the medical profession can do is summon its moral authority to argue that important questions bearing on the legalization of PAS and euthanasia should be looked at from a different perspective. The medical profession can take the lead in asking, not "How does the life of the elderly look to those in the prime of life?" but "How do the lives of the elderly, the sick or the infirm look to them?" It should draw on the experience of care-givers to testify that these lives can be rich and meaningful to those who lead them, however much they may look like lives from which the young and healthy would prefer a painless and quick exit.

Unfortunately this is not testimony physicians are currently well prepared to give. This is because they too often project their own current preferences onto their elderly and dying patients when they reason about how their lives must seem to them. Studies show that doctors regularly rate the quality of their elderly patients' lives lower than the patients themselves do and that they significantly underestimate their chronically ill patients' desire for resuscitation. Anyone who doubts that this confusion of points of view, or a vacillation between them, adds impetus to the movement for legalizing PAS need only consult the most forceful writing in favor of legalization. The anonymous author of the famous "It's Over Debbie" ended a "scene" s/he found "cruel" on the basis of a very ambiguous request. (Richard Uhlmann and Robert Pearlman, "Perceived Quality of Life and Preferences for Life-Sustaining Treatment in Older Adults," *Archives of Internal Medicine* 151 (1991): 495-97.) Timothy Quill's moving discussion of his grandmother's death in his book advocating legalization appeals, not only to what he takes his grandmother's wishes to have been, but also to his family's shame "about their helplessness in the face of [her] extreme suffering." (Richard Uhlmann, Robert Pearlman, and Kevin Cain, "Physicians' and Spouses' Predictions of Elderly Patients' Resuscitation Preferences," *Journal of Gerontology* 43 (1988): M115-M121.) These writings show that doctors are not immune to natural human responses to pain and death. Precisely because these responses are natural and ubiquitous, they raise worrisome questions about whose pain and indignity PAS would generally be employed to end. What matters for present is what this shows about the point of view from which doctors are naturally inclined to speak, that is, from their own points of view rather than the view of their patients.

One lesson of the debate surrounding *Glucksberg* and *Quill* is that testimony about the possibility of meaningful yet infirm lives may not carry the day, any more than Cardinal Bernardin's testimony about the possibility of a good death did. This is because moral authority in the contemporary world elicits respect far more often than it elicits agreement or imitation. It is also because some instances of suffering, infirmity, and death will appear meaningless from so many points of view. Thus prolonged dementia ending only at death does not appear meaningless only to those in the prime of life. Many at other stages of life find the prospect meaningless or horrifying as well. Many may also regard as meaningless painful deaths which are unconsoled by religious faith. Good deaths may seem unavailable to terminally ill patients who are lonely, abandoned, or neglected by their families. Larger social trends like the loss of faith in the religious view that suffering is redemptive, the break-up of families, and the mobility of nuclear families combine with the availability of technology that prolongs life to create situations in which euthanasia and PAS will seem attractive from many points of view. What can the medical profession do in the face of them?

Something it should not do is rely on the exercises of historical imagination that Callahan recommends to determine when life has reached its natural end and when life-extending treatment is no longer called for. Those exercises are to ask "if that person had died a hundred years ago, would it have been considered a tragic death?" and "a century ago, would one have invented technology precisely to keep somebody alive in that state?" Technological, surgical, and pharmacological advances may have blurred the distinction between natural and unnatural deaths. It is questionable whether even those naturally occurring deaths which we can identify are good ones. These are serious issues. Unfortunately asking Callahan's questions will not help us address them.

Context suggests that these questions are supposed to be asked only about demented patients and patients in persistent vegetative states. One reason using them as tests is a bad idea is that the link between the questions on the one hand and dementia and persistent vegetative states on the other is, to recall a phrase of Callahan, too "unstable." In fact, it is every bit as unstable as that between control and mercy. But it was the latter instability which led Callahan to reject the argument for legalizing PAS that proponents consider the most compelling. Let's look more closely at how unstable Callahan's own link is and at the danger of that instability. If his tests for the use of life-extending treatment were in general use, their application could easily be stretched beyond the demented to, for example, Down's Syndrome babies with birth defects which are now correctable. If the death of a Down's infant from an intestinal blockage would have been thought natural a century ago, it would follow that the infant should not be treated now. But when applied to this case, the test probably yields the wrong result and certainly picks out the wrong reasons for arriving at it. Even if the defect should not be treated now, which I doubt, this plainly has nothing to do with the fact that infants routinely died of similar defects during the reign of Queen Victoria.

The deeper problem with Callahan's tests is that they invite physicians to take the *status quo ante* – *ante*, that is, the enormous medical and public health advances of the last hundred years – as their standard in a limited class of cases. But it was arguably the refusal of physicians, nurses, researchers, and public health officials to acquiesce in prevailing standards of natural death that was responsible for those advances to begin with. It is an open question in medical psychology whether the passion to fight contemporary scourges like AIDS and Alzheimer's is compatible with even a highly qualified acceptance of hundred-year-old standards of natural death. This is because professional virtues are often rooted in the commitment to simple injunctions like "Do no harm," "Heal the sick," and "Combat disease." Perhaps the virtues and dispositions that can reliably be sustained in professional life are coarser grained than those Callahan seems to recommend. If they are, then we must decide which ones we want health professionals to have. Given the choice, the passions needed to fight the scourges seem the more socially desirable. They also seem the more desirable in the present connection. The movement to legalize PAS owes less to the fear of being over-treated for AIDS and Alzheimer's than to the fear of contracting them in the first place.

Something the medical profession *can* do is take a lesson from the fact that neither side thought it lost in *Glucksberg* and *Quill*. Neither side thought it lost, I believe, because those on each side were convinced that they denied their opponents the outcome they really wanted and that they did so by staking out their own positions as forcefully as they did. Thus proponents of legalization thought that by making the arguments they did, they persuaded the Court not to find PAS statutes unconstitutional and laid the groundwork for future decisions finding a right to PAS in the Constitution.(This is clear in Dworkin's interpretation of the decision, particularly in his discussion of Justice Breyer's opinion; see the article cited above.) Opponents presumably thought that without their arguments, the Court would have found a right to PAS in the Constitution. Americans are often said to be instinctive centrists – this is a prominent theme in Alan Wolfe, *One Nation, After All* (Viking, 1998) – but the story of American politics that emerges here is different and more nuanced. It is one according to which America sometimes reaches the middle position by compromise between the extremes rather than by consensus among those who were clustered around the political center from the start. Decision-makers like the justices of the Supreme Court strike compromises like that in *Glucksberg* and *Quill* as much to avoid polarization as to satisfy the moderate majority. If this dynamic is indeed among the forces that drives American politics, then stable centrism depends crucially upon some political actors taking positions at the far ends of the spectrum. This, in turn, suggests that the medical profession can testify about good deaths and can vigorously oppose PAS, while knowing that proponents of legalization will remain resolutely unconvinced. It can do so on the grounds that its vigorous opposition is necessary to keep policy from being pulled to the other extreme.

What can the medical profession do to oppose the legalization of PAS and euthanasia, besides saying that the lives of the infirm can be meaningful and that a good death is possible? The profession can use its moral authority to amplify the voices of a special group of its patients, those who do not think their control over their own lives will be increased by the legalization of these measures. They are patients whose lived experience suggests that their society regards them as burdensome even when they are healthy. They are patients who may see the affirmation of their right to end their lives when they are sick as further confirmation of their dispensability. They are the poor and minorities, the elderly, and the marginalized.

Among the reasons legalization of PAS and euthanasia will not empower these patients is that their health care and their dying are particularly ill-managed. Advance directives and DNR orders are routinely ignored so that many patients are treated with extreme measures against their will. (Hanson, Tulsky, and Danis, "Can Clinical Interventions Change Care at the End of Life?" *Annals of Internal Medicine* 126 (1997): 381-88; also "Doctors Ignoring Last Wishes of the Dying, Study Finds," *New York Times News Service* (November 22, 1995).) It is well known that under-medication for pain discriminates by age, race, and gender, as the American Medical Association acknowledged in the brief it filed in *Glucksberg* and *Quill*. ("Brief of the American Medical Association, the American Nurses Association and the American Psychiatric Association, et al.," pp. 7-8.) If it discriminates on these grounds, it probably discriminates by wealth and income as well. Furthermore, there are significant differences between the quality and intensity of medical care received by black and white Americans, even after differences in income and clinical characteristics are taken into account. (Council on Judicial and Ethical Affairs of the AMA, "Black-White Disparities in Health Care," *Journal of the American Medical Association* 263 (1990): 2344-46.) African-Americans are more likely than white Americans to report that their physicians did not discuss the results of their tests or examination, explain the seriousness of their illness or injury, or inquire sufficiently about their pain. (Robert Blendon, Linda Aiken, Howard Freeman, and Christopher Corey, "Access to Medical Care for Black and White Americans," *Journal of the American Medical Association* 261 (1989): 278-81.) As a consequence, sick, infirm, and elderly members of these groups may unfairly be placed in positions in which PAS and euthanasia are the most attractive options. Having placed them in positions in which previously undesirable options look attractive, we can hardly be said to increase their autonomy by assuring them that these are options they are legally free to exercise.

Speaking on behalf of those most at risk from the legalization of PAS and euthanasia therefore requires the medical profession to speak about the incapacity to manage death that Daniel Callahan spoke about in his Clarke lecture. This would not be, in the first instance, a confession of the medical profession's past moral failures or an expression of its future resolve. It would be an acknowledgment of limitations inherent in professional practice under current conditions, with all their disparities of power and wealth. Under those conditions and in the face of those limitations, the legal prohibition of PAS and euthanasia has much to recommend it. The recommendation grows stronger when we take account of how much those disparities favor physicians and how much power doctors consequently have over the lives of their patients. This power prominently includes the power of suggestion. The suggestion that seriously ill patients consider suicide as a form of medical care will carry special force because of the moral authority the medical profession enjoys. It is a suggestion doctors may well find themselves making, given the liability to natural human responses that Quill's writing betrays and the way the deaths of the poor and the marginalized are managed. The prohibition of PAS and euthanasia is therefore a safeguard doctors should favor imposing on themselves. It is one for which the medical profession should argue with force and vigor.

(According to a 1990 study in the Netherlands, 50% of Dutch physicians "suggest" to terminally ill patients. See Herbert Hendin, "Correspondence," *New England Journal of Medicine* 336, 19 (1997): 1385, citing Paul J. van der Maas, J.M. van Delden, and Loes Pijenborg, "Euthanasia and Other Medical Decisions Concerning the End of Life," *Health Policy* 22 (1992): 1-262. One reason for thinking the percentage would be higher in the United States than in the Netherlands is connected with the requirements of informed consent. Some hospital counsels warn that if physician-assisted suicide were legalized here, staff physicians at American hospitals would be required to present assisted suicide as an option to the terminally ill in order to obtain their informed consent to any treatment of their condition.   Or at least, they warn that physicians would be required to do so in the absence of prohibition by a legislatively imposed "gag rule."   It may even be that worries about informed consent account for the high incidence of discussion of physician-assisted suicide between Dutch doctors and their patients.   I am grateful to Maura Ryan for these points.)

THE MORAL INEVITABILITY OF TWO TIERS OF HEALTH CARE

H. Tristram Engelhardt, Jr.

I.   INTRODUCTION

Thank you very much for the generous introduction and the remarks about the book on humanism. (H. T. Engelhardt, Jr., *Bioethics and Secular Humanism* (Philadelphia: Trinity International Press, 1991)) Dr. Philip Clarke embodied the ideals of the humane physician. When I spoke with a surgeon friend of mine in Houston, Dr. Harold Haley, who knew Dr. Clarke, he told me how fully Dr. Clarke achieved this ideal. The humane person is not just a well-educated person, or a well-educated person without refinement and generosity. Had Dr. Clarke lived in the first century, he would surely have been recognized as a *humanissimus vir* – the title used by Cicero to address individuals who possess that special constellation of grace, energy, generosity, intelligence, wit, and capacity for friendship that characterizes the humane life. It is a distinction marking the physician who is a true member of one of the three learned professions. It is a pleasure and an honor to give this lecture under the aegis of his name. Indeed, his recognition of the humanities invites a recognition of the human condition and its finitude, which will be the focus of this lecture.

Today I will argue that we are morally constrained to accept a two-tier health care system, by which I will mean one that has a tier provided out of public resources and a second purchased out of private means. The force of this argument is that an arrangement such as the Canadian system involves a fundamental violation of human rights. It violates not only the right to dispose of one's own property, but also the right to achieve with others in free association a common understanding of human flourishing. This recognition is placed within a much larger challenge to our moral predicament: secular moral reasoning cannot disclose a canonical, content-full moral vision. Moral authority in a secular pluralist society such as ours must, by default, be derived from the consent of those who collaborate and is, therefore, always limited. Free and informed consent, contracts, the market, and limited democracies are the practices through which, given our circumstances, authority is garnered for common action. Through such practices, one creates – one does not discover – common responses to the human predicament. In the context of a limited democracy, appeals to justice, fairness, and rights to health care in fashioning health care policy are grievously misguided and misguiding. Such appeals presume a content-full normative view of distributive justice that cannot be established as canonical for a secular pluralist society. They inflate moral expectations so as to make limited democratic compromise difficult, if not impossible. Instead, one should focus on the creation of a basic health care insurance package for those in need, recognizing that individuals, given their own understanding of how to face suffering and death, may very well decide to purchase better basic as well as luxury health care. In short, given the limits of secular discursive moral reasoning, the moral authority of health care policy is limited. It does not allow the imposition of an all-encompassing, single-payer system from which individuals and communities could not escape by direct payments or through fashioning their own private insurance. The public provision of health care is best regarded as the democratic creation of a limited public insurance against losses in the natural and social lotteries.

II.   FACING FINITUDE

There is surely no more significant bioethical issue or set of issues than the ethics of health care policy. This is the case, not just because of the ubiquitous influences of medicine on ordinary life, but because of the very magnitude of our current expenses. As of 1992, about one out of every seven dollars in the United States was invested in health care. The rise in health care expenditures over the last seventy years has been dramatic and inexorable. In 1929, we deployed about 3.5 percent of the gross national product for health care – about what the former Soviet Union was investing when it went out of existence. By the year 1940, the American expenses had risen to 4 percent, by 1950 to 4.4 percent, by 1960 to 5.3 percent, by 1965 to 6.1 percent, by 1970 to 7.6 percent, by 1975 to around 8.6 percent, by 1980 to 9.4 percent, by 1985 to 10.6 percent, and by 1990 to 12.2 percent. (Katharine R. Levit, "National Health Expenditures. 1984," *Health Care Financing* 7 (Fall, 1985), 3; and G. J. Schieber, J.-P. Poullier, and L. M. Greenwald, "Health Spending, Delivery, and Outcomes in OECD Countries," *Health Affairs* (Summer 1993), 120-129.) Moreover HCVA promises us that if all health care cost containment measures in fact succeed, the percentage will only rise to 16.4 percent, which is about one out of every six dollars by the year 2000. Nearly one percent of the gross national product of the United States is deployed for critical care or intensive care alone. The very size of these expenditures makes health care policy a central focus of political and moral debate.

It is not just that we spend so much for health care, but that the purchases do not bring dramatic returns in the alleviation of mortality. We can see this if we compare the American expenses per capita with countries showing a comparable life expectancy. For example, in 1991, the United States invested about $2,868 per person; Canada $1,915; France $1,650; Japan, with the longest life expectancy for males and females on the face of the Earth (probably also due to their eating in sushi bars, not in fast food purveyors), $1,307; Great Britain invested $1,043; and the grand winner was Greece, with only $404 per person (Ibid.). Why do we expend so much and achieve so little? There are many answers. There are differences in diet and different exposures to various risk factors. In part, however, a major factor is played by the ways in which we invest resources in high-cost, low-yield diagnostic and therapeutic interventions. Of course, better access to health care can at least lead to morbidity relief. (S. J. Katz, H. F. Mitzgala, and H. G. Welch, "British Columbia Sends Patients to Seattle for Coronary Artery Surgery: Bypassing the Queue in Canada," *Journal of American Medical Association* 266 (1991), 1108-11: and S. Globerman and L. Hoye, "Waiting Your Turn: Hospital Waiting Lists in Canada," *Fraser Forum Critical Issues Bulletin* (May 1990), 5-38.) The point is that we must decide how much protection against death and suffering should be a part of a basic package of health care for those in need, bearing in mind that many countries achieve quite a lot with a very low investment.

One way to bring across the issue of how much protection to offer and at what price is to consider its portrayal by Woody Allen in the movie *Hannah and Her Sisters*, where Woody Allen develops a decrement in hearing. The sequence is more or less as follows. (Let the reader beware that I have laid the script of *Hannah and her Sisters* on the bed of Procrustes in the service of underscoring its moral for health care policy.) He goes to his local physician to have the matter assessed. After a history and physical, the physician tells Woody something to the effect, "You're getting older. You turn your Walkman up too loud; New York is a noisy place; you go to loud discos. Live with it." That would have been the *terminus ad quem* anywhere from Athens to Berlin and London. However, at that point in the film, Woody Allen turns to the physician and asks, "Well, could it be cancer?" At this juncture a herd of zebras scared by the thought of lawyers charges across the imagination of the physician. As a consequence, Woody Allen is CAT-scanned. You must presume that Woody Allen – even in the movie – possesses good insurance coverage. The data from the CAT-scan are ambiguous, so there's a repeat CAT-scan. Some many hundred dollars later, Woody Allen is returned to where one would have been to begin with in Athens, Berlin, or London. The physician more or less says, "I really don't know what's wrong with you; you'll have to live with it." In the mean time, there's been a major transfer of resources, not without benefit. If you recall, at that juncture Woody Allen turns his anxieties from death to his love affairs. This minimal but still real benefit is unlikely to be expressed in hard-core differences in mortality outcomes or easily measured morbidity outcomes. This story is meant to highlight the question as to which diagnostic and therapeutic interventions are only marginally useful and which should be a part of the standard of care.

In addition to the issue of how much should be expended for what amount of morbidity and mortality protection, there is the question as to whether health care must be provided equally to all. It must be noted that just because there is equality of input in health care, that is, equality of access to health care, this does not mean that there will be equality of output. Canada gives us a good example. Canada's differences in life expectancy between highest earning and lowest earning males and females remain quite large, though Canada has aggressively made sure that people have equality of input. (John Iglehart, "Canada's Health Care System Faces its Problems," *New England Journal of Medicine* 322 (February 22. 1990), 562-68.) Now there is little consideration, or at least little effective action, attempting to close the gap between life expectancy of the rich and the poor. If you look at higher earning Canadians and lower earning Canadians in that regard, the difference is 5.6 years for males and 1.9 years for females.

Having said all of that, we have our own well-known problems – a large proportion of our population has no direct health care insurance. Yet, even this problem is more complex than it might appear at first blush. Billions of dollars are invested in the care of the uninsured through non-obvious insurance systems, which include the various city, county, and state hospitals that provide care for the uninsured, as well as through unreimbursed care provided. Of those uninsured, many may be paying for their care out of pocket, since around half are between 18 and 39 years of age and almost a third have a yearly income of over $25,000. The population of persons with health care insurance whose health care costs are likely to exceed their resources is much less than the whole population of the uninsured.

The challenges that confront us are not just rising costs, dubious returns from high-cost, low-yield interventions, the questionable value of equal health care access, and the population of uninsured, but also the problem of facing the meaning of death. (In the eight years since presenting this lecture, I have turned to the importance of the transcendent in understanding health care policy. See Engelhardt, *The Foundations of Christian Bioethics* (Lisse: Swets & Zeitlinger, 2000).) The difficulty of fashioning acceptable health care policy is tied to the ways in which we confront finitude, an issue that is extremely hard to discuss in a secular society where death is highly feared and where the adage reigns, "You only go around once," and the corollary is, "How much should you invest to stay here for this life, if it's your only life?" Realize how different this attitude is from the Christian view of dying. In intact Christian communities, death is not the real downside risk. The significant risk of serious illness is not dying but dying without repentance. In the West until very recently one prayed, "*A subitanea et improvisa morte, libera nos, Domine,*" "from sudden and unprovided death, deliver me, O Lord." (Philip T. Welter (trans. and ed.), *The Roman Ritual* (Milwaukee, Bruce Publishing, 1952), vol. 2, pp. 454-55) I presume those praying in this fashion were often somewhat like people running for higher office from Arkansas or Texas; they had committed a number of sins in their youth, if not also later in life. They recognized that the major downside risk of serious illness is to die unprepared and as a consequence to burn in hell. The great risk is to die unrepentant. If one examines the reflections on death, at least in liturgies and litanies, the focus is rarely upon a long life, except in marriage ceremonies, but instead on a good death. ("May they both see their children's children unto the third and fourth generation, thus reaching the old age which they desire." *Ibid.,* vol. 1. p. 469.) In the liturgy of St. John Chrysostom, once before the creed and once before reciting the Our Father, one prays for a Christian ending to our life – "painless, blameless, peaceful; and a good defence before the dread Judgment Seat of Christ." (Isabel Hapgood (trans.). Service Book of the Orthodox-Catholic Apostolic Church, 7th ed. (Englewood, NJ: Antiochian Orthodox Christian Archdiocese, 1996), pp. 99, 112.) Our secular culture does not help us to relativize death by recognizing the transcendent. As a consequence, the prospect of accepting a reasonable chance of dying becomes formidable.

It is not just that we now face the issue of how much money we should spend to avoid suffering and death. We must also acknowledge that deciding how to deploy our resources is deciding when to expose ourselves and others to real risks of suffering more and dying earlier. If the most important thing is to avoid suffering and to extend life as much as possible, it is hard to come face to face with the decision that we must at some point judge that it is more important to have funds for some good Jack Daniels bourbon than to provide more health care. The framing of health care policy is encumbered by our disinclination to come to terms with our finitude, to recognize we must gamble with our lives, albeit prudently.

The magnitude of the challenge facing us is considerable. As we move to the future and increase health care spending from one out of every seven dollars to one out of every five dollars, we will likely increasingly limit access for some people under some circumstances to expensive health care. Second, in a society that has grown increasingly secular, it has become increasingly difficult to face the circumstance that limitations to health care spending involve choices to accept a somewhat increased risk of dying earlier or suffering more. Third, as we shall see, the greatest limitations we have are not those of money, but those of moral vision.

III.   FOUR APPROACHES TO HEALTH CARE ALLOCATIONS

The 1983 report of the President's Commission on Securing Access to Health Care outlines four ways one might consider establishing a health care system: (1) provide all health care that would benefit individuals; (2) meet all their health care needs; (3) secure equality of access for all; or (4) guarantee a basic or adequate package. (President's Commission for the Study of Ethical Problems in Medicine and Biomedical and Behavioral Research, *Securing Access to Health Care* (Washington, D.C.: U.S. Government Printing Office, 1983). See, especially, pp. 11-47.) In the last case, a health care system would not provide everything that people might want, benefit from, or need, but instead a basic adequate package, after which all would be at liberty to buy more. The last case was presented by the Commission in a nuanced fashion, but the fundamental insight they achieved is that we must face two unhappy elements of our condition: the finitude of resources and of our secular moral authority. We must recognize not just that our resources are limited, but that we lack the authority to impose an egalitarian system such as Canada's. In endorsing an adequate package of health care in a two-tier system, the President's Commission recognized that it would not be feasible to provide all care that might convey a benefit, because this would include MRIs for everyone who is worried about the cause of a hearing decrement, despite the financial costs. It would also include plastic surgery for all not pleased with their aging features. Second, the President's Commission recognized that shifting the focus from benefits to needs will not dispel this difficulty, since many are likely to hold that it is a basic need to avoid great suffering, not to mention an early death, such that one should provide treatment even at great cost and a low likelihood of success. The difficulty is that all choices are made with insufficient information and finite resources. Since the whole world is a gamble, and since medicine is part of the world, most medical choices have the character of a gamble; they involve possibilities of avoiding a particular death or form of suffering at a particular financial cost. Here concepts of futility will generally not help to determine when one should wager on a long shot. If one examines concepts of futility, one finds that they are usually not judgments that a treatment will provide no benefit. Instead, "futility" cloaks a very different judgment: a treatment is held not to be worth our while. That is, we will not provide care, not because the treatment is absolutely futile, but because it costs too much and the probability of success is too small. Consider, for example, if we had a cure for AIDS that worked one out of every 10,000 times and cost one dollar. We would use it in developed countries, because we would save lives at the cost of $10,000 per life saved. If it worked once out of every 10,000 times and cost $100,000, we would not use it, because it would save lives at the cost of one billion dollars per life saved. How, then, should we determine what health care should be available in a basic health care package?

The difficulty in discovering the content of a basic package of health care has deep roots. The secular philosophical hope has been to disclose a canonical, content-full moral vision, so as to understand how much we should invest in health care for all and under what circumstances. Many presume that philosophical reflection can show us which needs are more important and how competing life projects are best balanced. This expectation is a misguiding inheritance from the rationalistic aspirations of the Western Middle Ages that bequeathed a view that we can discover concrete moral direction regarding the important projects of life and of health care without embedding our questions in a particular community with a particular moral understanding. We have come to presume that we can discover a guiding moral view from nowhere and no history, that we can understand what a *recta ratio* requires outside of any particular moral tradition. In particular, the United States does not share a common view or moral tradition concerning what health care should be provided for all. To the contrary, there is no way to have such a guiding moral vision outside of a particular moral tradition.

Because we are a pluralist society, because we do not share one moral vision, we must create the compass of a health care policy by a democratic process which, in the end, will be arbitrary and limited in its moral authority. Let us now see why this is the case. Imagine that you have a dispute about how much health care should be provided to individuals and you have various plans from which to choose: Greece's, Germany's, the United Kingdom's, Japan's. How will you justify the choice? First of all, you might presume to appeal to your intuitions or to the intuitions of various people to give guidance. But obviously for any intuition you have, your interlocutor may have a contrary intuition. One can then appeal to higher-level intuitions *ad infinitum*. If one abandons an appeal to intuitions in favor of an appeal to consequences, the same problem recurs. Imagine you retort, "Well, at least we can examine the consequences of having a Canadian versus an American versus a German health care system; we can determine which has the best consequences." But to do that, one must already know how to rank outcomes. That is, to determine the consequences, one must know already how to rank interests in liberty, interests in equality, interests in prosperity, interests in security. One must already know how to rank interests in quality of life, and interests in quantity of life. One must in particular know how to compare morbidity and mortality risks. The challenge is something like the following: if you take a trip and you come back with receipts in Australian dollars, Canadian dollars, and Taiwan dollars, and you want to be reimbursed in American dollars, then you must know the exchange rate. The problem at the core of all of this is determining the appropriate exchange rate among outcomes. How do you know, for example, the exchange rate between liberty consequences and longevity consequences? One cannot appeal to consequences to answer that question.

Maybe you will say, "Well, I would accept what a hypothetical choice theory would affirm or what a disinterested observer would endorse." There is still a cardinal difficulty. If the disinterested observer is truly disinterested, the observer will not choose anything. It will not have moral interests. First, you must import a particular moral sense or a particular thin theory of the good so as to know how one should choose. Of course, that is the question at stake at the outset. The same is the case if you try to appeal to a content-full account of moral rationality. You must decide which concrete moral rationality should guide. Nor will it do to appeal to human nature: you cannot examine human nature and determine in a morally normative sense what humans are naturally inclined to do in a moral sense of the idea (e.g. inclined to do as good moral agents) without already imbedding human nature within a particular interpretative framework. The question is, which interpretative framework should guide and why. Human nature, considered simply as a biological, psychological, and sociological given, is a constellation of various diatheses and inclinations. To determine what is normatively natural presumes that one already possesses the normatively appropriate understanding of nature. This difficulty cannot be evaded by appealing to notions of health and disease, for one must first determine the appropriate goal of adaptation and the environment in which one should judge success. Worse than that, some socio-biologists argue that the human race may have developed by striking a balance between hypocrites and sincerely moral people. (For reflections on these matters, see Christian Vogel, *Vom Töte zum Mord* (Munich: Hanser Verlag, 1989) and Donald Symons, *The Evolution of Human Sexuality* (New York: Oxford University Press, 1979), especially pp. 144-158.) Evolution may have awarded success to groups that balanced those who cheated, killed, cuckolded, and fathered children out of wedlock, with those who judged such actions as immoral. It may have been the right balance between these two that led to successful adaptation. If one is interested in maximizing inclusive fitness, then one may discover that much of which we morally disapprove was integral to strategies that led to human evolutionary success. To discover the correct moral vision, one must already have moral guidance as to which behaviors are acceptable and under what circumstances. One cannot get started without begging the question or arguing in a circle.

The point is that, if one hopes to identify the needs that should be a part of a health care package, one will not be able simply to turn inside reason and discover its contents, somewhat like pulling a conceptual rabbit out of a philosopher's hat. Such answers are not available outside of a particular moral vision. It may be another matter if you live within an intact functioning moral community, as for example one would as an Orthodox Jew, Orthodox Christian, or a good ole boy or girl in East Texas. In such cases, you already have a concrete understanding of the good life and the good death.

Consider, for example, the famous phrase in St. Augustine's commentaries on the Gospel according to St. John: *"Non quia cognoscerunt ut crediderunt, sed ut cognoscerunt crediderunt. Credimus enim ut cognoscamus, non cognoscamus ut credamus."* "They believed, not because they knew, but that they might come to know. For we believe in order that we may know, we do not know in order that we may believe." (Augustine, "Homilies on the Gospel of John" in Philip Schaff (ed.), *Nicene and Post-Nicene Fathers,* First Series, vol. 7 (Peabody, MA: Hendrickson, 1994), Tractate XL.9, p. 228.) The point is this: once you believe, once you are within a particular moral framework, then you have guidance. You then know, for instance, which moral sense, which thin theory of the good to impute to disinterested observers. You know, in fact, how to rank outcomes. And if you are a preference utilitarian, you know how God discounts time, so that you can compare current and future satisfaction of preferences.

All of this has a crucial bearing on the moral justification of health care policy in a secular pluralist democracy such as ours. We have no common way to discover the contents of a just health care package without begging the question or arguing in a circle. To recognize this as our condition is to recognize that we live in postmodernity. That is, if there is no general, content-full, universal moral narrative to provide canonical guidance in determining the nature of the good life, then there will also be none to inform us concerning the proper compass of a health care system. This means we will not be able to discover how to compare needs.

The second approach suggested by the President's Commission, that is, to establish the appropriate health care package by discovering real needs cannot succeed. But so, too, we are morally barred from establishing a health care system that insures health care equality. As the President's Commission recognized, losses at the natural lottery with regard to health can render us in such deplorable circumstances that additional health care will often not appreciably increase the quality or length of life. Think of being quadriplegic, blind, deaf, and epileptic. One may do some things to make the quality of life of such a person somewhat better, but one will never restore the person to the *status quo ante*. One cannot achieve equality of health. The focus then shifts to equality of health care. However, given our financial limitations, the only way to have equal health care access is to have a closed menu. Everyone must receive the health care approved by the government. One must achieve equality by forbidding the purchase of better basic care as well as luxury care offering significant morbidity and mortality benefits. The difficulty is to account for the secular moral authority needed to impose such an egalitarianism by coercive force, given the difficulty of establishing a particular content-rich moral vision as canonical.

Because one cannot justify a canonical, content-full moral vision that could in turn justify the intrusive activities of a state, and since instead political authority must be derived from the consent of the governed, one is generally free, after having paid one's taxes, to buy a crash-resistant luxury car, and thereby purchase a greater chance of living longer, or to buy a compact car without such crash-resistant properties, investing the remaining funds in Jack Daniels and good books. If one then crashes and dies in the compact car, it is due to the risks one decided to assume. Similarly, after one has paid one's taxes to support a basic health care system, one has a very strong claim to be at liberty to purchase better basic and luxury health care, just as one can purchase better basic and luxury cars. Or, to take another example, David Solomon offered me only a coach fare round trip ticket for this conference. I was able to use upgrade stickers and come first class. I do not anticipate that he will reimburse these costs, though I would be overjoyed if he did. The difference between first and coach was not just greater comfort, but likely a decreased risk of dying from a pulmonary embolus due to cramped leg room. It takes a very strong argument regarding state authority to justify forbidding the purchase of better basic health care or safer cars.

Our discussions of health care policy are framed by the circumstance that the ways in which we can justify people's being in moral authority, as well as being moral authorities, are brought into question by the collapse of the modern philosophical project. In order to select the correct ranking of values and moral principles, we must already possess a normative moral account. We cannot establish the authority of a particular moral vision, including an egalitarian moral vision, without begging the question or arguing in a circle. It is for this reason that only limited democracies have a plausible claim to moral authority, and a limited democracy will lack the authority to impose a universal one-tier egalitarian health care system as in Canada. We entered the modern age expecting that philosophers could discover what rational persons should endorse. If that had been possible, then sound rational argument should have ended moral and public policy debates. For philosophers and not-so-limited democracies, this would have been superb. First, if one could discover what a rational person should endorse, one would at that point have the authority of rationality to impose that view as public policy. Second, one could then dismiss all those who disagreed as irrational. Third, if one used coercive public force to impose the policy, one would just be restoring those coerced to the deportment that rational men and women should have embraced. Among other things, one could have imposed an all-encompassing egalitarian health care system as in Canada. To do all this, one would have to possess a canonical, content-full vision of what men and women should do. As we have seen, this is not achievable in secular terms.

IV.   WHY ALL WE MAY HAVE IS A LIMITED DEMOCRACY
AND ITS HEALTH CARE POLICY

When we come to frame health care policy, we do so with all the problems of postmodernity. We possess neither a universal moral narrative nor the means to discover one by sound rational argument. In a large-scale, pluralist society like ours, we cannot appeal to God. Nor can we turn to reason to discover what we should do without begging the question of which moral rationality should guide. What then can we do? Despite these limitations, we can still secure a way to justify health care policy. Imagine all of us here being the only people to survive a worldwide cataclysm. At this point, we have to decide what we will do together. What is the authority of the *res publica,* the public thing, the common thing we might create as an organization for collaboration? Since we do not all believe in God the same way, or agree about what God requires us to do, an appeal to God will not resolve our controversies (after all, if we have two academic theologians in our group, we will probably have at least six divergent theological views about the role of the state). We might then think that philosophical reflection could establish a canonical approach. However, we already know that will not work. Again, there will be quite different understandings of how to rank liberty, equality, prosperity, and security. If you do not believe that we are separated by quite different moral visions in this matter, then consider the diversity of moral visions embraced by those running for public office. If we cannot agree about what God requires, and if philosophical reasoning cannot discover the canonical moral vision that should guide, then we can still draw authority from common agreement. This moral salience of the importance of agreement or permission accounts for the salience of free and informed consent, the free market, and limited democracies. This is not because people necessarily value these practices. It is because these are the procedures that moral strangers can engage so as to derive authority for common projects.

Consider why these practices are so central, not only for public policy generally, but for health care in particular. Free and informed consent authorizes a physician and a patient to do certain things together though the physician and patient may have radically different moral lifestyles, different religions, different views of human flourishing. They draw moral authority from their agreement. Also, people can enter the market and can trade together even if they hate each other. Across the world, there are exchanges taking place in markets between people who deeply dislike if not despise each other. Finally, limited democracies can justify political actions in terms of the plausible consent of their citizens without justifying a canonical understanding of the public good. The difficulty is that, since limited democracies draw this justification from consent, they are limited in what they may do to their citizens. Still, limited democracies can legitimately perform a wide range of functions. They may (1) use force to protect the innocent, (2) enforce recorded contracts, and (3) distribute commonly owned public funds (e.g. establish welfare programs). However, such a polity will not have authority to forbid the use of private resources for health care purchases because it is implausible that a limited democracy has the consent of its citizens to use force against their peaceable, consensual collaboration. Although a limited democracy can create a basic package of health care from its publicly owned resources, it will lack the authority to impose a particular egalitarian health care vision through prohibiting access to better basic and luxury health care. Moreover, since a limited democracy is a means for individuals with diverse moral visions to collaborate one with the other, it must create health care policy, not discover a just or fair policy to impose. It is for this reason that the health care provided through public means can best be understood as a limited insurance policy against certain losses at the natural and social lotteries.

Because of our finitude and the limits of plausible secular moral authority, America should forthrightly acknowledge the propriety of developing a two-tier health care system, where one tier provides a basic package for those in need and where citizens with resources may directly or through insurance buy better basic or luxury health care services. In other words, the United States should explicitly do what most countries in fact do and surely not do what Canada has attempted to do. It should acquiesce in a two-tier system of health care as the moral default position resulting from our not being able to establish the canonical authority of any particular moral vision that might legitimate the imposition of an egalitarian vision. Limited democracies must not only leave people free to use their private resources as they wish, but also recognize that they must democratically create the contours of any basic package of health care. Such a package cannot be discovered by appeals to justice, fairness, and health care rights. Such appeals will at best make difficult the task of agreeing to a basic health care insurance package against losses at the natural lottery (e.g. becoming ill or disabled) and at the social lottery (i.e. not having sufficient funds to pay for one's health care). One is better served by focusing further rights on the task at hand. To live in a limited democracy is to live with public policy constrained by the limits of secular moral authority. We are left with the expedient of creating through a limited act of solidarity a basic insurance package for health care, with the presumption that all will be at liberty, should they have the resources, to purchase better basic as well as extra luxury care.

In framing health care policy, we are considering a universe of unfortunate outcomes and deciding to denominate some of them as unfair by creating limited entitlements to be treated. Let me provide an example of what I have in mind. Once, a long time ago, I lived in Maryland. We had big, old trees. My wife loved those trees, and she said, "Tris, what we need is a tree doctor to come look at those trees and make sure they are healthy. I want to make sure we do right by those marvelous trees." They looked perfectly healthy to me, but I said, "Okay, get a tree doctor." The tree doctor came out, examined those trees, and said, "Those are healthy trees; that'll be $100." I gave him $100 and I got a little receipt saying, "Those are healthy trees, Dr. Engelhardt." A few weeks later, a research assistant of mine, after xeroxing various articles at the National Library of Medicine, brought them to me at my house. As she walked out, a big wind blew, and a tree crashed down. My first concern was that she had been killed. However, I should have known that all research assistants run as quickly as possible so as not to be asked to do more work. She was safe, but the wind had done thousands of dollars worth of damage to Chevy Chase City property. Like any good physician, I at once called my lawyer. I said, "Doris, what should I do?" I told her I had a little sheet of paper saying my trees were healthy. She said, "Well look, Tris, what this is, is an act of God. They will have to sue God, and God is judgment-proof, so you are off the hook." What she was explaining to me was that, although a very unfortunate circumstance had taken place, no one could be held liable to make others whole for it.

This story illustrates the foundations of Oregon's recent health care reform. Framing health care policy involves establishing a limited response to the unfortunate outcomes that can harm us. Health care policy creates a limited insurance against morbidity and mortality risks. As you may rightly conclude at this point, I am endorsing something like the Oregon plan, which has defined a basic adequate health care package for the poor, while allowing those who wish and can to buy more and better care. (For an overview of the Oregon Plan, see Martin A. Strosberg, Joshua M. Wiener, and Robert Baker (eds.), Rationing America's Medical Care: The Oregon Plan and Beyond (Washington, D.C.: Brookings Institution, 1992). I do so, not necessarily because I take Oregon to have produced results that I celebrate without qualification, but because Oregon was able to break through the American health care ideology of providing the best of care for all. Oregon has focused instead on the manageable and justifiable task of providing adequate care for the poor while forthrightly recognizing that there will be inequality of care. The genius of Oregon lies also in implicitly acknowledging that one cannot discover the contours of the health care package that should be guaranteed to all, in particular, the poor. Oregon has come the closest to recognizing that health care policy involves democratically creating a basic insurance package, not discovering what must be provided as a matter of justice or health care rights. We will do best if there were a number of Oregons. Before the United States have an actual nation-wide basic health care system, we should experiment with the ways we can come to terms with our nearly infinite expectations, the plurality of our visions, our limited financial resources, and worse yet, our limited moral resources – that is, reason's inability to discover the moral understanding that all should accept.

V.   CONCLUSION

A two-tier health care system is just, in the sense of morally unavoidable. It is the most we can justify, given our embarrassed philosophical circumstances. In secular terms, we are left with numerous moral visions, limited secular moral authority, private entitlements, and the very limited moral authority of those limited health care policies that can be established by limited democracies. The state remains, like all other undertakings of finite men and women, a finite undertaking. We may create a basic insurance package against losses at the natural and social lotteries, but people will be morally free to purchase additional and better care through various private systems. Our limited moral visions constrain us to fashion a health care system that takes limited governmental authority seriously. To act responsibly, given the human condition, we must face the limits of secular moral reason as we face the limits of our lives. We should be about this task as honestly as possible. Here physicians can make special contributions since physicians live with finitude. Indeed, this Clarke Lectureship reminds us that physicians can contribute to the body politic as members of one of the three traditional learned professions. Physicians can help our society face the inevitability of death, the costs involved in postponing it, the character all medical decisions take as forms of gambling with life and suffering, and the costs of attempting to preserve health and postpone death at all costs. These are the counsels of finitude. Facing finitude is difficult, for we humans have infinite aspirations. Our cardinal sin has always been hubris. The sin of Adam and Eve was to pursue deification on their own terms. Though we all have aspirations of gods and goddesses, unfortunately we have only the finite moral authority, vision, and resources of very finite men and women.

Response to
THE MORAL INEVITABILITY
OF TWO TIERS OF HEALTH
CARE

Joel James Shuman

(The ten years that have elapsed since Engelhardt first delivered his lecture do not diminish the impact of his analysis. Health care in the United States has continued along the same trajectory Engelhardt describes. If anything, his insights are more salient than in 1992.)

Professor Engelhardt's 1992 essay "The Moral Inevitability of Two Tiers of Health Care" presents a serious conceptual challenge to those who would advocate a comprehensive single-tier health care system in the United States. His insights into the current state of American health care and health care policy, and so with the difficulties that might be associated with the United States' adopting a Canadian-style single tier system, are so many and so striking that one is tempted to forgive the problematic aspects of his argument. As it turns out, however, that argument finally hinges on a rather contestable claim about what women and men properly are – that is, about what little is genuinely universal and natural about human life and thought. Although it must in the final analysis be left to the good people of Kentucky and Tennessee to decide whether to overlook his mistakenly calling Jack Daniels "bourbon," I believe his claim that we are on an inevitable trajectory in the United States toward a two-tiered health care system – and, more importantly, that it is necessarily appropriate to describe this trajectory as *moral* – cannot be overlooked. The United States may well adopt a two-tiered health care system in the not too distant future (some would argue that this is what we already have, but that is a conversation for another day), but such a system would not be necessarily moral in any fulsome sense.

According to Engelhardt, the United States will eventually adopt a two-tiered health care system in which so-called "basic" health care services will be made available to all – or at least to the "needy" – and paid for by public resources, while more elaborate services will continue to be availed privately to those who can afford them. This development is inevitable for two reasons. First, health care costs in the United States are spiraling out of control. Many of the most recent advances in biomedical technology are exorbitantly expensive and, at least in terms of their social utility, minimally beneficial. Moreover, health care in America has progressively embraced and institutionalized our inability to confront death and our obsession with vigorous longevity at any cost; Americans, more than any other culture in history, see medicine as offering something bearing a striking resemblance to salvation. The combination of these factors has exponentially elevated health care costs, making it harder and harder for the average American to pay for health care. A serious illness, as has often been observed, is for the working and middle classes now potentially a financial, as well as a personal, disaster. (An especially interesting account of the moral development of this possibility may be found in Wendell Berry, "Health as Membership" in *Another Turn of the Crank* (Washington, D.C.: Counterpoint, 1995), pp. 86-109.) The population of persons who are "needy" with respect to heath care is growing and likely soon to include a significant part of the middle class. Second, for contemporary American culture to adapt a single-tier health care system in response to spiraling costs would be a case of our reach exceeding our grasp. It would represent the imposition of what Engelhardt calls a "content-full morality" on a pluralistic secular society that is by (his) definition incapable of arriving at such a moral consensus.

This means, he believes, that the development of a two-tiered, as opposed to a single-tier, system, is not only inevitable, but also *moral*. Any attempt by the secular reason which properly characterizes public discourse in a country like the United States to arrive at the kind of substantive moral agreement requisite to a universal health care system is bound to fail on the grounds that it will do a kind of violence to at least some members of the society. A universal health care system presumes a significant level of agreement about the ends of human life – about, for example, what constitutes a well-lived life, a "normal" life span, and a good death – and such agreements exist only within content-full moral traditions. Such agreements are not available to a pluralist secular culture dependent on instrumental reason and bound by what Engelhardt believes should be a purely procedural account of justice. If the United States were to adopt a single-tier system, that adoption would represent the imposition of a particular, content-full morality on persons who have not chosen such. A single-tier system, in other words, would be a fundamental violation of certain people's basic human rights, "not only the right to dispose of one's own property, but also the right to achieve with others in free association a common understanding of human flourishing."

My primary disagreement with Professor Engelhardt's argument is with his contention that the development of a two-tiered health care system is *morally* inevitable, by which he seems to mean both that a two–tiered system best reflects the kinds of agreements properly produced by the secular reasoning characterizing what he has elsewhere called the "peaceable society" *and* that a two-tiered system best reflects the way things are. (Because of his skepticism about the limits of reason to tell us anything about the way things are, Engelhardt would probably be reluctant to assent to the latter of these conditions. Yet it seems to me that if he is going to make the kinds of claims he does about basic human rights and the good afforded by order, he must also at least tacitly concede that he is dependent upon a particular account of the way the world is. For his defense of the peaceable society, see both his *Foundations of Bioethics* (New York: Oxford University Press, 1986) and his *Bioethics and Secular Humanism* (Philadelphia: Trinity Press International, 1991). Thanks to Stanley Hauerwas for this characterization of Engelhardt's project. For a detailed theological critique of Engelhardt's distinction between the ethics of secular reason and the ethics of content-full moral communities, see Hauerwas' "Not All Peace is Peace" in *Reading Engelhardt*, Brendan Minogue et al, eds. (Dordrecht: Kluwer Academic Publishers, 1997), and my *The Body of Compassion: Ethics, Medicine and the Church* (Boulder: Westview, 1999), pp. 72-77.) That contention is first of all based, it seems to me, in his insistence upon a sharp distinction between two levels of morality. On the one hand, there is the "thick," content-full morality of tradition-bearing communities possessing a substantive account of the ends of human life. On the other hand, there is the procedural morality of secular reason, a (relatively) content-less morality based in the consent and deliberation of individuals and groups with disparate notions of the goods of life. These two are for Engelhardt radically distinct and incommensurable. Secular reason cannot and should not attempt to offer thick accounts of justice or of the ends of human life. It cannot tell us, as Wendell Berry would say, what people are *for*. (Wendell Berry, *What are People For?* (New York: North Point Press, 1995), pp. 123-125.) Yet, it seems that Engelhardt's secular reason does offer a significant account of what people *are*, and this account is indispensable to his argument.

It is apparently self-evident to Engelhardt that women and men are autonomous, rational, property-owning individuals who engage naturally and as a matter of course in mutually self-interested exchanges of goods and services. It is self-evident that women and men possess basic and ostensibly natural *rights* to conduct their lives as they see fit, to acquire possessions, and freely to dispose of or exchange those possessions. Should women and men *choose*, for whatever reason, to enter a moral community with a substantive account of the human good, thereby exchanging some of their natural liberty for the temporal – and perhaps also the eternal – security of a content-full morality, they are perfectly free to do so. However, nothing properly compels them to enter such communities. Until they make that choice, they mostly ought to be left alone to live and trade. This is what nature demands.

But this argument is contestable on two closely related grounds, the first of which is Engelhardt's insistence that the two levels of morality he describes are radically incommensurable. Content-full moralities properly exist only among the members of tradition-bearing communities, membership that those members choose for reasons apparently inscrutable to public reason. Such historical communities have a real, "thick" common good based in and derived from their preservation of particular, narrative accounts of the human *telos*. They prescribe for their members a concrete way of life, based in a set of common practices. Procedural moralities, on the other hand, which are essentially void of content, are available to "secular reason," which seems for Engelhardt to serve as a description of the logic of all human discourse outside particular, chosen, tradition-bearing communities. These moralities serve only to preserve the order requisite to what Engelhardt indicates is "natural" human intercourse, namely the orderly occupation of proximate (not genuinely common) spaces, and the exchange of mutually desirable goods and services.

On one level, this distinction is certainly viable. (Here see Alasdair MacIntyre, *After Virtue*, 2nd edition (Notre Dame: University of Notre Dame Press, 1982).) Moralities are fundamentally functions of particular narrative accounts of the ends of human life, sustained by the practices of the communities whose common life traces its origins and reasons for being to those narratives. What Engelhardt fails to see, or at least admit, however, is that his insistence that women and men are *naturally* autonomous, rights-bearing individuals, and that these rights should not be violated, is itself part of an historically contingent, and, more importantly, a content-full morality. The liberalism he posits as formal and content-less and in some sense "natural" is itself a contingent narrative tradition. (Here see MacIntyre's *Whose Justice? Which Rationality?* (Notre Dame: University of Notre Dame Press, 1988) esp. pp. 326-348.) Such a view of how women and men "really" are derives from the classical myths of Liberal political philosophy. (I admit to a certain speculation here. It is not clear that Engelhardt's account is explicitly dependent upon either a classical Enlightenment account of women and men living in a pre-social state of nature, such as was advocated by Hobbes, Locke, or Rousseau, or a Hegelian account of the dialectical emergence of human freedom in history. What does seem clear is that he believes that freedom is "just there," and that everything else is properly chosen.) Those myths may or may not be true; in my judgment, their emergence is part of the apologetic requisite to the establishment of secular, capitalist order in early modern Europe. (My judgment here is derived both from the later work of John Rawls in his *Political Liberalism* and from William Cavanaugh, "A Fire Strong Enough to Consume the House," *Modern Theology* 11:4, October, 1995, pp. 397-420.) However, they are no more self-evident to untutored reason than the equally contingent Christian claim that women and men are created for friendship with the triune God, and so with one another and the other creatures. If in fact, "everywhere is somewhere" – an idea Engelhardt seems willing to entertain – then he must concede that *everywhere* is somewhere, including the realm of autonomous, rights-bearing individuals. (Here see Humberto Materana and Francisco Varela, *The Tree of Life: The Biological Roots of Human Understanding* (Boston: Shambahla Press, 1987).) There is no a-historical, neutral perspective from which to make judgments about what women and men are like, no universal place of privilege from which to distinguish between content-full and content-less moralities. We are always and everywhere smack in the middle of things; as John Howard Yoder reminds us, "Any given wider world is still just one more place, even if what its slightly wider or slightly more prestigious circle of interpreters talk about is a better access to 'universality.'" (John Howard Yoder, "But We Do See Jesus: The Particularity of Incarnation and the Universality of Truth," in *The Priestly Kingdom: Social Ethics as Gospel* (Notre Dame: University of Notre Dame Press, 1984), p. 49.)

Here we encounter a second difficulty with Engelhardt's argument. Even if he is wrong to insist that his characterization of human being is self-evident to human reason, we must still give that characterization due consideration as a truthful description. But if women and men *are* in fact rational, self-interested, and acquisitive individuals who relate to one another only insofar as they freely *choose* to do so, is not clear *why* anyone in a position of natural advantage would consent to dispose of some of his or her resources to help establish even a health care system – even a minimal one. Perhaps such individuals might enter such agreements for purely pragmatic reasons – that is, in order to preserve public order in an otherwise violent world. (This is of course the Hobbesian version of the origins of liberalism. For an account of the ongoing existence of Hobbesian thinking, see Patrick Neal, "Justice as Fairness: Political or Metaphysical?" *Political Theory* 18: February, 1990, pp. 24-50.) But if the imposition of a single-tier universal health care system would represent a violation of the rights of such individuals, why would the imposition of a two-tiered system not also represent such a violation? Given Engelhardt's insistence upon the significance of consent in secular moral reasoning, is it likely that all the citizens of a secular polity would consent to such a system if they are genuinely rational individuals? Engelhardt would seem constrained by his own account to support nothing more that a libertarian minimal state. (Here see Robert Nozick, *Anarchy, State and Utopia* (New York, Basic Books, 1974).)

I would argue that the Liberal position Engelhardt advocates is not more or less rational than any other. It is no less particular than any other. It is content-full and substantive, based in an account of human flourishing that privileges individual liberty and participation in a laissez-faire market economy. Engelhardt's concerns over coerced egalitarianism probably have some merit, but they are no more or less "natural" than concerns about the coercive violence inherent in capitalist markets. Both are questions brought to a conversation conducted by women and men who find themselves living alongside, if not necessarily with, one another.

Readers should not mistake my critique of the particulars of Engelhardt's position for a vigorous or an optimistic defense of welfare liberalism or a single-tier national health care system. The social arrangements, including the health care systems, which derive from what he calls "secular" thinking are likely to be every bit as inadequate and impoverished as he suggests. We do live in a morally fragmented and frequently incoherent world. Yet, we are not absolutely strangers to one another. Although we should not in such a world presume that we will agree on matters like health care policy, it is not clear that we should presume that we will *not* agree. Admittedly such agreements as we do achieve or discover we will achieve or discover in spite of our differences – especially if we take those differences seriously, something liberal thought has been historically unwilling to do. As such, those agreements will be reached through painfully stammering deliberation, punctuated by confusions of language and conflicting (and sometimes incommensurable) views about human flourishing, and corrupted by the unwelcome politicking of special interests. And yes, they will in all likelihood be characterized by at least some violence against the preferences of at least some individuals.

Yet, at least from the perspective of my own moral commitments as a Christian, those of us living in the United States must continue to strive toward some level of agreement, however imperfect, about the provision of health care services to those for whom even mundane illness would prove their financial undoing. In our deliberations and our attempts to persuade one another about the shape of such a system, our first concern should be not with property rights of the wealthy, but with the welfare of those who would otherwise not receive care. For it is not more apparent to the impaired vision of reason that women and men are autonomous, self-interested, acquisitive individuals than it is that they are the neighbors for whose care we are finally responsible. The United States may well eventually arrive at a two-tiered health care system, but just to the extent that it leaves the marginalized of our society with inadequate care, we cannot rightly call such a system moral.

COMPASSIONATE CARE OF THE DYING

James F. Bresnahan

I consider the fact that Father Dick McCormick introduced me an additional gesture of kindness toward me because he is somebody that I have appreciated over the years. Also I think that many of you who are at Notre Dame and have an opportunity to study with him appreciate him. I remember the first time I met you, Dick. You were just coming back from your doctorate at Rome and you stopped at Weston. Do you remember being down by the pool at Weston? You talked to us about what was then considered a big moral problem. This, I suppose, is the joke for the evening. The big moral problem was teenagers' going steady. And you suggested that people ought to think more about why teenagers would want to go steady and what needs teenagers had that were not being responded to. But it impressed me greatly at the time and you have impressed us all since then. So thank you for your introduction.

I also want to thank the people who have planned these weekends, eight of these conferences, and who have invited me to them. I was invited in the first place, of course, because I was a friend of Philip Clarke. For two years in Denver, when I was teaching there – from 1972 to 1974 – Phil was my doctor. As I said two years ago, when we had the brief memorial service for Phil, the first time I met him he was taking my medical history and doing a physical on me. I realized very quickly that he not only wanted to know what was going on in my body he also wanted to know who I was and what my interests were. That was very important to me personally. It would prove to be medically important before I left Denver within that two years. Phil was a very dear person. It is a very special honor for me to be able to give this address which he,

together with his wife Doris, endowed. Doris is again with us and I
appreciate her coming. That, too, is a special honor.

I want to talk to you about compassionate care of the dying,
and perhaps as a subtitle – Catholic conscience and compassion in
health care. It seems to me that the compassion we need to show the
dying is something that we – those of us who are Catholics, those of
us who are Christians, those of us who are Christians and Jews – can
contribute to the culture in which we live.

I want to start this afternoon by evoking for you some scenes
from a movie that made a great impression on me when I first saw it.
It continues to fascinate me and, perhaps, it has fascinated you. It is
regarded now as a classic. It is a movie about medieval life and the
encounter of people with death. It offers some contrasts and, I think,
a springboard for our reflection on our own age and our own attempts
to deal with death. Some of you probably have suspected already the
name of that film. It is the 1957 movie, "The Seventh Seal," by the
Swedish director, Ingmar Bergman. The story in the film is about a
Swedish knight, Antonius Block, who is returning home after ten
years on a crusade in Palestine. As he lands in Sweden, Antonius is
weary and disillusioned and full of longing for his Scandinavian
home and, above all, for the loving wife whom he left behind a young
woman and who is faithfully waiting for him. Antonius is weary and
disillusioned. These life experiences have left his faith troubled. His
squire, Jon, is an out-and-out cynic and an atheist now. Antonius is
not like Jon, but, nonetheless, he is deeply troubled. Antonius longs
for answers from out of God's silence.

This is a very typical theme in Ingmar Bergman's films.
Furthermore, Bergman sets the story at the end of the medieval era
and before the Reformation. This was a time when Christianity in
Europe meant Catholic Christianity with all of the customs that those
of us who are Catholics are used to – customs of worship and
devotions. Bergman is quite faithful to that in his portrayals of life
in this film and another famous film by him about the medieval era,
"The Virgin Spring." (I always connect these films with the novels
of Sigrid Undset. I link her "Kristin Lavransdatter" and her "Master

of Hestviken" with Bergman's medieval films. They both portray human life and faith and the struggles of faith and love and hope in that era.)

After Antonius lands, he and his squire, Jon, are riding their horses along the beach when they encounter Death. Death – the Black Death, the plague – has accompanied them and is beginning to ravage their native land even as they wend their way homeward. Death is personified as a chalk-white faced man in a black monk's cowl and robe. Antonius says, "Have you come for me?" "Yes," says Death, "I have been walking at your side for a long time. Are you ready?" Antonius replies, "My body is frightened, but I am not." Antonius is a soldier. "But wait a moment," Antonius continues. "They all say that," says Death, "but I grant no reprieves." However, Antonius is clever. He entices Death. "You play chess don't you?" And, with that, Antonius produces a chess set from out of his saddle bag. "Yes," says Death, "I am quite a good chess player." So Death does grant a reprieve and they begin the chess game that will be played through to the end of the film.

Here we have a very modern theme – the game of struggle against death. At one point Death asks, "How did you know that I play chess?" And Antonius says, "Well I've seen it in pictures." Pictures, of course, painted in churches and in cathedrals. So this is a very old theme, the struggle against death, the attempt to trick death. But our contemporary games, of course, are different. We marshal science in an array of high technology medicine against death as an expression of what Father Dick McCormick has called "medical vitalism" – a single minded battle to preserve mere biological existence no matter what the cost.

Back to the film. Antonius and Death begin their high stakes game. They play the first few moves there on the beach and then they continue the game during the stops they make on the journey toward the home castle of Antonius. On the journey Antonius and Jon, shadowed by death, encounter a large number of people in different walks of life. These people are reacting in various ways to their realization that the plague is abroad in the land. They show human terror and desperation at the approach of death. (The coming of the plague, which wiped out so many people, is an historical moment of decisive importance in western civilization.) They meet a group of flagellants who are publicly chastising themselves by following a *pest kreuz* – a plague cross on which the corpus – the body – of Jesus is terribly deformed by the scourge and the crown of thorns. They also encounter a young woman who is about to be burned as a witch because she is being blamed for bringing the plague. They journey through a whole series of scenes portraying human fear and folly, and also human courage and goodness, in the face of impending death. And so the game goes on between Death and Antonius, the knight of the chess game.

Here, again, we have a modern theme expressed quite differently by a psychiatrist, Dr. Elizabeth Kubler-Ross in her studies on *Death and Dying* and *On Children and Dying*. In those books, she describes for us the stages that dying people go through as they struggle to come to terms with death. The first stage is denial and isolation. The second stage is anger, often lashing out at people around them. The anger is usually not personal, just a need to express anger. The third stage is bargaining – bargaining with God. If only you will let me live, I will ... this is the chess game. The fourth stage is depression. Finally there comes acceptance, and with acceptance, dialog about death.

Let's turn back to the film. There is a final climactic encounter as the film nears its end. Antonius is welcomed by a young married couple – Mia, the young wife, and Jof, the young husband – traveling players. Mia and Jof, with their infant baby boy, are camped next to their horse drawn wagon. Antonius finds himself able to speak to Mia. He speaks of the troubles he has experienced, the weariness of heart, the anguish of faith. She consoles him, and she and her husband share with him sweet wild strawberries that they have gathered and the bowl of milk that they have with them. (If any of you have been out camping at the right moment of the year, you know what I mean.)

Then Antonius moves a bit away from the couple and their child. They are in the background as Antonius begins the last stage of his chess game with Death. Death had not been doing well in the game up to this point, but he tricked Antonius into revealing his chess tactics. Death is one move from checkmating the knight. Death is so intent on winning the game against Antonius that Death does not notice the young couple and their little baby in the background. He doesn't look up and notice them. Antonius now realizes that he himself must die because he will not win the game. However, he also realizes that Death hasn't noticed this young family. So Antonius tries to keep Death's attention entirely focused on the game while the young couple hitch up their horse to their wagon and steal away into the forest. Now we begin to really know Antonius – who he is; the kind of person he is – the courageous soldier, the compassionate protector who puts himself at risk in order to rescue others even at the cost of his own life. (These traits are still characteristic of those called to be health care givers in our time. That self-risking is still an ideal of health care.)

The young family go on their way without Death noticing them or where they've gone. Checkmate. The game ends. The knight himself must die, but not immediately. Antonius and his squire, Jon, make the last short leg of their journey to the castle. A terrible storm builds up around them. The wind, marking the onset of death by the Black Plague, howls over the top of the forest. The weary travelers come into the castle. Antonius finds his wife Karin waiting, still full of love and longing for him. She is all alone in the castle because everyone else has fled the plague. Karin sits the knight and Jon and a few other folks who have followed them down to eat. She begins to read from the eighth chapter of the book of "Revelation" of St. John. She reads the passage where the seventh seal is broken and the avenging angels bring apocalyptic destruction upon the earth. As she begins this reading, Death pounds three times on the castle door and enters the hall of the castle to take them all away.

The film ends with a vision of a fantastic "dance of death" that Mia and Jof observe from afar. They have survived the storm and come out of hiding. They have been passed over by Death; they have survived the plague. In this vision, Antonius and his wife Karin and the squire and all the others whom they met on the journey home, all hand in hand, dance, led by Death, the stately long dance of death. Jof describes the vision. "I see them, Mia. I see them. Death tells them to hold each other's hands and then they must tread the dance in a long row. And first goes the master – Death – with his scythe and hourglass. They dance away from the dawn. And it's a solemn dance toward the dark lands while the rain washes their faces and cleans the salt of the tears from their cheeks." The Dance of Death! And so Bergman powerfully evokes feelings, responses to the experience of death, which, right up until the generation before yours, accompanied people, old and young, in their encounter with death.

These people from the past – from the medieval times right up to the middle of the Twentieth Century – were well acquainted with death. They knew death as a companion of young and old alike. They knew death as a familiar fellow pilgrim in this life. And in this way they are so very different from us.

The situation in our time and place is very different from that of Antonius, the hero of the "Seventh Seal." It is different, too, from that of Ingmar Bergman in the mid 1950s when he made that film. That was at the very beginning of the new era which we call (mistakenly, in my view) an era of modern high technology, science based medicine. So I do not claim that Igmar Bergman intended this movie as a parable about the way we live and die as we wage our war against death under the regime of modern high technology medicine.

We entertain, in our own way, the idea that it is possible to play a desperate game of chess with death. That, perhaps by doing so, we can ward off death. We hope that we can some day achieve earthly immortality, if we constantly stretch and strain our science-based, cure- oriented, high technology, medical interventions to the ultimate degree. And so the film says something to us about the encounter with death as we still experience it, that is, our obsessive mood and attitude toward death – our way of *denying death*. In our day, the game is played not with chess, of course, but with high technology which is based on what today we recognize as the only sacred science – the biological science. We seek to survive so desperately, so obsessively, that sometimes the struggle against death makes us forget or foreshortens our compassionate caring for those who suffer. That is our problem. We sacrifice sensitivity. Antonius the knight did not. But we do. We sacrifice sensitivity to suffering – the call to relieve suffering compassionately – in favor of making a greater quantity of life the end. We allow biological survival to justify what is too often an unspeakably, torturous, prolongation of dying. So we struggle with a loss of sober realism about human limitation, about human mortality, about the inevitability of death. And we get engaged in a game that becomes an end in itself.

There's an old Latin saying, *"inter arma silent leges."* "In the midst of war, the laws are silent." It means, of course, that ethical laws, as well as international law, in the ordinary sense, cease to mean anything, if winning is not only the main thing but it is the *only thing*. There are no restraints. Preoccupied with destroying this enemy, death, we succumb to the delusion that we can achieve control even over death. And so, we sin by immoral neglect of our duty to take appropriate, good, compassionate care of the dying. We have to learn anew how to respond well to human suffering, to the pain and grief which inevitably accompany every kind of loss in human life and, ultimately, the great loss in human dying. This is the problem on which I want to reflect in this lecture.

Let me present two practical theses about the challenge to conscience which we face in our time, the Twentieth Century, living in our high technology medical culture – the challenge to renew our dedication to good and compassionate care of the dying. The first thesis is that each of us must take responsibility, as an exercise of our freedom, for our own dying. And to do that, we must seek to provide for good and appropriate care for others, our sisters and our brothers, in their dying. The second thesis is that good care of the dying is the best response to current proposals for relieving the suffering of the dying by physician assisted suicide or physician inflicted death at the request of a dying person. Our response must be affirmative, not merely negative. We must practice good care of the dying and, by this practice, convincingly present what will be a "better way."

I.   My first thesis: we must exercise responsible freedom in preparing for our own dying. There are two practical ingredients to this first thesis. We must plan for our dying and we must provide good care for others in their dying. In preparing for our own dying, we need to do some planning for the probability that we will approach our dying under high technology medical care – in a hospital, possibly in an intensive care unit.   Under these circumstances, a person may not always be able to direct care givers about what kinds of treatment one will consent to and what kinds will no longer be acceptable because one reasonably judges them to be, under the circumstances "excessively burdensome" and, hence, unreasonable.   These phrases translate the traditional term, "extraordinary," by which Catholic moral theology has consistently described treatments which we are morally free to reject, may even be obliged to reject under certain circumstances, in spite of the fact these treatments may be claimed by others to be "life-prolonging."

Dying under high tech medicine means that we are very likely not to be awake and alert enough to give such direction. So, we must prepare an advance directive. Examples are, first, the living will in which we spell out for care givers in advance what we would consider appropriate and inappropriate medical interventions in circumstances that may exist as we are being treated for terminal illness or injury. The second example is the power of attorney for health care by which, besides spelling out what we would want and do not want, we designate a person or persons to act on our behalf to direct medical care givers concerning the use or the foregoing of certain medical interventions.

These medical directives, therefore, can and should be understood to be spiritual testaments, not just legal documents. We should thoughtfully and prayerfully prepare these directives. In them we can express our faith-inspired deep moral convictions about what we consider appropriate end of life care, and especially why we believe foregoing certain kinds of medical intervention as death approaches is really an expression of our hope in God and our trust in God's loving providential care of us in our dying and beyond our death. We can, thus, express our love for God and for others whom we are about to leave behind.

By such advance directives, we can indicate that we reject what Fr. Richard McCormick, S.J., has called "medical vitalism" – the notion that one must war against death in spite of all suffering involved.   We can express the religious reasons why we conscientiously refuse treatments that have become futile, and thus useless and wasteful of medical and financial resources needed by others in a world of limits. We renounce such treatments not out of ingratitude but out of our faith, our hope, and our love of Jesus Christ to whom we are willing to entrust ourselves in our dying, and also out of love for our human neighbors whose needs we respect even as we leave them.

My second point about preparing for our own dying is that we can and should do so by becoming involved, long before our own dying approaches, in caring for those around us who are now nearing their dying. We should support good palliative medicine and hospice type care of the dying. For some of us, I hope many, such support can take the form of becoming personally involved as volunteers in the hospice movement and practice wherein we learn to be with the dying right to the end.

Hospice volunteers, who need not be health professionals, visit the dying, especially those dying at home, and help professional health care persons offer every kind of psychological, spiritual, and very concrete practical support needed both by the dying person and also by those relatives and friends of the dying who are present. This response enables, in my experience, the dying person, even in great weakness, to care for care-givers – for his or her loved ones and even, wonderfully, for medical care givers and hospice volunteers.

Hospice enables a community of love to be formed anew around the one whose death nears. Hospice care provides not only pain control where needed, but above all the kind of personal support of dying persons and of those who are close to them that these last weeks and days and moments together call for. We learn how important it can be to show caring and love of neighbor in simply being with the dying and those dear to the dying who are grieving together at their approaching loss and so need to be able to treasure the time left to be with each other. Hospice professionals and volunteers support this community of love, and, indeed, enter into it. For those of you who are undergraduates, a term paper might allow you to research and reflect upon the meaning and methods of the modern hospice movement. A place to start would be provided by Sandol Stoddard's *The Hospice Movement: a Better Way to Care for the Dying.*

A few more reflections bearing on this first thesis, that we must prepare for our own dying and care for others in their dying: Why do I think that we need to do these things in our time and culture?

Since we live within this era and culture of high technology medicine, we become aware of a contrast between our situation and that of the people in the story of the Seventh Seal. We have been shaped very differently in our thinking about the approach of death from those characters whom I described. Death still sometimes comes suddenly to those around us; but in the medieval era, death came more suddenly, more inexorably, and much more often to younger persons--to the knight Antonius and his companions in the story of the Seventh Seal. In our time and place, we tend to struggle to maintain an illusion of immortality more unrealistically than they could. We erect barriers. When death attempts to enter the intensive care unit, death is thwarted by crash carts, ventilators, and dialysis machines. We live in an era characterized by, as Ernest Becker entitles his book, *The Denial of Death.*

There are reasons for this problem of ours. Through modern public health measures and improved dietary resources, which we complement by the techniques and tools of modern medicine, we have achieved notable postponement of death. In severe illness or injury, we can manipulate the dying process by interventions such as kidney dialysis, pulmonary support with ventilators, pharmaceutical treatments of failing hearts and falling blood pressure, and in the last crisis by cardio-pulmonary resuscitation. But, though we seem to be taking control of our dying by prolonging living successfully, we are brought up short when we begin to realize that sometimes we merely prolong dying itself.

Indeed, if we get beyond our illusions of immortality and pretensions to be in control of death, we may begin to suspect that sometimes we really make the kind of dying that often takes place in our hospitals harder, not easier, than it was in earlier eras. In some circumstances, we have erected barriers to a peaceful death. A sobering statistic that I have heard tells us that for each year we have been able to add to our life expectancy, on the average less than half of the survivors are able to care for themselves in ordinary tasks of daily living. Through our high technology we have achieved a quantitative increase in years of survival, but we have failed to match that with acceptable quality of life for those who survive, and we have introduced new kinds of suffering into the dying we all eventually experience.

The challenge we face, therefore, is to discern when these purportedly life-prolonging medical interventions do more harm than good – when they prolong dying rather than reasonably acceptable living. And with that, we need to have the courage to stop those interventions of cure oriented medicine which do more harm than good – not simply to give up on the dying but rather to turn our skill and efforts to provide palliative medicine to comfort and support the dying. We must have the wisdom and courage to let nature take its course – this Dr. Phil Clarke, so wisely and compassionately, was able to do for his patients.

In order to do that, however, we must prayerfully ponder our mortality. We act freely and with autonomy if we learn to submit to our dying, the unavoidable destiny of every human being. If we allow ourselves to acknowledge that we are poor, limited human beings who will finally be taken from ourselves by death, we will be empowered to begin to accept the deepest dimension of our responsibility as free but finite persons.

Our freedom does not mean that we are to be totally in control of everything in life including death. Rather, being free can and should include fostering a spirituality of submission to our limits and our mortality. Of course we cannot do that without a prayerful trusting in God's loving providence over us both in our living and in our dying. Pierre Teilhard de Chardin, the great Jesuit spiritual writer, urged us to learn freely to cherish not only our active creative powers but also our "passivities of diminishment." We must become willing not only to be active but also to be submissive, ready to accept our experience of human limitation and what that imposes upon us. When we accept limitation, contradiction, disappointment, and finally, death, we are being drawn into the likeness of the dying Jesus. This is a gift that can be given to us only by going through the diminishment that Jesus willed himself to undergo. As Jesus moved from, "Father, let this cup pass," to "No, for this I came to this hour," so too our submission, acceptance, and self surrender are necessary exercises of freedom. We allow God to draw us into the mystery of Christ's death and so into the mystery of Christ's resurrection.

We who are Christian believers do this by living in hope that God draws us by the power of grace into the mystery of Christ's dying and death, and so into Christ's risen life--that all loss is made gain by God's love for us. Karl Rahner, the late Jesuit theologian, insists that the more we submit to God, let God take over our lives, even unto our dying, the more truly free we become, the more we become who we really long to be. The paradox is that human control is not the primary expression of freedom. The more we let God take over our lives, the more truly independent and free we are. We become, in this free submission, persons who love. So, in our dying we must learn to say, with Jesus, "Into your hands I commend my spirit."

Such a spirituality is ours to practice if we are Christian believers. But, I believe that it can also be shared among all "persons of good will" of every religious (or non-religious) sincere conviction who, in various ways, accept the reality of their own humanity and its limitations. Good persons supported by hospice care, whatever their beliefs, are found to grow through something like those stages of dying that Dr. Elizabeth Kübler-Ross described in her pioneering study *On Death and Dying*.

II.   My second thesis: we are challenged in our time to confront and resist claims being made that a morally acceptable (even the best) way to deal with the dying and their problems must involve allowing those who want it to take complete control over their dying, even to the degree of inflicting death on self with the help of doctors or even having their doctors inflict death at their request. This is a claim based on the view that individual autonomy must always be respected.

I believe that we can meet this challenge effectively only by affirmative response. By fostering good hospice type care of the dying, we provide positive witness to the way in which we can best help people in their suffering to accomplish their deepest human desires to love those they are about to leave. This, of course, involves our acting decisively and skillfully to relieve pain, and to do so even when we may fear unwanted side effects that can include acceleration of dying – a risk in many cure oriented medical procedures as well as in hospice care. But, in our Catholic moral tradition, that is another manifestation of our being ready to accept death, but not willing to accept an action aimed at killing. We relieve pain in order to support the dying and their loved ones as they do the final work of dying, express love and care for one another, and finally, come to terms with death and the grief it brings. Only by such effective hospice care of the dying will we persuade others that deliberately inflicting death is really a self-defeating use of autonomy that fails to deal well with human dying.

I would argue, then, that we cannot merely demand that the legal *status quo* be maintained; presently, assisting suicide, even when done by physicians who claim to be helping the dying who request it, is a crime in all U.S. jurisdictions. True, it is being challenged in our time, though so far unsuccessfully, by ballot initiatives first in Washington state, then in California. How can we resist effectively these efforts without appearing merely to deny people who claim that their freedom and moral convictions about what is right should be recognized?

I certainly believe that we should be deeply troubled by all kinds of killing, even though we allow that killing in self-defense (in just war and in the self-defense of the person) has been recognized as morally right action--but, of course, only if the stringent requirements of the moral theory are observed. These require that lethal force be employed only: 1) in a just cause; 2) as a last resort; 3) with use of lethal force restrained to what is strictly proportional to the need to defend; 4) with reasonable hope of success. We should be deeply troubled by accidental killing through carelessness in the use of automobiles and firearms. We should be deeply troubled by deliberate killing inflicted by governments which continue to use the death penalty. I believe that in our culture, we are all too complacent about infliction of death – too reckless in our disregard of its meaning and its consequences.

When, therefore, claims are made that inflicting death should become an accepted medical treatment for the dying who request it, I believe that accepting these claims will lead us out onto what is already very thin ice. Sure, as a Catholic Christian, I believe it is simply morally wrong to inflict death in the name of mercy (we are talking about what used to be called mercy killing). But, we Catholics believe that what is really morally wrong is such because it is really self-destructive of the human; we believe that what is really wrong will bring with it evil consequences to individuals and to our society as a whole. We are not trying to impose our beliefs on others but to warn them of harm they will do to their own humanity.

151

What are some of those evil consequences we anticipate? First, to approve physician assisted dying as just another medical treatment will imperil the vulnerable aging who, in the often difficult circumstances they endure in too many nursing homes, will be subjected to subtle but powerful psychological pressure to ask for inflicted death whether they really want it or not. Further, I think that in our present health care system with its obsession about efficiency, pressures for "cost control" will grow, demanding that patients make a request, however reluctant, for physician assisted suicide. At present, a large proportion of health expenditures are made in the last six months of life. We can foresee hearing: "If you will ask us for physician assisted suicide, your health care insurance premiums can be made lower." Finally, to make available physician assisted suicide to whoever asks for it will advertise a new technological "quick fix" for the problems of pain and suffering when death approaches. We are members of a culture that searches desperately to find and use a "magic bullet" to fix any problem quickly and completely--even when the problems are much more complicated human issues than any quick fix can ever deal with appropriately.

And, there are more predictable evil consequences, but these are enough to mention here. They illustrate that the claims of individual autonomy should and must be weighed in a realistic way against the foreseeable harm these claims will inflict on others and on the common good.

Nonetheless, it seems to me that we will never successfully persuade people that physician assisted suicide is a bad solution to the difficult and complex human challenge of being mortal merely by predicting its bad consequences and then claiming that we simply have to retain criminal penalties against it. Convicting Dr. Kevorkian and keeping him in jail just won't be enough. No, successful persuasion requires that we demonstrate a better way for autonomy to be exercised.

So, we must live out in action what we believe. Let our *orthopraxis*, right practice of our beliefs (our *orthodoxy*), demonstrate that in relieving pain, consoling and supporting those who suffer, staying faithfully to the end by the side of the dying, we provide an affirmative argument against introduction of physician assisted infliction of death. If we learn to do this hospice thing well, we will revive and renew, individually and corporately, the spirit of compassion and humility and caring amongst us. We will show that people who are dying have a final work to complete their living, and that we can support them in doing it well. We will show that people can end their lives in a heartfelt exchange of love with those dear to them and with those who care for them. We will show that a peaceful death, a non-violent death, can be found among us.

So, let us pray to understand the mystery of our mortality. And, let us ready ourselves for our dying as a time of God's coming to us (as we pray in the Mass in the prayer after the Our Father). And let us ask for the courage and ingenuity to practice well our really good care of the dying. And, to conclude, if we pray and act thus, we will also be honoring the faith and moral ideals and loving service which, I believe, were lived so beautifully by our departed dear friend, Dr. Philip Clarke, and by others we have known like him.

Response to
COMPASSIONATE CARE OF
THE DYING

John Young

Over the nine years since Fr. Bresnahan spoke so compellingly of its importance, compassionate care of the dying has become increasingly fashionable. It is now a frequent topic of the ongoing scholarly conversation among clinicians and ethicists alike. To see this, one need only turn to a recent JAMA article (2002;287:749-754) by Bernard Lo and 12 others "for the Working Group on Religious and Spiritual Issues at the End of Life" offering practical suggestions for discussing religious and spiritual issues with patients and families facing terminal illness. The article serves as a thoughtful primer, marking the increasingly accepted importance of its topic as it whets and directs the reader's appetite for further reading, education, and experience.

The rising interest in caring well for the dying has several apparent causes. A prominent one for ethicists is the noticeable emphasis on autonomy that increasingly seems to mark recent writing in the field. This trend itself probably represents a natural swing of the social pendulum as reaction follows action only to give way cyclically to its own opposite over the years. There is also the noticeable rise of consumerism, with advertising reaching deeper and deeper into people's lives. We have come to expect freedom of choice as a kind of right. Patients are instead referred to as clients or even consumers (and "covered lives" in managed care schemes). Medicine is openly referred to as a business, giving me jitters when I open memos at the hospital requesting compliance by "the close of business" on a given date. Along similar lines, some of the best-regarded hospitals have (P. Cram et al: JAMA 2002;287:2945-2946) opened fast food franchises on their premises. And smoking banns were slow to come into force.

Other factors behind the increasing emphasis on the importance of quality care for dying patients are more localized. Some of the energy with which professionals react against the inroads of managed care is expressing itself by defending the terminally ill from its effects. Also, technology continues to advance in exciting ways, for example in the effectiveness of some life support systems and the ingenuity of transplantation procedures including the use of stem cells. These strengthen the prospects of benefit to the gravely ill where none had existed within easy reach of memory. The availability of new technology also stimulates appropriate worry that it may be inappropriately used because it is an attractive and exciting challenge.

The challenges of using new advances in technology well are at least equaled by those of making wise choices about when to use them. The way to this wisdom is through compassion. Compassion means sharing of suffering, being with the other in painful experience. We can best do this, as Bresnahan says, through recognition of the reality that we all die. If we can allow ourselves to share the experience of Antonius Block's awareness that our own death is constantly present, then we can also allow the best that is in us as caregivers to make us worthy. We will, especially with the help of God's ever present grace, find ourselves able to share intimately and appropriately our sickest patients' sufferings, and thus to act towards them with the compassion that is our ideal.

But, even with grace, the mere acknowledgement of our own death will not suffice; we must cultivate some important habits. The principal one is communication. Too often, our busyness facilitates a kind of taking for granted that we and our patients have heard each other more fully than is really the case. Especially for the terminally ill, it requires patient application of time to be sure of really knowing what each individual is ready to hear. We should know from familiar informed consent studies how little is retained when this principle is overlooked. Eric Cassell (*The Healer's Art*) gives a patient explanation of how to go about watching for signs of comprehension after giving a piece of information. When such signs are lacking the proper response is to come up with a smaller piece of information, give it, assess for comprehension, and repeat as necessary. This requires considerable patience. We also may need to rephrase what we are told in order to assure our own understanding of what patients are trying to tell us. Again, patience, but the smile of one who has just begun to feel understood can brighten like the rising sun.

Patients, after all, grant their physicians and other caregivers a great privilege of intimacy, letting themselves be prodded and probed, quizzed and studied, examined and re-examined almost at will. Among professionals, only the clergy come close to having such closeness. Great is the responsibility that goes with such a privilege! It is ours to use on behalf of the one who bestows it. When the patient is dying, the stakes for us to meet this challenge are high. Then, helping another human being to die well becomes an unavoidable dimension of the great privilege. It can become one of the ultimate experiences of communication.

There is a more pragmatic side to excellent communication, far beyond care of the dying. It is the best malpractice insurance – and assurance – a professional can have in any setting. For those who work in forensic settings with dangerous patients, it is the best security for their own safety and that of the patients as well. Each reader can find similar applications appropriate to their own situation.

Aside from communicating well, some specific skills are important. Patients vary widely in their capacity to make difficult and important decisions. Despite being close to death, many are calm and clearheaded enough to evaluate their condition, reflect on it with those closest to them, and make the appropriate choices as they are needed. Their processes and results reflect the fullness of their religious and their human experiences. But others are less fortunate and may, despite appearances, be vulnerable to making choices less than free and not fully their own. As caregivers, it is incumbent on us to discern the level of competence our patients have to make the decisions they face. This requires the humility to recognize the times when a consultant might be helpful.

Another important skill is the ability to navigate well through the current futility debates. At their present stage, there is room for legitimate disagreement so that the controversy is helpful as well as interesting. Significant humility, again, is required to maintain a proper perspective in order to distinguish what we would consider futile from the way it appears to each patient. Often we do not have the desired clarity as we consider prospects of benefit versus degrees of risk and discomfort. Our patients need our help in order to face uncertainty. Being ready to provide it demands continuous attention both to each patient's condition and to the ongoing technological developments that may prove relevant. Although it can be vexing, dealing with the issue of futility is best approached with a sense of excitement about the relief we can provide. Most often we do this by helping the letting go of what once offered hope but now has become an excessive burden. But at least occasionally we do it by finding genuine fresh hope.

Facing futility confronts us with the issue of physician-assisted suicide. Bresnahan is crystal clear on this point when he articulates "action aimed at killing" as a precise statement of what is forbidden. He explains well how misguided efforts to relieve suffering too readily are likely to have clearly unacceptable consequences. There is controversy here on the question of whether efforts to relieve intractable pain, as they increase, cross over the line of being genuinely not aimed at killing before they achieve analgesia. This concern has to do with those whose pain is the most extreme. Bresnahan's formulation helps here: as long as analgesia is not achieved, one can continue to aim for it, and thus not be aiming to kill. As a profession, we are finally – but only – beginning to respond to repeated studies showing the widespread under-treatment of pain in hospitals.

We enter a sacred space when we care for the gravely ill. Perhaps we need more ways of reminding ourselves of this, and we might do well to make fullest use of those we presently have. It is a great privilege to share so intimately in approaching that great divide all of us must face. To force this crossing prematurely, especially in the name of compassion is a grave disservice. The approach of Dr. Kevorkian, the best known violator of this privilege, shows in its very gruesomeness an absence of compassion. This absence is all the more apparent in his medical carelessness. One of his videos illustrates the struggle to suffocate, with a plastic bag, a victim of chronic obstructive pulmonary disease. As any competent physician knows, it would have sufficed to quietly turn down the oxygen flow during the victim's sleep.

Kevorkian, as Bresnahan suggests in his second thesis, could find so many clients despite the poor quality of his own care because there is a tragic shortage of compassionate care for the terminally ill. But the problem is more serious: the quality of care for the dying follows the quality of care for all patients, whatever their apparent clinical distance from death. Bresnahan reflects this fundamental connection as he reminds us that denial of our own death lies behind much of the difficulty we have in compassionately approaching the care of those close to death. He shared with me recently his horror at realizing, as a Medicare patient in an eye clinic away from home, that he was himself being treated as an old man whose life was valueless. As I listened to him, I could hear the vigorous young physicians securing their illusions of immortality by sharpening through their inconsiderate treatment of him the contrast between Jim and themselves.

When a person, unlike Jim in the eye clinic, finally comes to the terminal stage under insensitive and mediocre care, it is almost too late. What is needful can yet be done, thankfully, but now only with great effort requiring resources that seem ever more unlikely to be available. Therefore, our concern about compassionate care of the dying must lead us to pursue the same concern for the living – or rather, for those whose dying, as our own, happens for the moment to be apparently more remote.

Just as good care during life leads to compassionate care as death approaches, having a good death ordinarily couples with leading a good life. As a human act, dying well is a challenge for most; it involves difficult work preparing to end many long relationships, finishing business, making peace. As a Christian, Bresnahan takes care to point out, one has the possibility of dying a death joined with the death and therefore the resurrection of Jesus Christ. Most of us, as Schillebeckx reminds us, require time and help to accomplish this. Supporting this process is the high calling of those who work with the dying, narrowly if they are Christians and more broadly for other dying patients. Cutting it short or allowing it to be bypassed is disservice indeed. Patients must be helped to come to say, with Antonius Block, "my body is frightened, but I am not."

The work of giving patients compassionate care that helps them to die well demands still more than habits of giving quality care to all one's patients. It happens best – perhaps only – as part of a life generally well lived. In our lives as well as in our practices we need to promote and practice life-affirming values and priorities. The mentally ill and physically challenged, the poor and unattractive, and all such as these, need our support and protection. Dr. Philip Clarke clearly provided an example of such living and caring.

In this light we might ask ourselves about our sense of justice with regard to social priorities. What is to be said of a nation with both the most permissive personal firearms (and other weapons) laws and a homicide rate that far outstrips all others? What should be done about capital punishment? More globally, what of political and economic decisions that allow 15,000 people to die every day from AIDS, tuberculosis, and malaria when so much more could easily and cheaply be done? What of clearly unjust third world debt structures which in some cases has people starving to pay for loans made to their former oppressors? What of global warning, energy consumption, and the attention we should be paying to the needs of future generations? Owning up to some level of responsibility for these realities, I submit, can provide perspective and momentum for attention to compassionate care for the dying.

There are several ways to form a personal response in answer to Bresnahan's summons. Education is a natural place to begin. Some can exert a constructive influence on general education at all levels, talking and writing in ways that assist teachers in their noble task to impart wisdom for its proper use along with good knowledge itself. At the undergraduate medical education level some can strive to discourage and constructively replace that "medical vitalism" of which McCormick has so effectively warned. As medical students learn in increasing detail of the wonders of biological life they require encouragement to appreciate the meaning of the content they work so hard to master. At the graduate level, the chief lesson is that of how to prudently take and share the inevitable risks that we and our patients face. We need to teach the wonderful example that pervades Bergman's film, especially when Antonius bravely works to distract Death from the presence of the young family and thus saves them. We can also respond on a personal level. We could strive to take fully to heart the implications of Bresnahan's first thesis, that we must each take responsibility for our own dying. At the very least, this means making an advance directive, something that seems to be catching on more and more each time I see an informal survey of medical colleagues. Also, as he further suggests, some might volunteer to care personally for people facing the nearness of death who are not our own patients. Probably better, organize others to do so and provide them help and supervision, or provide similar supervision and support for Eucharistic ministers visiting in hospital.

As we confront these demanding issues, there are encouraging signs of hope. An example quite mundane is the Americans with Disabilities Act. Also, in an intriguing way, the direct marketing of medications to patients, in addition to the obvious profit motive mentioned above, gives a positive message by showing them that they are taken seriously and respectfully as decision makers regarding their own care. Such advertising also, a patient recently told me, offers fresh encouragement with the news that there are drugs available to help. The continuing proliferation of new technology, for example the automatic external defibrillator, can and should have a similar uplifting effect.

Our Christian tradition encourages an optimistic and even grateful attitude in the face of these uncertainties and challenges. The gift of faith enables us to make effective use of grace where we are otherwise prone to respond with something more like brute force. Where God is, that grace is at hand; and God, we know, is everywhere.

ETHICAL DIMENSIONS OF HEALTH CARE RATIONING

Charles Dougherty

As a graduate of the Philosophy program at Notre Dame, you may notice I have inherited some of the spaciousness of David Solomon's interpretations of reality. I appreciate the kindness of what he had to say about me. I am honored to be here. It is always a treat to come home to my *Alma Mater* and to be able to say a small thank you for what I have received. I know many of you feel the same way when you return. I am especially delighted to be able to give a lecture in honor of Philip Clarke and his family. I cannot say I knew Dr. Clarke well but I did have the opportunity to meet him over the last few years of his life at this meeting. He was awarded the Sorin Award, the highest award the University gives. He was instrumental in starting this conference. He was a man devoted to his patients, especially dying patients; something worth remembering at a meeting like this. Finally, I would observe that many of us have been to meetings where there is a main lecture, but rarely is it named for a family. This is not the Philip Clarke lecture; it is the J. Philip Clarke Family Lecture. I think that speaks volumes about Phil's own values. So for Philip Clarke and Doris and their children, I am pleased and honored to say what I can in his name and in the family's name.

Let me start with a brief anecdote that I think captures a problem we are facing in health care today. An airplane is moving through dense fog. The pilot comes on the intercom and announces: "We have good news and bad news. The bad news is we are in very dense fog and we have just had an electrical problem in the cockpit that has knocked out all our directional equipment. We literally do not know which way we are going." Panic begins to break out in the cabin. The captain comes back on and says: "But wait; there is good news. We are making great time." This, I think, is like our situation in health care today.

Think about the changes we have experienced with the dramatic technological developments in medicine over the last generation or so. Think too of the changes in the ethical context of health care. For example, the institutionalization of informed consent that we now take for granted was a moral sea change, and not so long ago. The first legal decision that touched upon informed consent was in the 1960s. The Karen Ann Quinlan case that changed our views on artificial respiration was only in 1975. It was in the same year that a Federal Trade Commission ruling triggered advertising by physicians, dentists, lawyers, and accountants – another dramatic change. The eighties and nineties have ushered in the massive changes of managed care, health care networks, and increased cost consciousness. Doctors of a generation or two ago were oblivious to the costs of what they did, not by accident but by professional commitment. Cost was none of their business, so to speak. It was business and business was not medicine. But now, like it or not, business has become a large part of the practice of medicine.

With all of these changes, we are making great time. Our directional equipment, however, if not completely out, is at least suspect. What should give direction to our lives – our moral values – are not receiving sufficient attention or not exercising sufficient influence in the debates about health care. As a consequence, these debates are being consumed by economics and politics, while very little of the values that are at stake enter the discussion. Today I want to consider a problem that has political, economic, and financial dimensions and that affects medical practice in a direct way. I want to introduce into discussion of this problem – not for the first time, perhaps not even in the best way either, but in my own way – an explicit value framework.

I want to reflect on the values at stake in health care rationing, and I want to do so within an explicit ethical framework. The framework I am going to offer is a Catholic one. I will cite some major tenets of Catholic social teaching that I think are relevant and then use them to ground some criteria – ethical guidelines – for health care rationing. I am not going to be arguing for any particular form of rationing but, as you will see, I believe that some form of rationing is inevitable. The real issue is what kinds of rationing we should accept and under what sets of circumstances.

Debates about health care rationing have been exacerbated because of conceptual disagreements about what health care rationing means. There are disagreements about the denotative sense of rationing. There are also disagreements about the wider connotative sense of what rationing means to us culturally and viscerally. In many cases, discussions about rationing generate more heat than light because of this emotional charge. For many, there is a very quick negative reaction to rationing, but others react positively. Those who have the negative reaction (typical in medical circles, especially among clinicians) do so because rationing means the withholding of potentially beneficial health care services. It means that some patients will be harmed. Or, to put it in another way – some people will not be helped as much as they might have been helped. Some patients will die sooner than they might otherwise have died. Some patients, if potentially beneficial health care is withheld, will suffer a diminished quality of life compared with the quality they might otherwise have had. There will be pains that could have been avoided or lessened. Opportunities in life for some will be diminished. Because of rationing, some people may face the indignity of being treated differently from others with similar health care problems.

Those who stress these negative consequences also point out the skewed priorities of our health care spending in general. How much do we spend on luxury items, vacations, jewelry, or clothes compared with our spending on health care? How much do we spend on costly unnecessary treatments? How much waste and fraud is there in the health care system? Of course, we cannot all agree about what exactly constitutes waste and fraud. One person's waste can be someone else's salary. But many feel that the high percentage of administrative cost in health care represents waste. This is money that should have been, or could have been, directed toward patient care. In addition, there are high levels of profits taken out of the health care system by passive investors.

A second major negative consideration is that duties may be violated by rationing care. I believe, and I think most philosophers and theologians agree, that there is no duty always to do the best for other people. In spite of how attractive this may sound, it probably goes well beyond what we are duty-bound to do. There is, however, something of a consensus among ethicists that we have a duty to perform what is called "easy rescue." A duty of easy rescue comes into play when the stakes for someone I might help are great and the risks to me from helping are small. In such circumstances, rescue is a duty. Depending upon how a system of rationing is set up, the duty of easy rescue may be violated. Rationing might cause us to avoid small efforts to help people in cases where our help might mean a great deal to them, perhaps even life or death itself.

A third major area in which there is reason for concern about health care rationing is the potential impact on the doctor-patient relationship. There is a real possibility of undermining trust in the physician-patient relationship in clinical settings. Patients, generally speaking, are vulnerable – not all, but most patients. It is important to remember that people often enter therapeutic relationships in pain and anxiety. They rely on doctors to put their interests as patients first. When doctors become rationing agents, however, they have to put economic interests on the same plane or sometimes ahead of the interests of the individual patient. These three concerns are the heart of the case against health care rationing: increased suffering, violation of the duty of easy rescue, and damage to the doctor-patient relationship.

How could anyone think health care rationing is a good thing in the face of these negatives? Contemporary debates on health care reform suggest one reason: health care rationing may be necessary. There are over thirty-five million uninsured Americans. Lack of insurance creates serious limitations on access to care. Lack of access has serious consequences for morbidity and mortality. At the same time, Americans spend more for health care than any other nation does, both in terms of absolute dollars and as a percentage of our gross domestic product. This year we will spend close to fifteen percent of the economy on health care, about one out of every seven dollars. More important is the rate of increase. Some have estimated that if we continue at the current rate of increase, Americans will spend one hundred percent of the gross domestic product on health care within the lifetime of our grandchildren. Clearly, this is an unsustainable rate of increase. But the imperative to spend more is also plain. President Clinton, as you know, has threatened to veto any health care reform that does not cover every American. I agree that this is a moral bottom line. There is an imperative to develop a system in which these thirty-five million uninsured gain coverage in some meaningful way. But this entails serious cost containment. How can we expand the system to cover more people and at the same time bring the rate of cost increase down to a more manageable level? It seems to me, and to many others, that the only way to accommodate these contrary goals is through some explicit form of health care rationing.

So rationing is necessary. Moreover, rationing can make a bad situation better. There is a commitment to equity built into the very meaning of rationing. Rationing is an equitable distribution of a scarce resource. Equity means fairness. The implication, then, is that rationing is a way of doing fairly what is likely to happen in some fashion anyway – scarce goods will be distributed. Therefore, rationing is not only necessary but, from a moral point of view, a good thing. It introduces fairness into an otherwise neutral or unfair situation.

Against this background of competing assessments, it is important to find a neutral definition of health care rationing, one that does not settle the moral issue of rationing by definition. Definitions that make rationing inherently bad or inherently good should be avoided. Instead, a useful definition should accommodate our competing intuitions. On the one hand, rationing seems wrong in clinical contexts because it can mean denying needed services to some people. On the other hand, rationing may be right if it can help to introduce greater equity into the distribution of health care.

Let me offer such a definition of health care rationing. It is taken from a recent study by the Catholic Health Association, a voluntary organization that represents about six hundred Catholic hospitals in the United States. Two years ago, the Catholic Health Association assembled a task force to examine the ethics of rationing. They arrived at this definition: "Health care rationing is the withholding of potentially beneficial health care services because policies and practices establish limits on the resources available to health care." Health care rationing is the withholding of *potentially beneficial* health care services. If what is withheld is actually wasteful or extraordinary or does not have the potential to help a patient then withholding is not rationing. The phrase *policies and practices* was employed because policies to limit resources are explicit, while practices generally are not. Hence, whether explicit or not, rationing is a response to established limits on the resources available for health care. This definition does not prejudge the question of whether a given program or a proposed program of rationing is good or bad. The definition is alert to the central moral concern that potentially beneficial services are being withheld. But it allows the possibility that the withholding might be justified on the basis of limited resources. This definition of rationing allows for the self-conscious examination of whether a given form of rationing is morally acceptable or not.

Another benefit of this neutral definition is that it allows us to see that rationing already occurs in the American health care system. Potential health care benefits are withheld from many Americans because of deliberate choices made at different levels. In the Medicare program, for example, we make no distinction among patients on the basis of income but we do use age. The social choice to cover wealthy people over sixty-five years of age in the Medicare program, but not poor people younger than sixty-five, has a significant rationing effect; it withholds benefits from some while it gives benefits to others. When state legislatures restrict eligibility in their Medicaid programs, rationing takes place. When counties deliberately create paperwork barriers to public assistance for health care, there is rationing. Rationing occurs when levels of Medicaid compensation to physicians and hospitals are set so low that they lead providers to shun Medicaid patients.

Health insurers also pursue policies whose effects, whether consciously intended or not, ration care. For those without health insurance, access to the system is limited if not foreclosed. Some are turned away when they seek care. Many uninsured people with genuine health care problems do not try to get health care, knowing they can not pay for it. Others, who do try, arrive too late for effective care. In addition, they are often treated in hospital emergency rooms, where service is neither comprehensive nor personal. Another factor causing rationing through health insurance is the move away from community rating: one package of benefits and one schedule of payment for all enrollees based on the statistical prevalence of disease and risk in a community. Increasingly insurers use experience rating, assessing the health history of particular groups and individuals, and matching coverage and premiums to that experience. In short, the sick and the likely to be sick are made to pay more. Experience rating leads to the exclusion of people who have preexisting illnesses. And it has led to the creation of that peculiarly American health care pariah, the "uninsurable" person.

So health care is rationed *de facto* in the United States on the basis of ability to pay in the open market, on the basis of employment (the link to insurance for most of us), on the basis of history of illness, and on the base of age and income. In the Medicaid program, there is also rationing on the basis of having dependent children. Furthermore, it makes a great deal of difference where one lives in America; geography, too, causes rationing. For example, someone in rural America, who has great distances to travel in order to reach a provider, faces health care rationing. One might even say that health care is rationed simply on the basis of luck. One third of uninsured Americans are children. These children were simply unlucky to be born into households without insurance. One of the cruelest bits of bad luck is to be born into a household with a working parent who has no health insurance – precisely the situation of many uninsured children.

Another recent phenomenon in the health care system leading to rationing is the development of organized delivery networks, especially managed care plans. These plans have the positive potential of transforming what is otherwise a fragmented non-system into a coordinated system of health care. To that extent they can be very good, helping to control costs while delivering care that might otherwise have been unavailable. On the other hand, in the absence of universal coverage, they may elevate competition in health care to a higher level. In such an environment, potential enrollees who cannot contribute positively to a plan's bottom line are undesirable. They will be avoided in the marketing of the plan. The net result may be further erosion in coverage for America's poor and seriously ill.

Current terms of health care rationing raise serious ethical issues, especially against the background of millions of Americans with no health insurance. In my view, the obligation to perform easy rescue is violated since the resources of the United States are clearly sufficient to cover all the uninsured without great sacrifice. All other comparable nations do so. Moreover, these forms of rationing cause serious harm. Lack of coverage causes barriers to care. Barriers to care cause higher morbidity and mortality. Consequently, the uninsured have significantly higher rates of preventable disease and death than the insured population. Even when needed care is secured, there are indignities associated with having to depend on the charity of others for the satisfaction of such fundamental needs.

Recently, there have been calls for explicit and systematic health care rationing. After widespread debates Oregon, for example, recently began a rationing plan in its Medicaid program. Although some hesitate to call the Oregon Plan rationing, I believe it is. The question is not whether what Oregon has done is rationing. From my point of view, the question is rather whether the Oregon rationing plan is ethically justified. There is also debate about whether the Clinton health care plan would ration care. I believe it must. It has to set limits in order to afford the cost of universal coverage. There can be no health plan that offers everything to everybody.

Now I want to introduce an ethical framework from Catholic social teaching that I think will give us some additional perspectives on rationing. It might strike you, or at least some people, as odd for a philosopher to grab onto Catholic Social teaching, as I will do, but I think it is simply a matter of truth in advertising. I cannot argue for everything right now. If I were a Marxist, you should know that. If I were a libertarian, you should know that, too. So if I am using Catholic Social teaching, I want to be explicit about it. There are four elements of Catholic social teaching to which I will appeal. They are, I hope, commonplace for this audience. First, every human being is sacred and possesses a dignity that is the basis for a comprehensive range of human rights. Human dignity entails human rights. Second, human persons are inherently social. This social nature is the basis for an obligation to serve the common good of our communities. Simply put, communities shape and sustain persons. Therefore, respect for persons requires care for communities. Third, because creation is a finite gift, persons must be responsible stewards of limited human and natural resources. This is an age of limits in a world of limits. Finally, while all human beings are equal in their dignity, there is a special responsibility to the poor – those who are of low socioeconomic status, the sick, the uneducated, the marginalized. We must be in solidarity with those who are least well-off. Let me say more about each of these four elements.

First, persons have dignity. Formulations of the Catholic tradition on this issue in the last century have displayed a great deal in common with Immanuel Kant's conception of dignity and the respect owed to persons. According to Kant, persons, unlike things, have an incalculable value or dignity that is intrinsic to their existence. Consider an automobile, by contrast. Its value is captured by a price that expresses its worth in relationship to other commodities. The price value of the automobile is relative. Moreover, the price of a car can fluctuate on the basis of things external to itself, such as how many similar cars there are and how many people want cars of this sort. Kant held that both of these characteristics of things are untrue of people. The value of a person is not relative; it is absolute or incalculable – too great to assign a price. At the same time the value of a person is not external; it is internal. Thus, to say that humans have dignity is to say that the value of persons is fundamentally different from the value of things. Unlike things, persons have an incalculable value that is intrinsic to their existence. This intrinsic, incalculable value is human dignity. It is not earned and it can not be alienated. One can not gain it or lose it on one's own. It is part of every human being's existence regardless of how exalted or diminished that existence is.

Because of this conception of dignity every person has rights. The most important right is the right not to be objectified, that is, the right not to be treated as or reduced to the condition of a thing without dignity. This general right can be articulated into a series of particular rights that protect a range of natural functions, including rights of speech, assembly, etc. In the Catholic tradition, the rights of human beings also include positive rights of access. These rights guarantee access to what persons need in order to live lives of dignity. For more than a hundred years, Catholic assertions of these rights have included a right to health care.

I do not want to lead you to believe that Kant's ethics and Catholic tradition are the same. Catholic tradition is grounded, as Kant's philosophy is not, in an explicit religious appeal. For Kant, human persons have dignity because each is an autonomous end-in-himself or herself. For the Catholic tradition, human life has dignity because it results from and participates in divine creation. Respect for personal autonomy can play a special role for Catholics, but is not the unlimited role that autonomy plays for Kant and in many other recent philosophical formulations. Metaphysically, Catholics see human dignity as ultimately heteronomous as opposed to autonomous. It comes from outside the person, namely, through creation by God. In practical relations with one another, however, respect for the autonomy of each person is broadly consistent with contemporary Catholic tradition.

Second, human persons are inherently social. As a consequence, the focus of concern about human dignity cannot rest exclusively on individuals. Practically, human dignity is realized or frustrated in association with others in the organic life of communities. It makes a difference, in terms of the practical realization of dignity, when and where a person is born, how he or she is raised, and who constitutes his or her circle of friends. Socioeconomic factors, institutional structures, and culture all help to make or break the reality of human dignity. Thus, respect for persons in the context of this social nature requires concern for the common good – a set of conditions that must obtain if all would have an opportunity to realize their potential as persons.

It is hard to define the common good precisely. It is an inherently vague notion and properly so. One thing the common good is not is a simple utilitarian calculus, an adding up and subtracting of people's preferences. The best society for a utilitarian is one in which the greatest good for the greatest number prevails. By contrast, the common good lies in the direction of creating communities of mutual concern and responsibility, communities that are willing to work, not simply for the majority, but for a conception of the good for all. This involves a certain kind of solidarity with others. It entails an ethical commitment to do what is necessary to build constructive humanizing forms of social, political, and economic interdependence, as well as a special sensitivity to relationships – roles and institutional structures – and their effects on individuals.

In this context, the Catholic tradition holds that health care is not simply a commodity that an individual sells or gives to another individual. Health care has important social dimensions. The knowledge and power of health care comes to us after centuries of scientific work and clinical experimentation. No individual owns health care. There is always a social or public dimension. The contemporary structure of health insurance, for example, would be impossible without government regulation and massive public support from the tax code for the provision of private health insurance as a fringe benefit. Health care infrastructures, hospitals in particular, have been built with large-scale public investment. In clinical contexts, doctors and other health care professionals must put their patients first. But in social policy the common good must take precedence.

A third element of the Catholic tradition is stewardship. For Catholics, nature is a gift from God. Therefore, the obligation to use resources wisely has religious roots. When resources are used inappropriately, more than economic efficiency is at stake; the waste of a gift is irresponsible. Responsible stewardship requires consciousness of costs, including opportunity costs. Many states, for example, are struggling with expanding Medicaid budgets and are beginning to find themselves in an ironic position. Medicaid budgets are growing so rapidly that the ability of states to invest discretionary money in education, housing, and economic development has become sharply limited. But many of these efforts – in housing, education, economic development – have more positive effects on a community's health status than the health care provided through Medicaid. Health care spending is creating opportunity costs that are diminishing our collective health.

Finally, there must be special concerns for the poor. There is a tension in the first three tenets of Catholic social teaching. All people have equal human dignity. Communities can enhance or frustrate the real expression of that dignity. Hard choices about spending priorities must be made in light of stewardship responsibilities. How should priorities be set? The answer in the Catholic tradition is that the poor and vulnerable have a special claim on our concern and resources. The religious roots here are obvious; I won't belabor them. A related secular point to be made is that the poor and vulnerable are least able to express and defend their own interests. In the current health care reform debate, for example, the American Medical Association, the American Hospital Association, the leading pharmaceutical companies, and the health insurers (in the guise of "Harry and Louise") will articulate and press their own interests. But will a reformed system be better for those who are least well served by it now and who are least able to press their own interests? This is the moral question that must be addressed.

With these four tenets of Catholic social teaching as a background, I want to move to an explicit consideration of the ethics of rationing. I will offer eight criteria for thinking about rationing from a moral point of view. These criteria will not of themselves determine whether or not the Oregon Medicaid Plan, for example, is morally acceptable. They will, however, provide a framework for articulating what is at stake ethically. There is one other point important to add by way of a preface. If we are rationing implicitly right now, as I believe we are, and an explicit health care rationing plan is proposed, ethical assessment is not simply a matter of analyzing the proposed rationing plan. The rationing that is proposed must also be compared to the rationing that is in place.

Here are the eight criteria. First, rationing must be justified in any particular case. There should be a demonstration of the necessity for particular kinds of rationing. I have already made the general case for rationing. We cannot sustain the present rate of spending increases. Yet, we have to cover more people. Therefore, we have to ration. But while the general case is easily made, it must be made again in application to specific cases. Do we have to impose this kind of rationing on this particular population? For example, there are states that spend comparatively little money on their Medicaid programs. Perhaps some of these states simply cannot spend more. They do not have the economic infrastructure. In other states, however, it is plain that limited Medicaid spending is either a political expedient or a public preference for lower taxation. It is important to remember that when such decisions are made values are being prioritized and health care limits set. In my estimation, the Medicaid programs of some states are so poorly funded that the consequent rationing is irresponsible. Citizens and corporations should pay a level of taxes sufficient to provide a reasonable benefit package to the Medicaid population. Obviously, inefficiencies and waste have to be taken out of the system or reduced. Administrative costs and profits should be evaluated. Every effort should be made to use available dollars for necessary care, before we approach the hard decision of having to deny patients potentially beneficial care. Although we will never have a system wholly free of waste, unnecessary administrative costs, and unconscionable profits, we have to be morally sure that a particular form of rationing is really necessary. The first criterion, therefore, is that rationing must be justified.

Second, health care rationing must be oriented toward the common good. This may seem a simple thing to say, but it is worth remembering that the Hippocratic tradition is oriented toward the good of individuals. The motivation of the clinician must be the good of the patient. But health care is also a social reality. In allocating resources, therefore, the motivation must be what is good for all of us, what is good for communities. Here I note a remarkable feature of moral psychology, noble in many cases but troubling in others. We are often willing to spend virtually unlimited dollars to aid identifiable victims of a particular catastrophe. At the same time, we are reluctant to invest in prevention or the kind of statistically significant efforts that might have avoided the catastrophes or minimized the problems. Several years ago, for example, a little girl fell into a well in Texas. There was no end to what we were willing to do to get that girl out of the well. I wonder how much money has been spent since capping open wells in Texas so that others do not fall in. Psychologically, it is much easier to react to need than to anticipate it. But different standards are needed at the social level of health care. Resources should be allocated in terms of what is good for the whole community. This requires the use of statistical reasoning and health services outcomes studies. In practical terms, service to the common good may mean a de-emphasis on expensive technologies that serve only a few in order to provide more rudimentary, less expensive things for all. It may mean, for example, fewer MRIs and more vaccinations. This is not to suggest a preference for the value of the public good over that of each individual. The value of each individual person is incalculably great. But the resources available for health care are not incalculably great.

The value of each person is priceless but the value of the goods and services we provide them is not. If we must ration, explicit reference to the well-being of the community as a whole must be a criterion.

The third criterion is an implication that follows from the dignity principle: a basic comprehensive level of services should be available to everyone. Defining the elements of a basic comprehensive package of coverage is difficult and controversial. My own view, after considerable struggle with these complexities, is now a simple one. I support any plan that provides universal coverage, regardless of the perceived adequacy of its coverage. The possibility of bringing everyone into the health care system is an opening in our political history that comes rarely. Whatever plan we choose, no matter how comprehensive its benefits may look at the time, will be revised through our lifetime and the lifetime of our children and grandchildren. Technology, economics, and politics will continually adjust our notion of basic and comprehensive care. By contrast, I believe we should not leave to our grandchildren the task of covering all Americans.

Again, the elements of a basic package of health care are difficult to determine. By its very nature the right to health care has to be a limited right. It cannot be a right to everything. No one or group can make an unlimited demand on a community's resources. Given the general affluence of our country, limits need not be set unreasonably low. Without overtaxing our individual and collective budgets, we can provide basic and comprehensive care for all Americans. As a strategy for opening this discussion, I would propose covering everyone with a middle of the line, moderately priced Blue Cross plan – one that average Americans would identify as close to what they have now. We could begin with an assumption that such coverage is basic and comprehensive. Then political dickering would add to and subtract from the coverage.

The fourth criterion is that rationing should apply to everyone. When the Catholic Health Association was developing these criteria, this was the one most hotly debated. It raised the most divisive issues. Yet in some respects it is the most morally obvious.

The reason why it is so obvious is its close connection to the Golden Rule. That Rule makes it hard to hold that it is just to impose rationing on other people while escaping it oneself. This moral presumption of reciprocity or equal standing and treatment is not simply a Judeo-Christian belief. In her influential book *Lying*, Sissela Bok claimed that the Golden Rule is part of every major moral and religious tradition. The world over, people have had the Golden Rule insight. It thus appears to be a hallmark of morality to hold oneself to the same standards to which others are held. By contrast, a distinctive mark of immorality is to hold others to high moral standards while making exceptions for oneself. For example, there is an obvious immorality in claiming that lying is wrong while excusing one's own lies.

The difficulty with this criterion for acceptable rationing is that it anticipates a large change in the health care system. Applying it literally would require a reform that creates a system sufficiently unified so that all could share the sacrifices of health care rationing. Right now our American system is too fragmented for such a result. It is hard to imagine how such a unification could be achieved practically. For example, it seems inevitable that in any system in the near future, some Americans will be able to buy outside of or above any common health care system. I do not wholly lament this. The problem is an expression of another important value, freedom. It is hard to conceive of a system in which Americans would not be free to buy more health care or purchase more insurance than what is included in a basic national plan. Our historic commitment to the value of personal freedom is such that some inequalities in health care will have to be accepted.

The key political consideration that makes this ethical criterion practical is that the vast majority of Americans should face rationing constraints together. If, for example, ten or fifteen percent of the population of the wealthiest Americans were able and willing to buy additional coverage, equity in the system would be diluted, but the overall justice of the system would not be imperilled. However, if forty or fifty percent of Americans left the public system for private alternatives, whatever common system was left would devolve into a welfare program. Then, a death spiral would begin. People would not want to pay for a system that is not their own. The consequent loss of tax support would result in diminished quality and additional flight from the system.

This is, in effect, an admission that a two-tiered system of health care is inevitable, given the values of our culture. However, two tiers can mean two profoundly different things. On my account, having two tiers is ethically tolerable if the first tier is a broad-based, comprehensive plan with a second, much smaller luxury tier. By contrast, a two tier system in which there is a comprehensive luxury model for most and a highly rationed welfare program for the poor is morally problematic. The first kind of two-tier system is a reasonable political compromise between fundamental values. The second kind is an injustice to the poor and a potential assault on their dignity. An important implication of this criterion is that Americans should not begin explicit and systematic rationing of health care for the poor while the middle class and the wealthy continue to use (and overuse) the health care system without constraint. This is my major objection to the Oregon Plan. Certainly, there are many good aspects of the Oregon Plan. When all is said and done, however, it is a system of rationing only for the poor.

If you have followed the twists and turns of the debate in Oregon, you may know this instructive story. Just before final passage, an Oregon senator who opposed the Plan offered an amendment mandating that all Oregon senators drop their existing coverage and enroll in the newly rationed Medicaid program. Of course, his amendment failed, as he knew it would. Through a bit of political theatrics, the senator was making a point about shared sacrifice. The same point is being made today by a great many people. Within the last month, two bills were introduced in the United States Congress mandating that all Americans receive the same coverage that members of Congress have. My own U.S. senator, Bob Kerry, an activist on health care reform, sometimes wears a lapel button that says, "Give us what Congress has." That expresses the moral intuition that both the benefits and restrictions of our health care system should be shared by all.

The fifth criterion is that plans to ration health care should result from an open participatory process. The process should allow for public discussion on limits and who shall bear the burden of them. Oregon provides a good example. Their process started with public town hall meetings across the state. People were asked to define what they want from health care; what values should drive allocation; and how are those values to be prioritized. The results showed that the people of Oregon generally valued quality of care and prevention over acute care interventions. That information about values was then put together with health care services outcomes data. Next actuarial considerations were added: how many Oregonians would use which services and at what unit cost. A prioritized list of hundreds of health care services was then developed, with the intent that less important services would be cut in order to expand the number of people covered for the remaining more important services. Whatever its flaws, this was a significant accomplishment in the making of public policy.

A sixth criterion is that health care for the disadvantaged must have a special priority. Low socioeconomic households have the highest morbidity and mortality rates in this country. There are unmet needs among African Americans, Hispanic Americans, and Native Americans. Over the last couple of generations, children in America have gone from being among the least poor to being among the most poor. The reason for this transition is the shift of public money into Social Security and Medicare, that is, toward the elderly. There is also inequity in addressing the health care needs of rural Americans. As we move towards explicit health care rationing and begin setting limits, we must be prepared for affirmative action in health care. Not everybody has benefitted equally from the successes of the American health care system. Before we impose restrictions across the board, we may have to add services where access has been limited historically.

A seventh criterion is that rationing must be free of wrongful discrimination. All of us are against "wrongful" discrimination. The problem of course lies in defining "wrongful." Clearly, health care rationing that discriminates on the basis of gender, race, religious beliefs, and sexual orientation is unacceptable. There are two areas, however, in which there is no similar consensus: age and lifestyle. Can we use age as a criterion for rationing? Ethicist Daniel Callahan raised the age issue explicitly and was pilloried for it. His view, simply put, is that when a certain age is attained, say eighty-five, curative care should take a backseat to social support and custodial care. My own view – far from an original thought – is that age as a criterion for rationing is not morally troubling when it is a factor in prognosis, that is, when age helps to determine if a patient will likely benefit from an intervention. For example, I would have no problem with the claim that eighty-five year-olds are not fit candidates for heart transplantation if it were statistically true that eighty-five year-olds do not do well after heart transplants. On the other hand, it is morally troubling to use age to ration without a basis in health outcomes. This would suggest that the value of a person's life is age dependent.

The other issue is lifestyle. To what extent is it legitimate to take lifestyle into account when rationing health care? Framed as an issue of freedom versus determinism, this is a problem that has haunted ethicists for generations. Should we hold patients accountable for the health outcomes of their choices? If we do, we respect their freedom and responsibility, but we might be tempted to limit their access to needed care due to their own bad choices. Alternatively, should we stress the circumstances that determine and influence choice – parents, genes, social environment, culture, etc. – and disregard lifestyle choices in determining access to care? This would ignore or deny personal freedom, but expand access to needed care since no disease or injury would be anyone's fault. My own view is stereoscopic. In public health and educational contexts – anywhere that information and incentives are thought to shape choice – we should regard people as free and responsible. We should presume that people want to live healthier lives, and they can choose to do so. In clinical contexts, by contrast, we should ignore the assumptions of public policy and regard patients as victims of circumstances. We should assume that something unfortunate has happened to them; we do not know fully how or why. Judgments about freedom and responsibility should be suspended in clinical contexts. People who are suffering from health conditions should be treated irrespective of their role in the etiology of their disease or injury.

Eighth and finally, the effects of rationing must be monitored carefully. The effects that we can anticipate – the ones already laid out here – include people not getting the care they need. There are obvious negative consequences to that. But there are other consequences to which we should also be attentive. One is the impact on the doctor-patient relationship. I believe the medical profession should play a key role in establishing rationing policies. Medical specialty groups and individual practitioners can help to develop reasonable criteria for rationing. At the bedside, however, doctors should not make direct rationing decisions. Doctors should remain fiduciary agents for patients, fighting system limits when they harm patients. Asking doctors to make decisions to ration for individual patients would undermine trust. If patients knew or suspected that their care was being limited because another patient or potential patient was being preferred, they would lose trust in their doctors. I believe that the threat of undermining patient trust by putting rationing in the hands of clinicians is so great that I would prefer to use medical expertise for rationing only at the social level, determining policy, and not at the individual level, determining limits on patient care.

There is a final issue that bears watching. It is large and important. As we move into the rationing arena, the economics of health care will become more insistent and more unavoidable. In economics, we are prone to pay attention to the quantifiable, to things that can be counted. Less tangible things may come to be considered less important. For example, if we attend only to things that can be measured, time spent with patients establishing a relationship – caring for someone in a personal way – could be lost from the system entirely. It is worth remembering that the value of caring for patients has animated health care from its very beginnings. For centuries, doctors could do very little to cure people. But they stood with patients while they suffered and while they died. That kind of caring was and remains immeasurably important. Rationing could very well undermine this aspect of care. We must be vigilant to protect the care in health care from an overemphasis on the economic.

In conclusion, we are making great time in health care. There have been dramatic changes in our recent past and more to come in our immediate future. There will be more stress on systems and providers to make hard choices – some explicit, some not, but all involving decisions to ration care. This can portend a bad future in which we simply deny care, increase suffering, and increase indignity. Or, it can usher in a better future in which we create more equity in the health care system and serve our communities better. The key to determining which future we experience lies in the use of our moral directional equipment. We must remind ourselves of our most important values and insist that they be used to steer through the health care rationing choices that lie ahead of us.

Response to
ETHICAL DIMENSIONS OF
HEALTH CARE RATIONING

Todd David Whitmore

Charles Dougherty provides a clear prescription for the ills of the contemporary health care system in the United States. He begins with the metaphor of an airplane in fog to describe the present situation. The pilot informs the passengers, "We have good news and bad news. The bad news is we are in very dense fog and now we've just had an electrical problem up here in the cockpit that's knocked out all of our directional equipment and so we literally don't know which way to go." The good news is, "We're making great time." In keeping with the metaphor, Dougherty's task is to reinstall new directional equipment. He sets out four overarching principles which generate eight criteria for getting the plane to the terminal safely.

On first read, Dougherty's equipment appears to do the job. There does not initially seem to be much to argue with regarding his principles and criteria. The four principles, in order, are: 1) human dignity as a basis for human rights; 2) human sociality affirming the common good; 3) the fact of the limited nature of creation requiring stewardship of the goods of creation on our part; and 4) the "special claim" that the poor have on our attention, and thus our "special responsibility" towards them. The eight criteria provide further specifications of the principles.

My own reading of Catholic social teaching would articulate the concept of the common good first. Catholic teaching certainly affirms rights, but they are subsumed under the common good. Leading with rights tends Catholic teaching more towards classical liberal political thought than I think is warranted. Dougherty's presentation of rights and individual human dignity prior to human sociality and the common good appears indebted, as is much interpretation of Catholic social teaching in the United States, to David Hollenbach's 1979 book, *Claims in Conflict*, and, to a lesser extent, the U.S. bishops' 1986 document, which Hollenbach had a key hand in drafting, *Economic Justice for All.* (Hollenbach later places more emphasis on the common good.)

The ordering in the presentation of rights and the common good may seem to be a small matter. After all, Dougherty, like Hollenbach in *Claims in Conflict,* follows the emphasis on the dignity of the individual person with an affirmation of sociality. Individual human dignity, according to Hollenbach and the U.S. Bishops, can only be "realized in society." In Dougherty's words, "human dignity is realized practically, or frustrated practically, in association with others."

However, I want to suggest that this reversal of ordering leads to a faulty analysis of the situation and to problematic prescriptions. My argument, in short, is this: when one begins with the rights of the individual person as the starting point for reflection, then the tendency is to move too quickly in one's prescriptions to the state because the state is the guarantor of those rights. The direct nature of the move to the state includes a tendency to bypass or, at best, to pay insufficient attention in one's initial analysis to other levels and spheres of society where there is social plurality and even fragmentation, but perhaps also potential for responsiveness to the problem of health care provision. In brief, the rights-driven predisposition to prescribe federal government remedies shapes the original description of the situation in a way that downplays other forms of social reality and response and offers inadequate tools for explaining why the federal effort has failed.

This is most of all evident in the controlling metaphor in Dougherty's account: the plane with a pilot but in need of a guidance system. Again, the idea is that with Dougherty's principles the pilot could direct the plane with the support of all the passengers to a destination that all of the passengers indeed would desire if they could see through the fog. The pilot in this scenario would be the President of the United States. At the time of Dougherty's writing – 1994 – the prospects of such a scenario where there is a singular plan, whether his or anyone else's, are in serious question. Dougherty, however, remains confident: "There is a debate about whether the Clinton health care plan rations health care. I think the Clinton plan is a serious contender. I think it is a good plan. I think we will rediscover it in this debate. The conventional wisdom right now is that the Clinton plan is dead. I understand that. However, I think as we really examine the alternatives, we'll find out why that structure looks like it does."

I write in 2000, with the hindsight of six years. Still, I think that Dougherty's assessment of the situation was wrong then, and could have been seen as such with a different – and I think more accurate – read of Catholic social teaching, one that began with the common good and did not move first to the state for its prescriptions. Beginning with the common good would have highlighted more the degree to which persons in the United States do not share the same values, or to the extent that they do, the values are centered around self-interest and thus are not the one's Dougherty offers the pilot. It is noteworthy that even though Dougherty provides at one point the qualification that what he is offering is a particular set of values, those of Catholic social teaching, throughout the rest of the article he refers without qualification to "our values." The problem, according to Dougherty, is that "our values – what gives direction to our lives – are not receiving sufficient attention or not exercising sufficient influence in the debates about health care." Whose values? The idea is that the plane is ultimately guided by the President of the United States and that the passengers are from all religious and secular persuasions. So the values may be originally Catholic, but everyone agrees with them. Such a view seems to presuppose the kind of argument that John Courtney Murray gave in *We Hold These Truths*: There is an American consensus regarding one God and one nation, and the Catholic tradition has been and is best at articulating it.

However, there appears to have been and to be presently a kind of dis-sensus, a pulling apart, either because we do not hold the same values or because the values we hold are selfish ones. An approach beginning with the common good could have brought this fact – by its very contrast – to the fore. The problem, then, is not that the guidance system has gone out, but that monkeys have escaped from the cargo bay, pushed aside the pilot, and are in the cockpit pulling every which way on the controls, trying to steer the plane to the airport closest to their own home. We can view these monkeys as commercial interests. It is notable that the presumed father of contemporary capitalism, Adam Smith, did not trust persons who worked in the commercial sphere of society with the common good of a nation. Such persons constitute, "an order of men whose interest is never exactly the same with that of the public, who have generally an interest to deceive and even to oppress the public, who accordingly have, upon many occasions, both deceived and oppressed it." For the monkeys to be at the helm is indeed, for Smith, for them to have escaped their bounds. We can further imagine that some, even many or most of the passengers, having seen what is happening up front, join the fray to help the monkey of their choice. The people and the monkeys are in cahoots. The problem was and is much more than the fog outside.

Developments since 1994 only reaffirm this reading of the state of affairs. It is noteworthy that as I write – less than three weeks prior to the 2000 presidential elections – the issue of health insurance is all but off of the political map. The number of uninsured people in the United States stands at 42.6 million – only in the last year, for the first time in 12 years, has it begun to show significant decline. This is all against the backdrop of an unprecedented economic boom. At the time of the 1992 and 1993 proposals for health care, the annual budget deficits were at their zenith, around $300 billion. Now there is a surplus, yet, because of the lack of public support for bolder plans, Al Gore's and George W. Bush's proposals are minuscule in comparison to their predecessors. The latter's proposals are, according to one expert, "simply dwarfed by his father's plan."

Moreover, even though Gore's plan is much more modest than Clinton's, his opponent still gains politically by likening it to "Hillary-Care." Discussion on health care has moved to prescription drug coverage for seniors. Robert Blendon of Harvard comments in *The New York Times*, "The elderly are a powerful vote. And not only do seniors vote more, but their ability to organize, to hold forums, has garnered their cause a great deal more attention than the uninsured." The American Association of Retired Persons monkey is at present the strongest. The "special claim" of the poor which Dougherty upholds does not seem to have much hold on the public imagination at all. The good news is that the candidates have plans. The bad news is that the plans are feeble and the pilot is knocked out cold.

There are places in his article that Dougherty seems to acknowledge this state of affairs. He discusses at some length how rationing is in fact going on at present: "So health care is rationed *de facto* in the United States on the basis of ability to pay in the open market." Those who cannot pay, do not get covered. Even at the time he is writing, Dougherty indicates that "we've seen much" of a situation where "those who cannot contribute to the bottom line are the least desirable to be covered and the ones first avoided by any kind of marketing approach or any kind of implied or explicit programs inside the network." In such a market context, health care provision is so "fragmented" that "it would be hard to think about how (rationing) might be done practically."

The question that arises, then, is that of why, in the face of this evidence, does Dougherty press ahead with guidelines for a federal policy? One reason may be opportunity. "This is an opening in our political history which comes rarely." The Clinton plan, while "dead" might resurrect in "the debate." Perhaps the vested interests – for instance, the insurance companies – can be caught off balance. A second and related reason is that it seems that Dougherty thinks that there still is an American consensus concerning "one nation under God" and that the disinterested debate – that is, rational exchange with concern for more than oneself – necessary to arrive at this other-regarding consensus is still, under present circumstances, possible and even likely.   One of his eight criteria states that "rationing has to result from an open participatory system . . .. An open participatory system will put limits on all of us and we should discuss together how we shall set these limits." The emphasis on participation echoes *Economic Justice for All*, which states, "Basic justice demands the establishment of minimum levels of participation in the life of the human community for all persons." Dougherty cites Oregon – with its town hall meetings on health care – as a case where such participation has taken place.   Such settings allow people to discern their agreement on basic value orientations – to agree, in other words, all to fly to the same airport and not join the monkeys up front.   The rights-driven predisposition towards the state allows Dougherty to read 1994 as a rare opportunity (despite the acknowledgment that the Clinton plan is "dead") and the Oregon case as replicable nation-wide such that efforts to install a federal policy remedy for health care appears to be worth the primary focus and energy of the Catholic community.

This is a good point at which to make some clarifying points so that my argument is not misread. First of all, I do not think that Dougherty's case for the Catholic community's primary focus and energy to be on federal policy is unreasonable, that is, that more or less cogent reasons cannot be given for it. On the contrary, it is precisely the *fit* between his read of Catholic social teaching, the present situation, and his prescription that I find problematic. Dougherty's argument is cogent, but wrong in a way where that very cogency reinforces mistakes in reading all three Catholic social teaching, the present situation, and the proper prescription for Catholic focus and energy.   Second, I think that he is right in indicating that to discern whether a consensus of an unselfish kind exists or not will require, among other things, public forums for exchange and debate. Third, I do think that a national plan of health care is needed. Where I disagree is on the point that Americans at present would settle on priorities and a plan that would reflect the same unselfishness that Dougherty's principles and criteria do once the specific implications of those principles and criteria for self-sacrifice were made clear.

If I am right, then the place to focus Catholic energy in moving towards making a national plan is less on broad public discussion than on the formation of a Catholic community that exemplifies what it would mean to undertake the sacrifices necessary to make Dougherty's plan plausible. If there is to be a move towards the kind of plan Dougherty wants, then people have to know not only what the sacrifices will be, but that they will not be alone in making them. Thus the priority of exemplifying the sacrifices on the part of those communities – including and especially the Catholic community – calling for them. In *Evangelii Nuntiandi*, Paul VI insists on the priority of what he calls "silent proclamation" and "wordless witness." His point is that moving towards publicly articulated proclamation is doomed to failure without a community that, granting sinfulness and finitude, already is embodying those words. And the popes are clear that putting forward principles and criteria of Catholic social teaching on health care or any other social problem is a form of proclamation. John Paul II writes in *Centesimus Annus* that "to teach and to spread her social doctrine pertains to the church's evangelizing mission and is an essential part of the Christian message." The concept of the common good, unlike that of rights, not only is better able to disclose the degree to which the America is fragmented, but also illuminates equally the full range of social organizations and institutions and so does not focus on the state at the expense of churches and other intermediate associations as starting points for addressing – and perhaps as obstacles to solving – the national health care problem. It is with these associations that silent proclamation – the precondition for successful articulated public proclamation – begins.

With these clarifications in mind then, let me fill out what I think the implications are of starting with the concept of the common good. Again, the first implication is that the concept of the common good can disclose the degree to which American society is fragmented, or to the degree that there is a consensus, it is one built around selfishness. The first question arises is that of "Which is it, fragmentation or a consensus of selfishness?" My answer here is "Both." An American consensus that selfishness best contributes to one's own flourishing (and perhaps that of others) leads people to pursue primarily and even exclusively those things associated with their own good. Because persons' individual goods, narrowly construed, diverge, and there is little or no sense of an other-regarding good, there is fragmentation. For a sixty-eight year old, spending the budget surplus on covering prescription drug costs for seniors is good; for two minimum wage working parents of an uninsured family, there are other priorities.

Much liberal political theory acknowledges and even affirms and celebrates the fact that people pursue primarily and even exclusively their own good, and tries in response to regulate that selfishness. I think that other traditions – namely the classical republican emphasis on citizenship and the Calvinist stress on the body of Christ – promoted social cohesion in early American history. Yet the geographical and social stability that is the primary condition for sustaining and fostering what I have called "traditions of communal commitment" has not been manifest. Unfettered economic and political liberalism – which identifies rights to adjudicate our interactions – thrives in a society marked by a mobility which turns us into strangers to each other. On this account, liberalism is not a villain tradition; the read is simply that in the absence of traditions with different tendencies, its strengths have become excesses. Also, in this view Americans are not uniquely selfish; rather unqualified economic and political liberalism is the more or less unique form that their selfishness takes. But rights language, as Mary Ann Glendon has pointed out, has become overextended, and Catholic contributions to conversation on health care not only misread the Catholic social tradition when they begin with rights, but also, however unintentionally, further this over extension.

The prescription offered in light of the common good would begin, as indicated, by not focusing on one type or level of institution or association at the expense of others. It does not move, without further explanation, directly to the state and the state alone. The principle regulating institutional interaction and prioritization in Catholic social teaching is that of subsidiarity. The key insight of subsidiarity is that those persons and associations most proximate to a situation are those best able to respond. This is because they can read best the nuances of the situation. They, therefore, have the first responsibility to respond. For instance, the primary responsibility for caring for and educating children rests with parents. However, subsidiarity is not a recipe for a form of libertarianism, as some Catholic neo-conservative writers seem to imply. The Latin root *subsidere* means "to support," and larger and more remote institutions – whether political, economic, or cultural – are to "support" the more proximate associations in the effort to address the situation at hand. The public school system, whatever its failings, is designed to aid parents in the education of their children. *In extremis* situations where the more proximate associations fail allow for direct intervention by more remote institutions – for instance, the state in the case of foster care when the parents fail. However, care needs to taken that the direct intervention be as short in duration as possible so as not to lead to the atrophy of the more proximate associations. Foster care, when it works well, helps the parents get well and returns the children to their parents when the latter are again capable of parenting.

The concept of the common good illuminates the full range of institutions and associations regulated by the principle of subsidiarity. Two points follow. First, it is clear by now that what Catholic social teaching puts forward is not an in-principled anti-state posture such as that found in the work of Stanley Hauerwas, author of *Against the Nations*, and, in its Catholic version, in the work of my colleague Michael Baxter. The state has a positive subsidiary and sometimes direct role to play in response to social problems. Second, however, where, when, and how the state, and particularly the federal government, is to be involved requires careful prior assessment of the capacities of the full range of social institutions and associations. By beginning with the language of rights, Dougherty, in violation of the principle of subsidiarity, bypasses this process of discernment and moves directly to the role of the federal government. People may have town meetings, but they are town meetings about how the state ought to regulate health care.

And what is my read of the situation? It is much like that of some social conservatives after the Monica Lewinsky affair. Prior to that, such conservatives held, like Dougherty does in his article, that the majority of Americans agreed with their views on what America should look like, if only certain interests – economic interests for Dougherty and left-of-center interests for the conservatives – were restrained or removed. The Lewinsky affair – and the simultaneous rise in Clinton's popularity – made clear to the social conservatives that most Americans do not think at all like them. The primary task then, should not be to enter the political arena of public suasion – which relies on the listeners having some basis for empathy – but to focus on other levels and spheres of society to build communities of empathy. These social conservatives were, and to some extent still are, involved in national politics, but now the primary energy for many of them is not on that level. Rather it is on other forms of association.

I think that American response to health care in 1994 – and certainly after then – warrants a response by the Catholic community that parallels these social conservatives. Catholic position papers on federal policy are not out of the question, but the prior issue is whether Catholic communities themselves – from the parish to the Archdiocese – are undertaking the kinds of practices that can make it possible for Catholic health care facilities to live in accord with the kinds of principles Dougherty sets out. What kind of practices do I have in mind? They can be summarized by the works of mercy carried out on a daily basis. I would add tithing and material as well as spiritual simplicity.

Two objections might be raised. First, it might be countered that Catholic health care facilities must cooperate – and thus compromise – in order to survive. Second, it might be added that the sociological data indicate that Catholics in the United States are becoming more and more like other Americans in their beliefs and practices. To expect them to radically alter, for instance, patterns of consumption, is to expect too much.

My answer to these objections is that they may well be correct. If that is the case, then the game is lost. My only point is that this – with the more proximate communities – is where it must begin. Without such communities of belief and practice, no appeals at the level of national political debate will take hold. In *Evangelii Nuntiandi*, Paul VI writes that the church itself must be "evangelized by constant conversion and renewal, in order to evangelize the world with credibility." Silent proclamation is "the initial act of evangelization." He goes on, "We are being asked: Do you really believe what you are proclaiming? Do you live what you believe? . . . The witness of life has become more than ever an essential condition for real effectiveness in preaching. Precisely because of this we are, to a certain extent, responsible for the progress of the Gospel that we proclaim." Amen.

REFORMING HEALTH CARE ETHICS

Jorge L.A. Garcia

(My thinking on these topics was influenced by my participation in the seminars, conferences, and lectures of the Kennedy Institute of Ethics at Georgetown University, my involvement in the annual alumni conferences on Ethical Issues in Medical Practice at Notre Dame, and by my year as both Visiting Fellow in Harvard Medical School's Division of Medical Ethics and Fellow in Ethics in Harvard's university-wide Program in Ethics and the Professions. The views expressed are my own. I am grateful to Laura Garcia for discussion, suggestions, and comments.)

I am very honored by this invitation. I did not know Dr. Clarke very well but it was a pleasure to work with him in starting up these conferences some years ago. I did come to know Dr. Pellegrino at the Kennedy Institute rather better. Dr. Pellegrino was the first lecturer in this series and there is really no one in medical ethics, and perhaps no one I've met in any context, whom I admire more than him. My predecessors, most of whom are here today, are mainly physicians and theologians – people who examine bodies or ponder God. However, since my training is in philosophy – a field that has no real subject matter – this presentation may be a little different. I will take that professional liberation from responsibility really to know what I am talking about as license to wander over many topics

– current events, recent history, Black Studies, multiculturalism, and religion. If some of what I say on controversial matters nettles you or strikes you as outrageous, at least I may have brought you to agree with me about one of my theses – that people generally, and especially those in your profession of health care, would do better if, for a while, they took somewhat less guidance from people in mine.

I.   INTRODUCTION

The principal social point of medical ethics must be to help us achieve a more ethical medicine, one more fully informed by the moral virtues. Once, we expected doctors to cultivate the requisite virtues in interns and to pass on traditions of behavior and habits of sentiment. Recently, however, this sort of moral education, while perduring, has been eclipsed. A new, academic model of medical ethics – as an interdisciplinary field of study led largely by philosophers, lawyers, and physician/humanists – has developed. We are unlikely to achieve a more ethical medicine without the cooperation of these new "ethicists," as they like to be called, for the culture now looks to them for guidance on the direction, aims, and procedures of medicine. My view is that we need to reform health care and that, to do that, we need, first, some radical reform in medical ethics.

Several recent events, such as Dr. Foster's nomination to be surgeon general, have made reforming the medical profession an urgent matter. The last few decades have seen an aggressive push to legitimize death-directed medicine – especially abortion, euthanasia, and assisted suicide. I am not here interested in the political question of whether Dr. Foster should be confirmed or whether his serving would be best for the country. What is of concern is what is the face of American medicine when the nation's most prominent physician – the people's doctor – sits on the Board of Directors of the leading provider of medicalized death, when that organization lists him as a member of its group – Physicians for Choice – organized to oppose "any legislation restricting abortion," when he stands accused by even a sympathetic feminist of performing "hysterectomies on retarded women for sterilization and hygiene," and when he is the principal investigator in national clinical trials of a self-administered, home-use suppository that, as a Nashville newspaper quoted him as saying, was designed "to eliminate abortions as we know them in this country by providing a non-invasive pregnancy termination procedure."

Now again, I am not interested here in the political question. I am not trying to make a judgment, one way or the other, on the larger question of whether his service would be good for this country. What I do want to direct your attention to is whether it is a good thing for medicine – what will medicine be like in years to come? Dr. Foster's nomination is just a starting point for that inquiry. Notice that phrase, "eliminating abortions as we know them." What about just eliminating them or severely curtailing them? Dr. Foster is said to abhor abortion. Mrs. Clinton thinks them wrong, even if not something to be criminalized. The President wants them to be rare. Yet today there are powerful forces at work to make abortion, already one of the most common medical procedures, even easier and more frequent. The Accreditation Council for Graduate Medical Education (ACGMA) just voted – unanimously – that "prospective obstetricians . . . include abortion training in their programs," and that their hospitals must provide abortion and sterilization training or arrange that they receive it elsewhere. The *New York Times* editorially responded to this (possibly illegal) coercion only to praise Planned Parenthood for its willingness to supply this training and to complain that the city's hospitals will find it difficult to provide it until they get on the ball and start terminating pregnancies more routinely.

One writer finds it unexceptional when physicians "consider . . . [abortions] . . . an ordinary and integral part of the [obstetrician's] job," and she condemns "the stigmatization of doctors who do abortions." (*New York Times* editorial, "The Hospitals Abdicate on Abortions," February 27, 1995, p. A14. In a letter of February 9,1995, the general counsel to the NCCB noted that the 1993 Religious Freedom Restoration Act, as well as laws in half the states, exempt conscientiously-opposed hospitals "from referring for abortion, artificial contraception, or sterilization," and reminded that

Council that some states provide for damages "against any person that discriminates against a hospital for exercising its right to refuse to participate in or refer for these procedures.") A member of the medical student group that pressed for more training is forthright about their aims: "We're trying to destigmatize abortion." (Ellen Willis, "Foster's Taint," *Village Voice*, February 21, 1995, p. 8. The medical student is quoted in Susan Gilbert, "Clinic Violence Sets off Push for Wider Abortion Training." *New York Times*, January 11, 1995, p. C11.) Stigma or de-stigmatization? Even for people who try to combine a "pro-choice" public policy on abortion with private moral opposition, however, it makes no sense to try to de-stigmatize what they think immoral. You cannot think something wrong and abhorrent without thinking it warrants the stigmas of immorality: shame, guilt, remorse, and so on. How do we make abortions rare if we make them easier to get, and are reluctant even to distance our most prestigious medical positions from those who ply this grisly trade? How will the face of American medicine look to a poor, Black mother when *soi-disant* conservatives succeed in cutting off AFDC childbirth assistance to mothers on welfare, while so-called liberals succeed in retaining state funding for the poor to get abortion on demand? A *Village Voice* writer correctly calls the current controversies a war over "the role of medicine in U.S. society." (James Ridgeway, "Doctor No," *Village Voice*, February 21, 1995 p. 19.) Courts, legislatures, citizen initiatives, and insurers push medicine towards the new model of the death-dealer rather than the healer, but the ACGMA action, like the AMA's recent rush to defend the nomination of a putative abortionist to be U.S. Surgeon General, show that the corruption of our medicine is not driven entirely by external factors.

It is easy for someone in my position to say to you physicians that you need to reform your profession. What about mine? What have the "ethicists" to say about the dangers of medicine's further degradation? Nothing much, and, surely, little to reassure us. When the prestigious "ethicist" Peter Singer says, "Philosophers are back on the job," we should stand warned. (*New York Times Magazine*, July

7, 1977 .) Hegel wrote, "Philosophy paints its grey on grey" only when "a shape of life" has reached maturity; "the Owl of Minerva spreads its wings only with the falling of the dusk." (G.W.F..Hegel, *Hegel's Philosophy of Right* (1821), translated by T.M. Knox (New York: Oxford University Press, 1952), preface, p.13.) By this he meant that intellectuals come on the scene late, to rationalize practices and structures that other social forces have already put in place. Nowhere is this more evident than in medical ethics, where for the past two decades "ethicists" have done little but argue that this or that principle or value can be reconceived so as to counsel retreat from medicine's traditional self-restraint and justify each new advance in our medicine's decline. A press report indicates that a list of the prominent and well-placed ethicists proposed for the revived National Bioethics Advisory Commission is filled with partisans of assisted suicide, fetal and embryo research, abortion, and passive euthanasia of the comatose and the brain-damaged. (Mary Meehan, "New Bioethics Panel: the Usual Suspects," *National Catholic Register*, February 5, 1995, pp. 1, 7.) Today, one of the chief obstacles to your profession's undertaking the reform that it needs is the willingness of mine to serve as house chaplains, giving the blessings of reason to awful deeds performed in health care institutions increasingly tied to centers of higher education.

II.   THE DECLINE IN THE NEW MEDICAL ETHICS

How did we come to this pass? I am no historian, but let me hazard a few speculations. College campuses these days buzz with talk of diversity: multiculturalism, pluralism, critiques of "Eurocentricity," and so on. I think the diversity movement teaches important truths about our need to listen to voices long suppressed or ignored. What is interesting for our purposes is that medical ethics has actually gone from being more diverse to less. Indeed, in its first appearance, the revitalization of medical ethics in the Sixties could almost serve as a model of civil and responsible pluralism. Back then, priests and rabbis, along with some ministers – people familiar with long traditions of theologically informed reflection on the mission and practice of medicine and its proper role in human life – were first out of the gate in addressing new controversies, especially those about "pulling the plug," as it came to be known. This was almost a paradigm of the theorist Alasdair MacIntyre's vision of thinkers, each steeped in a particular tradition, bringing the fruits of its reflection to bear on new matters, encountering new intellectual difficulties internal to it, and cautiously venturing to extend it by offering innovations for testing and critique. (I am careful to say 'his' here, because this first generation of medical "ethicists" was almost entirely male, a fact that came back to haunt and undo them. (For MacIntyre's views, see *Three Rival Versions of Moral Inquiry* (Notre Dame: University of Notre Dame Press, 1987).) Those were the days when Paul Ramsey tried to integrate elements from Catholic moral theology into Protestant ethics and, on the other side, Joseph Fletcher assimilated the Scripture's "law of love" to a "situation ethics" that even he ultimately saw as a version of the secular philosophers' utilitarianism. (See Ramsey, *The Patient as Person*; and in *Ambiguity in Moral Choice*; Fletcher, *Situation Ethics*; and "Situation Ethics," in *Encyclopedia of Bioethics*, ed. Warren Reich, (New York: Macmillan, 1973). Hoose maintains that today's revisionist proportionalist Catholic moral theology had its origins in Fletcher's situation ethics. (See Bernard Hoose, *Proportionalism* (Washington: Georgetown University Press, 1987.) Utilitarianism has for two centuries been a secular philosophy. However, its origins seem to lie in the efforts of Protestant thinkers to develop a theoretical understanding of Scriptural moral teaching to replace the medieval moral philosophies of natural law and Aristotelian virtues, which they saw as corrupted by excessive faith in reason.)

This was not a golden age, but it was in some ways a better epoch in medical ethics. Today, we see little comparable diversity. The most prominent and influential thinkers, especially the most promising ones in early middle age, are not ministers, priests, or rabbis, but primarily secular philosophers and lawyers. Moreover, there is little deep difference among them on the controversial issues. Some want to move a little faster, some a little slower; some are considered "principalists," some fancy themselves "casuists," some are Rawlsians, some feminists, and some are utilitarians. What they largely share, however, is a commitment to the same general direction of medical change. A direction that, of course, I deplore.

So far, I have urged that things were not always as they now are in medical ethics. Let me briefly speculate about some of the factors that may have brought us to the present situation. Some of you may be able to illuminate me on these matters and to correct my mistakes.

First, the appointment of national and presidential commissions on human experimentation, care at the end of life, and other matters created a demand for thinkers of a certain type, thereby establishing a new model. It accomplished these things by exerting pressure on participants, who had been selected in part to serve as representatives of different traditions of bioethical inquiry, to identify and reason from intellectual common ground, and ultimately to reach consensus. Stressing in this way what is common to differing religious traditions need not be a bad thing. It can sometimes even serve to remind those in each tradition what is most central within her own approach, as when Roman Catholics converse with Eastern Orthodox or with Episcopalians. However, as the range of conversants increases to include the resolutely secular, the need to identify and to reason from common intellectual ground holds the danger of focusing the religious thinker on what is peripheral to her own tradition, and treating that as the basis of what she says and, ultimately, of what she thinks. Whether or not one believes that any of the religious "ethicists" who served had their thinking affected, i.e. distorted, in the way I described, these commissions established a new model of ethical thinker and created a market demand for people conforming to that model. The ad might have read like the following:

> HELP WANTED: Highly educated ethical thinkers, who stay within the common intellectual methods of our academic elites, who find it easy to reach consensus with secular intellectuals and with similar thinkers of other

faiths, whose views nicely fit into position papers and final reports written in the secular voice of the federal government, and who will help to sell the commission's consensus to their co-religionists.

Whereas the first group of medical "ethicists" were largely people who operated primarily from and within certain religious contexts, demand arose for "ethicists" who, even if religious, had few religious rough edges.

Second, this was the age of ecumenism. Vatican II nudged Catholics into it, helped by the widespread theological dissent over artificial contraception, and the resultant unclarity over what might count as meaningfully Catholic moral thinking. Moreover, the interdisciplinary and public character of the new disputes in medical ethics exerted similar pressure toward common ground and consensus independent of the pressure from the government commissions.

Third, controversies over important and slow-moving legal cases (from *Quinlan* through *Cruzan* and beyond) contributed to secularization and homogenization. The "ethicists" were understandably and honorably motivated by the desire to contribute to the legal reasoning in these cases, and even to influence their disposition. However, expert testimony, legal briefs, and media commentary are more effective when sharp religious differences – the rough edges – are elided. More important, as the cases moved through the various levels of courts in various states, it became important to have experts who had mastered this new legal literature rather than old religious texts. (Even for masters of both, there were advantages to reducing religion to a credential, and speaking primarily within the legal paradigm.) So lawyers flowed into bioethics, and they proved more congenial than the religious first wave – more relevant, easier for courts to understand, more skilled in making legal predictions and identifying legal issues, better at building a compromise or a consensus within a panel and less constrained in defending it outside.

Fourth, the Sixties saw mounting criticism within philosophy of the arguments and assumptions that had restricted respectable moral philosophers to the study of moral language. This teamed with social and peer pressure within the universities to contribute to the wrenching national arguments over warfare, pornography, civil disobedience, and other social issues. In 1971, the publication of John Rawls's book, *A Theory of Justice*, and the first volume of the Princeton journal, "Philosophy and Public Affairs," secured this new movement that soon flooded medical ethics with thinkers who were trained in the analytical methods of Anglophone philosophy. These thinkers, typically free from religious commitments and attuned to the values and movements of the times, were often clever at finding and defending previously unnoticed or ignored possibilities, and adept at finding problems, inconsistencies, and puzzles in the reasoning of the lawyers, the courts, and religious writers. (My impression, based on an outsider's observations at Notre Dame in the early and mid-Eighties, earlier as a graduate student at Yale, and later at Georgetown, is that the leading graduate programs in religious studies and in theology stressed breadth of knowledge (of different denominations, traditions, epochs, cultures, languages, literatures, and disciplines), while the leading philosophy programs were content to let their students by with little or no knowledge of foreign languages, of different cultures, or of even the history of their own discipline, so long as they mastered acute skills in dissecting others' arguments and in framing their own, and clarity of exposition and defense.) These skills well served these new "ethicists" in staffing the new medical ethics establishment, which consisted in a network of research institutes, centers, programs, offices, and divisions in practical and applied ethics (most university-affiliated, but some free-standing) that inherited the mantle of the federal panel.

Fifth, the academic model of the new medical ethics took its toll. Even the religious writer who submitted her paper to a mainstream bioethics periodical was held to contemporary scholarly standards. That meant that it would not do for her merely to repeat objections raised within her religious tradition to some element of the new medical agenda. She had to be an original, creative researcher. Predictably, even those who wrote from within religious traditions were encouraged to be different, offbeat, *un*traditional. Some came to blend old with new in the easiest way – by devising novel rationales for the new agenda by reinterpreting the materials from within their religious traditions.

Sixth, various social forces, and perhaps some economic ones as well, combined to restrict how the researchers could make their work attractively novel. Defenders of traditional medical restraint were open to accusations of insensitivity to women, and to the rights and needs of the dying, and of protecting the subordination of the patient's will to the physician's habits. In addition, certain foundations, which supported medical initiatives that advanced their own agenda of social programs, such as widespread contraception for population control, gave money to the new centers. Several medical ethics institutions have received crucial financial support from groups whose members or sponsors have a financial interest in abortion "services" and fertility techniques. (Meehan, "Who's Watching the Watchdog?" *National Catholic Register* February 5, 1995, p. 7. She quotes Arthur Caplan as faulting medical "ethicists" for insufficient concern over these conflicts of interest. In 1991, a fertility professional society funded and established a "national" reproductive ethics advisory panel, with promises of independence but housed in the society headquarters and evidently intended to give ethical scrutiny (and approval?) to new technologies from which the funding society's members could profit.)

III.   WHERE WE STAND

I have speculated about some forces behind the homogenizing and secularizing trends that have brought American medical ethics to its current, degraded state. Mainstream medical "ethicists" scarcely notice the gutter in which they swim. Indeed, during my year at Harvard's professional ethics program I, several times, heard the burgeoning numbers of applied ethics centers, journals, conferences, newsletters, and professional societies cited as evidence of our culture's ethical growth. Surely, there was no heed paid to the possibility that the two phenomena are inversely related, as I think they are. After I left, I wrote to the lawyer who became acting-director of the program that one of my most disappointing failures that year at Harvard was the failure of,:

> [M]y effort to get people [the other Harvard fellows] to entertain whether, in the current state of professional ethics discourse, we need much more often to have recourse to *moral* criticism of our positions. To remind a colleague that this or that proposal would be monstrous not only to adopt but even to suggest is simply "not done" in the current climate; to do so would be to violate the rules of a kind of *politesse* . . . Elsewhere in the . . . [academy] . . . we hear calls for a new sensitivity to the marginalized and the voiceless. It is a sad and revealing irony that it is in the campus *ethics* programs . . . that we still hear some people derided as "vegetables," others classed as "marginal humans," the needs of some dismissed as parts of lives "not worth living" (and, by implication, not worth saving), and [even] suggestions made that we should vivisect [some people, specifically, those in a persistent "vegetative" state.]

The above is from my letter to Martha Minow, dated September 27, 1993. I think that both the content and the rules of discourse in professional ethics merit more reflection and attention than they have heretofore received. The degradation pervades this field, and professional ethicists need to be reflective *about*, and not just reflect, the cultural elements in which they operate. At one ethics center I know, one presentation defended the claim that we should prefer to perform mutilating and even lethal medical experiments on those brain-damaged people the speaker considered "marginal cases" of humanity rather than on healthy higher animals. This bothered some in the audience, but the center's governing board showed no support for a proposal, not even that the center censure that past speaker, but merely that it warn prospective speakers against using similarly degrading language and that it make provision for some occasion for moral rebuke of those who voiced comparably vicious and dehumanizing opinions in the future. Maybe the proposals went too far. My point is simply to illustrate the moral rot, usually voiced with the expectation of impunity, that pervades the discourse of bioethics.

And the list goes on. Prominent thinkers of the last few decades have advocated active and passive euthanasia, performing mutilating and even lethal experimentation on disabled people (including children) in preference to healthy animals, and compulsory organ "donations" for transplants, even killing helpless and unconscious patients to "harvest" their organs. For starters see Dan Brock, in *Hastings Center Report*; Peter Singer, *Practical Ethics*, 2nd edition, Cambridge: Cambridge University Press; Peter Singer, *Rethinking Life and Death*, New York: St. Martin Press, 1995; John Harris, "The Survival Lottery," *Philosophy*, 50 (1975): 81-87; James Rachels, *The End of Life*, New York: Oxford University Press, 1986; Richard B.Brandt, "The Morality and Rationality of Suicide," *A Handbook for the Study of SUICIDE*, ed. Seymour Perlin, New York: Oxford University Press, 1975, pp. 61-76; Michael Tooley, *Abortion and Infanticide*, Oxford: Clarendon Press, 1983.

IV.   REFORM IN MEDICAL ETHICS – LEARNING FROM MINORITY PERSPECTIVES

I do not counsel despair; there are hopeful signs. Some feminist scholars have begun to see that assisted suicide disproportionately victimizes women, who are socialized to see their lives as worthless when they can no longer provide services to others; and there is growing awareness of ways in which abortion and even contraception can also degrade women. (See Celia Wolf-Devine, "Abortion and the Feminine Voice," *Public Affairs Quarterly*, 3 (1989): 81-97; reprinted by and University Faculty for Life in *Life and Learning III*, edited by Joseph Koterski, pp. 45-71.) Some advocates for the disabled have decried the devaluation of their lives implicit in some arguments for infanticide and euthanasia, and in Germany they have organized protests (sometimes, unfortunately, excessive ones) against the peddlers of mercy-killing. Predictably, in the United States, this protest against euthanasia and its advocates is derided as an "Anti-bioethics movement," as if there nothing to bioethics but rationalizing medical homicide. (See Singer's self-pitying account in "On Being Silenced in Germany," *New York Review of Books*, August 15, 1991; reprinted in *Practical Ethics*, end edition pp. 337-59.) Given the current degraded state of the field in the Anglophone nations, and its almost uniform support for medical homicide, of course, these writers have a point. However, we should not concede that the study of medical ethics must be anything like what we have here today. That is to accept despair, and to close off the prospects for the kind of reform I here advocate. Most promising, we hear calls for a wider and more diverse range of voices to be heard in medical ethics, calls to view these issues from perspectives other than those of the liberal individualist paradigm of the white males who dominate the field. Robert Veatch has even called for replacement of the old medicine and its attendant medical ethics with 'postmodern' medicine and medical ethics. (Veatch, "Postmodern Medicine and the Decline of Modern Medical Ethics," a paper presented at the Kennedy Institute of Ethics in 1990.) What he has in mind is that deceptively uncontroversial notions such as 'medical necessity' should no longer be used to mask deep moral differences about who should be saved and at what cost, about whether an abortion is appropriate, and so on. In Veatch's vision, people of different faiths, commitments, and lifestyles will consult different "ethicists" and patronize different physicians, "ethicists" who share those commitments, and physicians who sympathize with them. Then, patients will not feel pressured – let alone, be coerced – to remain on life-support they deem worthless, to have abortions they find repugnant, or to undergo transfusions they think sinful. This "postmodernist" vision is not entirely acceptable, of course, but I think it offers opportunity for a break in the hegemony.

Elsewhere, I have sketched some suggestions for one way of understanding one type of ethical perspective, specifically, an African-American one. (J. Garcia, "African-American Perspectives, Cultural Relativism, and Normative Issues," pp. 11-66, in Harley Flack and Edmund Pellegrino, eds., *African-American Perspectives on Biomedical Ethics*, (Washington: Georgetown University Press, 1992). In addition to this work, some other sources on African-Americans and health care include: Annette Dula and Sara Goering, eds., *It Just Ain't Fair:' the Ethics of Health Care for African Americans*, (Westport, CT: Praeger, 1994); and Marian Secundy with Lois LaC. Nixon, eds., *Trials, Tribulations, and Celebrations*, (Yarmouth: Intercultural Press, 1992). Also see W. Michael Byrd and Linda A. Clayton, "An American Health Dilemma: A History of Blacks in the Health System," *Journal of the National Medical Association*, v. 84: 189-200.) On the model of perspective I offered there: (1) ethnic perspectives are individual, not shared; (2) they consist primarily in having one's ethical thought affected by certain types of experience and behavior (especially, types characteristic of those assigned to the same ethnic group) not in holding specific substantive views; (3) the ethical perspective's content need not be unique to those assigned to the ethnic group; (4) such a perspective need involve no special modes of inference, no special ways of conceptualizing things, etc.; (5) an ethnic ethical perspective is not one common to all assigned to that group. Rather, there are many ethical perspectives people assigned to any given ethnic minority group will take, and these will be influenced in different ways, not all of them desirable, by different political ideologies, religions, personal experiences, sensitivities, and commitments.

What can those in medicine and medical ethics learn from listening to these new voices? They might first learn how life, health, and medicine look to the neglected. According to one researcher's statistics, the death rate for African-Americans aged 25 to 44 was 250% that of Whites. Blacks accounted for 54.6% of AIDS deaths in children between 1984 and 1991. One third of Black Americans are hypertensive, compared to one fifth of Whites. University of

Michigan epidemiologist Sherman James has defended what he calls the "John Henryism" hypothesis.   According to James, the combination of what he calls an 'active coping strategy' and low socioeconomic status in an individual was found to predict high hypertension. (Sherman James, "'John Henryism' and the Health of African-Americans." Lecture at the Harvard Medical School. March, 1993.) To offer just one example, in a study conducted in 1990-1991 at UCLA, Hispanics were found to have been denied pain medication disproportionately in emergency rooms: 55% of Hispanics with extreme fractures received no analgesics, compared with 26% of non-Hispanic Whites. The researcher concluded that "Hispanic ethnicity was the strongest predictor of no analgesic." (Knox H. Todd, Nigel Samaroo, and Jerome R. Hoffman, "Ethnicity as a Risk Factor for Inadequate Emergency Department Analgesia," *Journal of the American Medical Association*, v. 269 (March 24/31, 1993): 1537-1539.) They might also learn how things look from the lower institutional rungs. If I may interject a personal note, one of my brothers and both my parents were hospital service-workers, the latter two in the non-profit neighborhood hospital that owned the tenement where we lived. My earliest picture of the hospital, from what I heard over the dinner table, was of an inefficient bureaucracy where supervisors scrambled to spend unused funds, lest the excess be lost in the next budget, and where the parking lot that was just paved last month would be torn up this month for new construction. More tellingly, my first knowledge of the hospital was as unjust and union busting employer, bad neighbor, and absentee slum landlord.

    Not all people assigned to a certain ethnic minority group have the same experiences and, in any case, people react to their experiences in different ways. Permit me to suggest, however, that one whose thought has been significantly shaped by serious reflection on minority experiences should, as a result, find herself better sensitized in certain ways. Among them are the following.

    (1) Someone who adopts or reflects upon such a perspective should be sensitized to the inequities of efficiency and maximization. Robert Veatch has argued that a priority principle of the sort

utilitarians favor, one assigning such scarce resources as donated organs to those likely to derive greatest medical benefit from them, will sometimes work in a predictable way to the disadvantage of black people, even in the absence of racist discrimination. There are several reasons. Those who are economically disadvantaged or who are acculturated into dysfunctional behavior patterns may be in worse health by the time transplantation is considered, because they may not be in the habit of frequent medical check-ups and healthful life-styles. Moreover, because of distrust of or unfamiliarity with medical institutions, they may be unlikely to serve as donors, thus making donor-recipient matches less common. There can be further difficulties as well. When, in general, a black person is harder to assign to a tissue type than is a white one, then she is less likely to be identified as a good match, that is, less likely to be designated as one in whom the transplanted organ will probably thrive. Veatch emphasizes that his point is not restricted to racial minorities in the following:

> So, attending to issues of ethnicity should make us more careful not to allow the magnitude of the good we can do to be decisive in social situations where we know that some may stand to gain less from our help precisely because of unjust past treatment or its results such as poor diets and insufficient exercise, for example.

(2) Members of long subjugated groups know all too well that respected, educated people can and do treat those they deem "unworthy" or "marginal" with contemptuous dismissal. Reflecting on their experiences ought to sensitize "ethicists" to treat even the marginalized and despised with the respect owed any human being. Maybe, then, the day of reform will dawn and "ethicists" will begin to clean up their acts, their mouths, and their minds, repudiating talk of the "veterinary aspect" of neonatology, of people who are not "persons" because they are too young, retarded, or mentally inactive, of "replaceable people," and so on. (These examples are from

medical ethics literature, or from my recollection of medical ethics group discussions at Harvard or Georgetown.)

(3) Someone who takes such a perspective seriously should find herself disinclined to situationism. African-Americans have much to fear from health-care decisions that flow from some individual's or group's seat-of-the-pants judgment. Some physicians complain about meddling from institutional or state bureaucrats, and these physicians would prefer to have their own goodwill and expert judgment trusted. However, the medical decision-maker is likely to share little of her black or Latina patient's personal experiences, social or economic stratum, interests, tastes, or educational level. That patient, to put the matter bluntly, is at the medical decision-maker's mercy, and the patient is entitled to the protection afforded by announced and codified procedures, policies that have had to be defended in open fora, before varied interest groups, and on grounds that even the inexpert can share. This can literally be a matter of life and death when physicians become empowered to advise and assist in the termination not only of a patient's treatment but of her life itself, as legislation in the Pacific Northwest proposes. When a patient, already poor and sick, also has had her sense of self-worth eroded by experience as the object of racist attitudes and practices, she needs to be assured that her life is important, and that others value her, in spite of the burdens that caring for her may impose on them. Instead, it is now expected that medical personnel should present themselves to this desperate, needy soul and offer their services to help speed her down the path that illness has already marked for her.

V.   REFORM IN HEALTH CARE ETHICS: LEARNING FROM RELIGIOUS PERSPECTIVES

A bioethics worthy of the name – one that honored the moral virtues in its commitment to life – would stand forthrightly against the dehumanizing and, sometimes, homicidal new medical agenda and the "ethicists" who serve it. That is, an ethical medical ethics would take up the cause of the despairing against those whose idea of mercy is to "assist" them in suicide, of the unwanted against those eager to dispatch them before birth, of the severely brain-damaged against those who can see in them non-persons fit only for experimentation or an organ-harvest, of panicked poor women against those who offer them only the cruel "choice" between reduced public assistance and subsidized abortions. Unfortunately, we can expect the opposite. The academy's most celebrated "ethicists" are sure to weigh in on the other side, brushing off the lives and needs of the least fortunate and the voiceless with condescending rhetoric about people whose lives are of insufficient "quality," with rigged and insulting criteria of "personhood," with an assortment of specious "principles," with hubris-driven fantasies of "autonomy" and "self-creation," and the rest of the intellectual apparatus that those privileged in health and education employ as they vindicate our neglect and victimization of the worst-off. I think the best hope for a renewed bioethics lies in using the opening afforded by the current demand for diversity to reintroduce a variety of religious viewpoints into the debate. Let me offer some suggestions on this needed resurgence, concentrating on Catholic medical ethics.

Notice, first, that the lessons I suggested we should learn from reflecting on the experience of the oppressed are familiar in Christian thought. The follower of Christ is called to love everyone as neighbors, not just the majority or those most easily or efficiently aided. Christians already know the absurdity of thinking that love cannot be expressed in rules (the loving God lovingly gave us His Commandments), and they should know that human dignity resides in each person: the brain-damaged and the despairing are no less human than the lowly carpenter's son and no less human than the mightiest prince.

There is, we know, controversy over just what counts as authentic Catholic ethical thinking. Which theologians really speak the truth that God has entrusted to the Church? What I want to do here is side step the issue. We can partially obviate the practical problem of which theologian to rely upon by concentrating on teachings from the bishops themselves, here and abroad, and those authorized to speak in their name. I shall take that course here.

Catholics understand the role of medicine on the model of love. John Paul II writes:

> The parable of the Good Samaritan . . . indicates what the relationship of each of us must be toward our suffering neighbor . . . Everyone who stops beside the suffering of another person, whatever form it may take, is a good Samaritan. His stopping does not mean curiosity, but availability . . . Man cannot fully find himself except through a sincere gift of himself. A good Samaritan is the person capable of exactly such a gift of self . . .. How much there is of the good Samaritan in the profession of the doctor, or the nurse, or others similar! Considering its "evangelical" content, we are inclined to think here of a vocation rather than simply a profession. (John Paul II, "On the Christian Meaning of Human Suffering," (1984), para. 28, 29.)

Medicine is a profession of love. Love is a concern for someone's welfare, and in health care, the specific aspect of that welfare at which the professional as such aims is the maintenance of health. The 1994 *Catechism* teaches that "Life and health are precious gifts entrusted to us by God." (*Catechism of the Catholic Church* (1994), para. 2288. (Hereafter, CCC.)) The 1994 "Directives" of the American bishops begin, movingly, by tying the health care profession and, with it, modern miracles of medical technology to Christ's own miraculous healings and love of the afflicted. (NCCB, "Ethical and Religious Directives for Catholic Health Care Services," *Origins*, v. 24, # 7 (December 15, 1994), part one, pp. 450-451.) Life consists in a certain degree of health, that is, of proper functioning. Death is a state approaching the limit of the loss of organic function.

Since medicine by its nature aims at the patient's health, it can never properly aim at her death for any reason. That would simply be antithetical to the mission of medicine. For the physician to aim at death would be unprofessional and unethical for the same reasons that abandoning a patient would be, but in an even more grievous way. "Even if death is thought imminent, the ordinary care owed to a sick person cannot be legitimately interrupted," the bishops write. However, "The use of pain-killers to alleviate the sufferings of the dying, even at the risk of shortening their days, can be in conformity with human dignity if death is not willed as either an end or a means. . . . Palliative care is a special form of disinterested charity. As such, it should be encouraged." (CCC, para. 2279.) This teaching is eminently sensible. The pursuit of health normally takes precedence. Pain is a bad thing chiefly because it distances the patient from the peace of mind that is part of mental health. Insofar as greater pain leads to greater distance, it is worse. (Bernard Gert once complained to me that my view that pain is bad only as the absence of mental peace absurdly commits me to the view that increasing the pain of someone already in such pain as to have no peace is unobjectionable because it makes the sufferer no worse off. This does not follow. The badness of pain need not be a function of how much it probablizes the sufferer's loss of peace. If it were, then, of course, Gert would be right, because the added pain leaves the sufferer who already has no prospect of peace no less likely to achieve peace. However, the added pain may leave her *more distant* from peace in that she has further to go , i.e. more pain to lose, before she can attain peace of mind.) Palliation is not of itself as important as restoration of health and prevention of illness, but it may sometimes be more urgent. Since dying can only be a diminution in health, it is grotesque to suggest the health care professional ever pursue it, even as a means. However, when little or nothing can be done to restore health, then the physician can legitimately pursue lesser goals, such as the alleviation of pain. In extreme cases, she can even pursue these other goals in such fashion that, without her meaning them to, they diminish health and even lead to death. She can justifiably withdraw treatment to end the discomfort or harm, even financial harm, a treatment causes the patient, independently of its success. However, she cannot licitly withdraw treatment simply to spare the patient the harms she suffers because the treatment succeeds in keeping her alive and the patient's medical ailment continues to harm her. Of course, this teaching is intricate, and it can be hard on us. However, it cannot be plausibly denied.

VI.   IS BIOGRAPHY WHAT MATTERS?

Why is intending to cause or allow death always a grave evil, an evil whose pursuit cannot be licit except in light of some ill-desert? The answer, I think, lies in the fact that, as organisms, it is part of our mission, our *telos*, to be alive. Indeed, it would be absurd to speak of the functioning (the health) of a dead organism. Our supernatural destiny lies beyond this life. But it does not follow that biological life, without what some "ethicists" call biographical life, is worthless or pointless. (Rachels, *End of Life.*) That is elitist thought. It treats life as valuable only to the extent it is filled with the sort of incident that makes someone's biography a good read. However, the life-story of most of us might not make such exciting reading. Our consolation is that this failing is not important, because the value and importance of a person's life does not derive from what interests someone who might read about it. (Ronald Dworkin criticizes the elitism of what he calls the "impact" view of the importance of a person's life in "Foundations of Liberal Equality," *Tanner Lectures on Human Values* XI (Salt Lake City: University of Utah, 1990.) His own preferred model, however, which stresses the extent to which one succeeds in living according to one's values, is still elitist in the way it favors the healthy and rational. In some unpublished papers, Thomas Loughran has persuasively argued that a truly equalitarian conception of the value must proceed from what we all share, our common humanity.) This emphasis on biographical life is also dualistic, in that it treats the body's life as nothing in the absence of mental processes. However, we are not minds temporarily trapped in bodies. Again, as John Paul II has written, "In fact, body and soul are inseparable: in the person . . . they stand or fall together." (John Paul II, *Veritatis Splendor* (1993), para. 48, 50. Hereafter: VS.) We are ensouled bodies – bodies brought to life, normally even to mental life. The life of the ensouled body which is a human being, a human life, is a matter of awe and wonder, and something precious. Indeed, believers should remember that we are in no position to look down on the life of someone severely brain-damaged or permanently comatose. After all, we are quite likely to be putting our time and energies to infinitely worse use than is she, as we go about our usual sinful ways while she passes her time giving passive glory to God. The life of a human body is the life of a human being, whether or not there is superadded to it the conscious life of the mind. Of course, the life *in* a human body need not be the life of a human being. It might be merely the life of surviving cells. In some unpublished work, Linda Emanuel suggests that death is a continuum, we gradually die as more and more cells lose life without being replaced, and we asymptotically approach total extinction of all vitality. I think this approach incorrect. The life of a human being is the life of the system *qua* system, not the total life *in* the organism's body considered merely as an territorial expanse. There is always reason to preserve it, even if not always reason to save it at all costs.

A reformed health care ethics, then, should reject the perverse view that medical care is fruitless when all it does is keep the human body alive and partially functioning. That is not everything we could hope for, but it is a great service, and one to be discontinued only for very strong reason. To think one needs some further justification for life-support other than that it sustains life, even if only biological life, is, I think, deeply wrong.

We also need to guard against the temptation to optimize the results of our use of resources. When care sustains life, it is therein beneficial. Sometimes, in triage situations, we may want to conserve resources by withholding or withdrawing them from patients who will benefit less and giving them to those who will profit more. This need not always be immoral, but as Veatch reminded us, it can be unfair. Even when it is not, we should remember that it will always be permissible to give, instead, to those who stand to benefit less, rather than to those who will benefit more. We should not automatically think it better to try to save or restore the conscious rather than the comatose, nor the normal, or exceptional, rather than the retarded. It is good Christian behavior to help the worse off, even when that act is not the most helpful. We should be moved by need and the urge to help someone needy, not to effect some maximally efficient utilization of resources. We should take care not to compound the injuries nature inflicts by insisting that our policies favor the more fortunate and abandoning those who can gain only life itself.

At one time, proponents of euthanasia based their claim on the evil of pain. This argument fails intellectually, I argued, whatever its popularity. It fails because the relief of pain is always of secondary medical importance to health, and the physician as such should never deliberately destroy health to eliminate pain. Of course, patients are not physicians – at least, they are not *qua* patients – and they may legitimately have other priorities which the physician may not properly override by imposing unwanted treatment. More recently, pain-management has become easier to achieve, and, moreover, effective employment of its techniques would probably do something to temper popular support for euthanasia. There need be no moral objection to this. Lately, however, enthusiasts for euthanasia have based their defense less on the desirability of sparing the patient unnecessary pain, and more on the moral importance of respecting the patient's dignity and autonomy by deferring to her wishes about life and death. I will offer a few observations about dignity and autonomy.

VII.   BEYOND THE NEW *FREEDOM* AND *DIGNITY*

Contemporary medical ethics makes a fetish of both autonomy and dignity. To offer just one example, a German intellectual protests what she, incredibly, sees as Western culture's recent exaltation of the fetus, and proudly takes "a stand that I would also wish for my friends: to ruefully smile at this phantom [i.e. the fetus]. Then one can speak an unconditional NO to life, recovering one's own autonomous aliveness." (Barbara Duden, *Disembodying Women: Perspectives on Pregnancy and the Unborn*, Trans. Lee Hoinackip (Cambridge: Harvard University Press, 1993, p. 110.) A reviewer offers a mordant comment on this remarkable conclusion to Duden's book: "The only way to be alive is to say no to life. A more succinct summary of what C. S. Lewis calls the philosophy of hell can hardly be imagined." (Laura Garcia, "Review of 'Disembodying Women,'" *New Oxford Review* (1995).) Consider the legal scholar Ronald Dworkin's influential book on euthanasia and abortion. Dworkin correctly sees human dignity as linked to freedom. (Ronald Dworkin, *Life's Dominion* (New York: Knopf, 1993), esp. chap. 8) He writes, "A true appreciation for human dignity argues decisively . . . for individual freedom. Because we cherish dignity, we insist on freedom." He willingly follows this freedom straight to homicide. Premise One: "The value of autonomy . . . derives from the capacity . . . to express one's own character – values, commitments, convictions, and . . . interests – in the life one leads." Premise Two: "Decisions about life and death are the most important, the most crucial for forming and expressing personality, that anyone makes . . ." (Dworkin, pp. 224, 236, 239.) So the conclusion: decisions to die and even to kill willing victims – suicide, assisted suicide, voluntary euthanasia – must be legally permitted and even constitutionally protected.

As arguments go, this one leaves something to be desired. Notice the crucial switch from the first premise's tying autonomy to the morally rich notion of *character* to the second premise's talk of death-decisions as expressing not character but *personality*, which is morally empty. This is crucial because the form of Dworkin's argument is to claim that the moral importance of human dignity transfers to individual character, because of their supposedly close ties, and that personality transfers it onto death-decisions, because of the tie between the latter two. Plainly, this argument requires that character be identical with personality or closely connected with it.

This is implausible, since we attribute many traits to personality, grumpy, giggly, persnickety, etc., that we neither ascribe to character nor consider of moral weight. Note, too, the difficulty of explaining why we respect autonomy in letting people kill themselves, or have others kill them, when such decisions end all their decision-making. Recall that it was out of this sort of concern that John Locke, even in his enthusiasm for liberty, stopped short of endorsing the freedom to enslave oneself.

All this kind of thinking stands in stark contrast to Catholic thinking. *Gaudium et Spes* says, "Genuine freedom is an outstanding manifestation of the divine image in humans. For God willed to leave them in the hands of their own counsel, so that they would seek their creator of their own accord . . . Their human dignity therefore requires them to act through conscious and free choice . . . They achieve such dignity when they, . . . in a free choice of good, pursue their own end by effectively and assiduously marshalling the appropriate means." (Vatican II, "Pastoral Constitution on the Church in the World of Today," para.17, in *Decrees of the Ecumenical Councils*, vol. II, translated by Norman P. Tanner, S.J. (Washington: Sheed & Ward and Georgetown University Press, 1990), p. 1078.)

What is most striking in Dworkin's writing is his absolutization of freedom. John Paul II warns against this. In 1993, in *Veritatis splendor*, the Holy Father condemns, "Certain currents of modern thought [which] have gone so far as to exalt freedom to such an extent that it becomes an absolute, so that it becomes a source of values." (VS, para. 32.) In contrast, he identifies the genuine moral autonomy of humans with participated theonomy (theonomy = "law from God") because our "free obedience to God's law effectively implies that human reason and human will participate in God's wisdom and providence." (VS, para. 42.)

This is appealing. Autonomy is "law from the self" and this is a disturbing idea, conjuring images of someone behaving as a law unto herself. Kant, the Enlightenment thinker who exalted the term and gave it currency, was able to allay some of these concerns by insisting that autonomy is consistently dutiful; that it is an exercise of pure practical reason; that it therefore is no mere expression of subjective desires, interests or personality; that it works the same in all people; and that, ultimately, it issues in those objective principles he called laws – the moral law. For Dworkin, and several others who fancy themselves neo-Kantians, autonomy is none of these things. Autonomy is all a matter of what the subject happens to commit herself to, of what interests her or serves her interests, of her own ideas about things.

Kant's autonomy, if it were something real, would clearly merit moral deference; the problem is that it is probably illusory. Neo-Kantians' autonomy, in contrast, is something real, but it is hard to see why we should take it so seriously. The Pope is suggesting that human autonomy is something real, respectable, and also, something unfrightening, for it is a matter of making God's law into the rule by which one governs one's life. Autonomy, as participated theonomy internalizes what originates externally; it is not making the moral law, but making the moral law one's own rule of conduct. So understood, autonomy ties us to God, to our own nature as God's freely-choosing creatures, and to all creation governed by the same eternal law that genuine autonomy internalizes. Human freedom and God's law meet and are called to intersect in a human person's "free obedience to God."

The capacity for such reasoned, freely-chosen obedience is not a part of human nature. Human nature is in every human being, but not all have such a capacity. However, it is part of our nature to develop such capacity unless blocked by internal or external obstacles. That is why we think there is something the matter with a human who never becomes capable of rationality and freedom. She is disabled, while we do not think there is something the matter with a wolf or cat no more capable. The human lacks the capacity because her internal developmental principle, her nature, is blocked; not so the lower animal. This natural inclination to develop a capacity for rational and freely-chosen obedience really grounds the dignity – indeed, is the glory – of humanity. "Human freedom . . . is an essential part of that creaturely image which is the basis of the dignity of the human person." (VS, para. 86.)

Freedom matters, not as an end and not as an absolute value, but as a component in our highest earthly accomplishment: the free choice of actions fulfilling our real roles and missions in life. "Hence obedience to God is not, as some would believe, a heteronomy [= "law from another"] as if the moral life were subject to the will of something all-powerful, absolute, extraneous to man, and intolerant of his freedom . . . [O]nly through this obedience does it [human freedom] abide in the truth and conform to human dignity. (VS, para.41, 42.) This is not freedom from obedience, but for it. This freedom liberates the human person to be what she is and liberates her from any reduction to a mere creation of local culture, habits, and conventions: "Human nature . . . is itself the measure of culture." Moreover, I should say that, even when some inborn malady or later misadventure blocks human nature in some individual from flowering into rationality and freedom, this natural orientation itself still grounds the human dignity that self-proclaimed neo-Kantians distort and cannot explain. This participation in God's law-making is "the condition ensuring that man does not become the prisoner of any of his cultures, but asserts his personal dignity by living in accordance with the profound truth of his being." (VS, para. 53.) Autonomy does its job when it confronts the person with, and enables her to realize, those truths about our creatureliness which the Pope calls splendid. This understanding of autonomy, unlike Dworkin's, comports well with the traditional view that our proper freedom over how to live does not extend to questions of whether to live or how long to live. Only when human dignity is rooted, as I have suggested here, in our innate tendency towards freedom is it a truly human dignity – a dignity that extends to all people. To deny that dignity to those held back by some physical or mental shortcomings is to privilege the lucky and to compound the woes of the afflicted.

People talk of assisted suicide as sparing the patient the supposed indignities of dependence, invasive treatment, or living by others' choices. However, there is no greater indignity than being dispatched because people agree that your life is worthless or feel they cannot fault your reasoning in reaching that conclusion.

VIII.   REPRODUCTIVE AND ANTI-REPRODUCTIVE MEDICINE

Modern medical ethics needs its thinking about death and disability informed by the kind of corrective that Catholic teaching can provide. I make no claim here that only Catholics can provide the needed corrective. Modern medical ethics needs that corrective at least as much in those areas where health care professionals are implicated in how others conduct their sex lives. This implication holds the danger of formal cooperation, when the health care professional immorally "intends the object of the wrongdoer's activity," or material cooperation, when she unintentionally assists. (See Appendix to 1993 NCCB Directives.) I will not get into substantive matters about the extent to which one may permissibly get drawn into sexual or reproductive practices that Catholic teaching regards as sinful: sterilization, *in vitro* fertilization, artificial contraception, and so on. Let me, however, offer a few caveats about the way in which people think about these matters.

Many of these, notice, are not properly medical matters at all. Medicine is centrally concerned with the maintenance of health, especially of organic functioning, and several of these procedures are not meant to correct improper functioning, nor are they ways of bypassing some dysfunction to protect other functions. For the most part, they involve not restoring a patient's health, but the morally shadier business of giving someone what she happens to want. These days, when Catholics talk of sex, they almost immediately get into discussions of authority, conscience, and dissent. This is odd since, in principle, questions of sexual ethics involve conscience and authority no more, and no less, than do matters of justice or pride or truthfulness. Still, we must take the world as it is, so I will go along, offering some remarks on authority that may strike some as simplistic and countering some ideas on conscience that strike me as simplistic, and suggesting that dissent, except in its most radical forms, matters much less than some people suppose. My education is not theological, I should point out, and my remarks here are not meant as theological scholarship. Rather, I wish to reflect philosophically on these three concepts, drawing distinctions, unpacking them, and tracing out some implications.

Let us treat authority first. The root idea behind an appeal to authority is that of authorship. To accept something on authority is to accept it because of who says it. There are two main types. (My discussion here derives from my "Moral Reasoning and the Catholic Church," *New Oxford Review* (1992) 59: 13-17.) When you have directive authority, then we can say that your commanding me to do something gives me a certain sort of reason, though not necessarily a conclusive reason, to do it. Note that when someone exercises authority, the reason she gives us to act or believe must be a reason *of a certain sort.* The armed mugger exercises power over me when she warns me to hand over my wallet, but not authority, though she obviously gives me reason to comply. When you have assertoric authority, then we can say that your asserting something to me gives me a certain sort of reason, not always a conclusive reason, to believe it. The Church does claim some directive authority, but it is assertoric authority that she exercises when she speaks on moral topics. We can speak of "obedience" here only in a broad sense: heeding Church moral teaching is not following orders, but it is acting *ob-audire* – from hearing. If the Church teaches morals authoritatively, then, like any assertoric authority, she must be in a privileged position to know. Indeed, Paul VI, when he spoke at the United Nations, called her an "expert in humanity." (VS, para. 3.) What privileges the Magisterium's teaching is that the Holy Spirit guides her, leading her in a certain direction, toward a certain destination. This suggests that the Holy Spirit's influence will be more evident in the conclusion of a piece of moral reasoning, than it is in the reasoning itself. The point of that guidance is to keep the substance of the Church's teaching free from error, not to keep its thinking cogent. Providing rational defense for what the Spirit guides the Church to teach is not a part of her magisterial mission, even as it was not a part of Christ's.

To accept the Church's assertoric authority to teach in morals is to accept that one has some reason to believe that teaching, independently of the persuasiveness of any arguments the Vatican chooses to offer, and independently of any arguments one reads elsewhere or devises by oneself. For the Church to have authority is, *ceteris paribus*, for us not to need arguments to accept what she says. Of course, often things are not equal. There are sometimes good arguments against what she teaches. Still, if authority means anything, it means that if the arguments for and against a doctrine are equally cogent, then one ought to believe the doctrine. Some will find this claim simplistic, but to deny it is simply to deny authority altogether; if it cannot even break ties, it must count for nothing. The hard question is when doctrine should be believed, even though opposing arguments are stronger than those in its favor. How much should authority count for? I will say only that this is the question of who is more likely to be right: (a) one's own limited knowledge and fallible reasoning, subject as it is to prejudices, self-delusion, and temptations to see oneself in the best light, or (b) the teaching office of the Church, where fallible humans act, but under the guidance of the Holy Spirit?

That is perhaps simplistic, but I doubt that the further complications that completeness requires really change the central point. In any case, let us move on now from authority to conscience. We are often told that, in the end, one must follow one's conscience. There is an important truth behind this, but it is simplistic for several reasons. (A) Conscience needs to be adequately informed. Following one's conscience contrary to Church teaching when that conscience is ill-informed by study of the doctrine is a moral violation, not a duty. (B) In addition to being informed, conscience also needs to be adequately formed, in the sense that the psychological mechanisms by which we come to hold beliefs should be operating properly. (For a discussion of this, see Alvin Plantinga, *Warrant and Proper Function* (Oxford: Oxford University Press, 1993).) They sometimes may be disposed to malfunction, after all, and, more important, even be morally corrupt. All Christians believe in sins against the virtue of faith. (My discussion in this section is heavily indebted to Robert Adams, *The Virtue of Faith* (Oxford: Oxford University Press, 1986), chap. 1.) What is important is that, even when a Catholic with a well-educated conscience finds herself simply unable to bring herself to believe what the Church teaches, she still may not be blameless in this. It may be her own fault that she resists. Her unbelief may be owing to her stubbornness, prejudice, or pride. It may result from her making an exception for herself, or allowing herself to be swayed by passions. She needs not only to educate her conscience, but also to cultivate habits of mental openness and docility. One who refuses adequately to open herself to be taught, will not learn. Her disbelief, however, is not innocent. Of course, assent to what the Church teaches may also be badly motivated or infected with vices. That only reinforces my point that following conscience need not exculpate. (C) In short: when someone cannot get herself to believe what the Church teaches, she should keep trying. She ought never to give up on herself, but always work on, recognizing that the Magisterium can mislead, but also that she is more likely to be wrong. During that time when she cannot bring herself to assent, she is, by definition, in dissent. What then? Here the theologian Fr. Raymond Gula is helpful. Gula usefully distinguishes three types of dissent: internal, private (i.e. shared with a few advisors), and public dissent. Within public dissent, he distinguishes individual from organized and, within organized public dissent, scholarly from popular. Popular organized public dissent strives "to influence public opinion . . . [which in the extreme] promotes its own judgments as an alternative pastoral norm." Fr. Gula thinks this goes too far. (Raymond Gula, *Reason Informed By Faith*, (New York: Paulist Press, 1989) p. 212.) John Paul II agrees: "Dissent, in the form of carefully orchestrated protests and polemics carried on in the media, is opposed to ecclesial communion and to a correct understanding of the hierarchical constitution of the People of God." (VS para. 113.) Few health care people would be tempted to that sort of event. It is more likely that they might be tempted to open and contemptuous disregard of some Magisterial teaching.   This would be a mistake for many reasons, some of which I treat below.

This leads us to dissent. Fr. Curran, sensibly, distinguishes core teaching from peripheral and, more problematically, uses this distinction to downplay the importance of dissent on such peripheral issues as details of sexual morality. (Charles Curran, *Faithful Dissent* (Kansas City: Sheed & Ward, 1986).) I will return briefly below to the question of whether these issues should really be relegated to the periphery in such a way that one can reject them without disturbing anything central. Here, I want to suggest that Curran's distinction is one-dimensional. When someone dissents from Magisterial teaching, even if only on a peripheral doctrine, it must nonetheless matter how she dissents. How far is her thinking removed from what the Church teaches on the subject? How much of that teaching does she reject? Permit me to elaborate a bit.

I think dissent is of little practical importance except in quite extreme forms. Notice, first, that dissent is merely lack of agreement. I dissent from what you say provided that I remain unconvinced that it is true, even if I am also unconvinced that it is false. Obviously, that someone is unconvinced by, say, Magisterial teaching on contraception gives her no reason to act differently from the way the Church teaches. So this sort of mild dissent raises no crisis of conscience and one in such a predicament need not at all act out of conformity with that teaching. Notice, second, that dissent is by its nature a passive and internal matter.   It is intrinsically passive because my dissent is simply the state I find myself in when I cannot get myself to agree. This is not an action of mine at all. It is intrinsically private because, as the etymology implies, my dissent is a matter of how I feel or how I think about some matter. In this, the central sense of the term, one can no more publicly dissent than one can publicly think or feel something. Real dissent from Magisterial teaching, because intrinsically private and internal, is thus never in direct conflict with maintaining public silence about, and even actively cooperating with and supporting, that teaching. Because of this crucial difference, there can be no easy argument from the unquestioned legitimacy of this central, and minimal kind of dissent to the legitimacy of the very different matter of actively disregarding Magisterial teaching, let alone, publicly expressing one's dissent in protests.

Now recall that Magisterial teaching on sexual matters can reasonably be characterized as quite stringent. Intentionally employing artificial contraception in anticipation of sexual activity, engaging in homosexual, or otherwise unnatural intercourse, having oneself temporarily or permanently sterilized, and participating in extracorporeal conception, for example, are all taught to be sinful mortally, intrinsically, and without exception. Because the teachings are so stringent, dissent can take many forms.

These reflections should caution us against one danger in the conduct of our professional lives in relation to sexual matters: sexual exceptionalism. By this, I mean the rather too comfortable view that one can properly accept all or most of the rest of Church teaching and just make all that sex stuff an exception. The British Catholic journalist Clifford Longley is said to have written: "I share none of the Roman Catholic Church's attitudes on contraception, divorce, abortion, and religious education of my children." (Quoted in Piers Paul Read, "Wine and Kisses," *Crisis*, March, 1995, p. 32, quoting from *Why I am Still a Catholic*.) Many of us sometimes feel tempted in this direction, but I think that this increasingly is becoming an untenable position. Some say the Church unreasonably fears sex. Surely, there are many church people who have. Most of us my age or even older can remember brothers, nuns, or priests who fretted over Elvis's hips or centerfold pin-ups or women in stretch pants. Much of this was silly, but it is not clear, to me at least, that very much of it has infected Magisterial moral doctrine. More important, even those of us who reject the cultural reactionaries' insistence that entertainment and the arts generally echo the Christian call for sexual moderation, and who welcome some ways in which the last few decades have eroticized the social environment, should recognize the Church's emphasis on restraint as a helpful corrective and as an aid in negotiating our way through the new milieu without succumbing irretrievably to its temptations.   Plainly, going to the opposite extreme by treating sex as just harmless fun has brought widespread devastation and misery, not least among some of the economically worst off.

In any case, sexual exceptionalism is becoming untenable because Vatican teaching, and especially John Paul II's own writings and addresses, continue to develop a religious anthropology of some depth which weaves a certain understanding of human self-giving and sexuality into its fabric. (See, for example, *Donum vitae*, *Veritatis splendor*, CCC, and the "Wednesday Sermons" collected in *The Original Unity of Man and Woman*, and subsequent volumes.) Whatever the validity, in principle, of Curran's distinction between core and peripheral doctrines, it becomes less suited to his purpose of legitimizing dissent on certain sexual matters as the sexual teachings are integrated into a comprehensive vision of human life and love that cannot plausibly be relegated to the margins of faith. Another danger is scandal. Part Six of the NCCB's 1994 Directives address this topic better than anything I can say. The danger is all around, as Christians occupy institutional roles or get drawn into partnerships with others. The temptations may become great to do things that compromise, especially with those sexual matters the world considers it flaky to object to: permanent sterilization, temporary sterilization (i.e. artificial contraception), prophylactics for sodomy, artificial insemination, and so on. Let me remind you only that we Catholic professionals, like it or not, represent the Church to others. Like Charles Barkley, we are taken as models, whether or not we want to be, and whether or not it is fair to us. Given that fact, we should take care lest it be said of us, as a reviewer wrote about a prominent Catholic writer recently, that our "Catholicism is lightly . . . worn."

> Sheed's account of his illness is underlaid by two conditions that shaped his nature. One is his Catholicism, and lest the secular reader be put off by this, it has to be said that Sheed's Catholicism is lightly and gracefully worn, skeptical, anti-pietist, and nowhere offered as

inspiration. It's not even affirmed exactly . . . (Robert
Stone, "Looking the Worst in the Eye: review of Wilfrid
Sheed's 'In Love with Daylight,'" *New York Review of
Books*. April 6, 1995, p. 4.)

However such a comment is meant, it is no compliment. It is, in fact,
an accusation of a nonchalance, an insouciance, about sacred things
that we must see as sin – maybe acedia, maybe even something
worse. Even if sexual morality is peripheral, surely the more
important metaphor needs to explain not how close it is to the core
doctrines, but how tightly it is tied to them. If humanity's imaging of
God consists especially in our gift of self in loving communion, and
if marriage is one of the highest arenas of self-giving, and if the
marriage act falls fatally short of this self-gift when the partners
distance themselves from one another whenever they contracept or
engage in sodomitic behavior or procreate asexually, then rejecting
Catholic teachings on sexual morality, no matter how far it is
removed to the periphery from the core doctrines, may seriously
distort a person's understanding of herself and her life in Christ.

IX.   CONCLUSION

All this goes very much against the spirit of the times. That
is to be expected. Christ himself pictured our modern times in
striking terms:

> The days are coming when they will say, "Happy are the
> sterile, the wombs that never bore and the breasts that never
> nursed." Then they will begin to say to the mountains,
> "Fall on us" and to the hills, "Cover us." If they do these
> in the green wood, what will happen in the dry? (Luke
> 23:29-31.)

Today, we cherish our sterility and work feverishly at it, lavishing
millions on chemicals and devices to render our sex acts barren.
Surgical sterilization is now the leading form of contraception. As

the Scripture predicts, our flight from life does not stop there. We are far beyond calling to deaf nature to bring us death. We invent new technologies for the purpose and even pervert the arts and sciences of healing to the service of *thanatos*. Right now the "ethicists" applaud all of this, fussing only over whether the mercy killers have done their paperwork, getting their consent forms duly completed. Even here, we do not succeed. Recent research indicates that physicians frequently terminate life-sustaining care on their own initiative and judgment. "In a recent survey of 879 doctors in adult intensive care units throughout the country, Dr. David Asch . . . found that 14 percent said they had withheld or withdrawn treatment that they considered futile without informing the patient's family. More than 80 percent had withdrawn care over the objections of the family members. Indeed Dr. Asch added, most of the time doctors call the shots. 'When you get patients to agree, there's so much subtle and not so subtle coercion . . . Patients are sold something.' We all know doctors who are good at 'quote' getting the DNR order." (Gina Kolata, "Withholding Care from Patients: Boston Case Asks, Who Decides?" *New York Times*, April 3, 1995, pp. A1, B8.)

The "ethicists," I am sure, will not long lag in justifying this abandonment too, though it is often driven by concern over expense. I heard one "ethicist" at a Harvard conference a few years back, fearful lest those contemplating abortion be exposed to facts about what the procedure does to the fetus, proclaim her discovery of a right *not* to be informed about certain medical procedures. Nor should we expect that any such red tape on which the more fastidious proponents of the new agenda insist will long hold the center. If we do all this in the "green wood" of prosperity, what will those paltry restraints avail us in the "dryer" age sure to come?

For Catholic institutions and professionals to stand as signs of contradiction to our age's homicidal and sexual viciousness is neither an easy nor a welcome calling. But it is ours. The health care professionals themselves may need to lead by the example of their lives. Perhaps the "ethicists" will learn and will eventually follow. I heard a priest remind his audience that someone who marries the spirit of the age will wind up a widower (or widow) in the next. I think this has two readings. On the first, it is a warning against tying oneself too closely to intellectual and lifestyle fashions, for it is their nature to change and we may soon find ourselves out of step. This is sage advice. Still, the second reading is deeper. We all live two ages. We live twice, because when this life is over there is still a life, an age, to come. If we marry the spirit of this earthly life, we may find ourselves in the next life not merely out of fashion. Anyone who weds this life will soon be bereft, and in the life to come the loneliness will be deep. Our faith is that those who spurn the worldly temptress and remain faithful to the Church's bridegroom will find bliss beyond imagining.

R e s p o n s e   t o
REFORMING HEALTH
CARE ETHICS

Joseph M. Incandela

In remarks both wide-ranging and provocative, Professor Jorge Garcia reestablishes himself as one of the most articulate contemporary defenders of the sanctity of life. That such even needs defending these days is already to lend credence to his diagnosis of our cultural and philosophical maladies. True enough, as he (and Hegel) point out: "the Owl of Minerva spreads its wings only with the falling of the dusk." But that leaves undetermined whether those who write in the wake of the rustling feathers are mere harbingers of a coming darkness or heralds of a new dawn.

Prof. Garcia surely intends and hopes for the latter, but there is much in his Clarke Lecture that gives ample cause for alarm, with a great bit of it directed against members of the very philosophical and ethical academic guilds that Garcia himself inhabits. Philosophy itself, says he, is "a field that has no real subject matter"; and academic medical ethics, now made up of a loose, interdisciplinary amalgam of "philosophers, lawyers, and physician/humanists," seems populated by those who have a subject matter but no real fields. These new "ethicists" (always enclosed in irony-laden quotation marks in the text of his lecture) promote "moral rot" which has left mainstream medical ethics in such "a degraded state" that its practitioners "scarcely notice the gutter in which they swim."

Compounding the problem of people inside the academy saying all manner of strange and injurious things is that people *outside* the academy are actually listening to them. Academic ethics has in the last thirty years moved from a kind of parasitic relationship on the medical profession (which largely used to deliver moral education in a company store housed within the profession and passed on by its practitioners) to a much more mutually destructive symbiotic one such that, today, "to reform health care ... we need, first, some radical reform in medical ethics." Garcia speaks of the willingness of those in his own profession "to serve as house chaplains, giving blessings of reason to awful deeds performed in health care institutions" and thereby legitimizing what he calls "death-directed medicine" as it pertains to physician assisted suicide, embryo research, abortion, and passive euthanasia of the comatose and brain damaged. All of which leaves this particular Clarke lecturer in a very precarious rhetorical stance: to unmask the dangers and ethical cul-de-sacs of the discipline out of which he speaks while also convincing an audience that the clear and rigorous thinking he most prizes about that discipline can point to a way out of these various cultural dead-ends. This is not unlike the challenges attendant on persuading the mistakenly captured animal that – to use C.S. Lewis's words – "moving the paw farther back into the trap is the way to get it out." (C.S. Lewis, "On Obstinacy in Belief," in Louis P. Pojman, ed., *Philosophy of Religion: An Anthology* (Belmont, CA: Wadsworth, 1987), p. 376.)

In the section of his lecture entitled "The Decline of the New Medical Ethics," Garcia cogently and insightfully describes six "homogenizing and secularizing trends" that have led us to the current deplorable state of American medical ethics. (Add to these homogenizing trends the impact of mass media, hospital mergers, and the proliferation of Ethics Committees and Institutional Review Boards.) In the remainder of my own comments, I'd like first to reflect – largely *with* him – about the consequences of such homogenization and secularization. Then from my perspective as a theologian, I'd like to try to challenge him a bit about how these themes play themselves out in the closing sections of his lecture where he unfolds the Catholic "corrective" in thinking about death and disability.

I.   DIVERSITY AND UNIVERSAL VALUES

Almost thirty-five years ago in Bampton Lectures later published as *The Religious Significance of Atheism,* Alasdair MacIntyre described an unpleasant dilemma which captured much of the drama and despair of twentieth century theology: *either* theology could attempt to "acclimatize itself" in an era dominated by empirical science and its cognate values of evidence and rationality (think Bultmann's demythologization and Tillich's ground of being); *or* it could refuse to do so (think Kierkegaard and Barth).   The consequence of the former course was to give modern culture less and less with which to disagree, thereby losing theology's distinctive voice or *raison d'être* and, in some cases, making it virtually indistinguishable from atheism. The consequence of the latter was to insure theology's own segregation from secular intellectual disciplines. In short, theology becomes either redundant or irrelevant to the host culture, "a realm apart, a discipline which legislates for itself and which disowns the current badges of intellectual legitimation . . .." (MacIntyre, *Religious Significance of Atheism* (New York: Columbia University Press, 1969), p. 11.)

This story along with these choices is not unlike the one Prof. Garcia tells about the fate of medical ethics in the United States and may be useful in contextualizing his narrative. Though he's careful not to label it a golden age, Garcia tells of a time in the fairly recent past when theologians like Paul Ramsey and Joseph Fletcher contributed to a public conversation with little attempt to hide their religious 'rough edges.'   This was a pluralism that respected differences and drew from their riches. What has replaced this diversity in Garcia's eyes is a moral Esperanto that only a bureaucracy could love, as the new ethicists found their energies engaged in drafting position papers in the secular idiom of governmental study commissions, testifying or filing briefs in landmark legal cases concerning the right to die, or establishing centers for applied ethics which trained the next generation of scholars to do the same things. (I borrow the apt phrase "moral Esperanto" from Prof. Jeffrey Stout, *Ethics After Babel: The*

Languages of Morals and Their Discontents (Boston: Beacon Press, 1988), pp. 72 & 74.) Medical ethics, then, on this telling of the story, has suffered the same fate as portions of contemporary theology in MacIntyre's account: differences have been elided in the attempt to 'fit in.' As a result, medical ethics has gone from "being more diverse to less" such that "there is little deep difference among [the most prominent and influential thinkers] on the controversial issues. Some want to move a little faster, some a little slower.... What they largely share, however, is a commitment to the same general direction of medical change."

Such a lack of diversity is certainly an arguable claim, but as a broad statement of a general trend, it is not easily or obviously falsifiable. The criteria for membership in the group of new medical ethicists is not specific enough to allow adequate assessment of Garcia's claim. Nor, outside of Peter Singer and Ronald Dworkin, are any of these people actually named. Certainly, though, it is the case that many who attend the annual Notre Dame conferences in medical ethics (including many other Clarke lecturers) have participated in the most suspect of secularizing and homogenizing conversations while managing to come out morally unscathed. But let us, for the sake of argument, accept Garcia's claim that there is a group of secular, influential thinkers who have largely taken over the field of medical ethics and imposed on it a kind of uniformity that puts at risks several categories of patients who had been heretofore protected from threat of death or untoward intervention on their lives. What follows?

One, more meta-ethical way to respond is with an utter dearth of surprise that a secularized morality lacks the ability to place any reliable firewall against legitimizing all manner of dreadful things in which some human beings are used or dispatched for the (perhaps even *sizable)* benefit of other human beings. (See William L. Craig, "The Indispensability of Theological Meta-ethical Foundations for Morality" available online at <http://home.apu.edu/~CTRF/ papers/ 1996_papers/craig.html>) This is not unlike the response of John Paul II in *The Gospel of Life.* When transcendent values and a transcendent value-er are removed, then all that's left is what the pope calls "pure materiality" which in turn breeds "individualism, utilitarianism, and hedonism." (All of the quotations from the pope in this paragraph come from John Paul II *The Gospel of Life* (New York: Random House, 1995), §23.) It promotes individualism because, "The only goal which counts is the pursuit of one's own material well-being." It produces utilitarianism and hedonism because others can no longer be valued for who they *are,* but for what they can do or produce. In this light, Prof. Peter Singer's views may be objectionable, but they are certainly not surprising. Singer renders personhood functionally – one is a person to the extent that one can do certain things. That's why, for Singer, killing a disabled infant (which is often "not wrong at all") is not killing a person. (Peter Singer, *Practical Ethics* (Cambridge: Cambridge University Press, 1993), p. 184.) Again, using or dispatching vulnerable people in aesthetically pleasing ways would hardly be surprising for John Paul, who explains that on this perspective:

> The so-called 'quality of life' is interpreted primarily or exclusively as economic efficiency, inordinate consumerism, physical beauty and pleasure, to the neglect of the more profound dimensions – interpersonal, spiritual and religious – of existence. When [suffering] cannot be avoided and the prospect of even some future well-being vanishes, then life appears to have lost all meaning and the temptation grows in man to claim the right to suppress it.

On a functionalist rendering of personhood, lives with impaired capacities must have diminished worth. To the objection that his view "suggests to disabled people living today that their lives are less worth living than the lives of people who are not disabled," Singer responds that "it is surely flying in the face of reality to deny that, on average, this is so." (*Ibid.*, 188.) The suffering of others comes to represent an inconvenience rather than an occasion of compassionate solidarity or an obligation to maintain vigil at the bedside of a dying loved one. Calls now come for the efficient termination of the patient's life, all with an irony Garcia nicely captures as a self-righteous moral blindness claiming to preserve the dignity of the one about to be dispatched.

In truth, there is a worrisome elitism operating here. As Peter Berkowitz points out in a recent essay on Singer in *The New Republic,* views in which rationality and self-consciousness define the morally significant person frequently feign egalitarianism but encourage the aristocracy of the astute. Berkowitz asks, "then why shouldn't greater rationality make you more of a person, or a more valuable person, an individual entitled to a greater proportion of society's scarce interests?" (Peter Berkowitz, "The Utilitarian Horrors of Peter Singer: Other People's Mothers," *The New Republic,* January 10, 2000, p. 33.) And surely, this is also the Pope's meaning when he wrote:

> In the materialistic perspective described so far, interpersonal relations are seriously impoverished. The first to be harmed are women, children, the sick or suffering, and the elderly. The criterion of personal dignity – which demands respect, generosity and service – is replaced by the criterion of efficiency, functionality and usefulness: others are considered not for what they "are," but for what they "have, do and produce." This is the supremacy of the strong over the weak. (John Paul II, *The Gospel of Life,* §23.)

I think, too, that this is how we should understand the many parts of Garcia's essay (as, for example, his discussion of organ donation) in which disadvantages incurred by birth or circumstance are only compounded by policies designed by the new ethicists to insure fairness. When in reality, these policies "privilege the lucky and … compound the woes of the afflicted."

And here, at last, we encounter the real dangers of a lack of diversity and a surfeit of homogeneity. As another Clarke lecturer,

Stanley Hauerwas of Duke University, has explained in many of his writings, assertions about universal values and mainstream morality often comprise a tale told by the dominant class to mask its utter historical contingency and to hide the body count of its own less-than-edifying rise to power. (See, for example, Hauerwas's essay, "A Christian Critique of Christian America," in Hauerwas, *Christian Existence Today: Essays on Church, World and Living In Between* (Durham, NC: They Labyrinth Press, 1988), pp. 171-190.) If there is a new dominant class in medical ethics today and if "homogenizing and secularizing" forces feed its growth and bolster its authority and confer an air of the obvious on its conclusions, then accounts like Garcia's which uncover its moral blind spots and ability to oppress are exactly what we need.

Despite his many concerns, Garcia remains hopeful, and his reasons for this are first articulated in Section IV of the lecture, which is subtitled "Learning from Minority Perspectives." For him, minority perspectives reintroduce diversity and broadcast the voices of the marginalized and disempowered who are particularly at risk, *especially* in the field of health care. For example, one frequently hears the concern voiced that physician assisted suicide could be a 'choice' foisted upon those who have least status, power, and privilege in society and thereby give new meaning to the phrase, 'the last shall be first.'

From Garcia's perspective, increased diversity breaks the monopoly perspective of "the liberal individualist paradigm of the white males who dominate the field." Moreover, for those whose thought has been shaped by reflection on minority experiences, it may afford greater sensitization to inequities, injustices, and all forms of treatment suggesting a diminished humanity. Experience has been called 'the plasma of theory,' and Garcia very competently narrates the benefits accruing to medicine and medical ethics by the kind of passing over which this transfusion of perspectives implies. Learning from and listening to the neglected has the power to expose elitism and the oppression of so-called objectivity. It may also challenge and render more robust one's notion of personhood against the critiques of those who would construe it functionally.

Finally, the demand for diversity can be used "to reintroduce a variety of religious viewpoints into the debate." It is the latter which Garcia labels "the best hope for a renewed bioethics." In the remainder of my response, I'd like to reflect on how well or uneasily some of the things he says about the value of diversity in the earlier parts of his lecture sit with some of the things he says in the later sections about authority and conscience.

II.   DIVERSITY AND A UNIVERSAL CHURCH

Thus far we've seen the value Garcia attributes to diversity as a helpful supplement to perspectives dominated by white males who share precious little of the "personal experiences, social or economic stratum, interests, tastes or educational level" of racial or ethnic minorities. When, towards the end of his essay, he articulates a corrective afforded by Catholicism, I find conspicuously absent any similar ringing endorsements of diversity. He does acknowledge the controversies (and presumably the pluralism) over what exactly counts as authentic Catholic moral teachings, but only to "side step the issue ... by concentrating on teachings from the bishops themselves, here and abroad, and those authorized to speak in their name." By the end of his lecture, however, this side stepping seems more like a flamenco dance upholding an almost exclusively vertical and hierarchical notion of Church authority flowing down from the Spirit to the Magisterium to the lay faithful. Though Garcia does admit that "the Magisterium can err," and that "for the Church to have authority is, *ceteris paribus*, for us not to need arguments to accept what she says." Of course, often things are not equal, and here he all but eliminates the possibility of public dissent.

I'm not concerned here so much with theological nit-picking on these issues themselves (since Garcia is clear that he doesn't speak as a theologian), but with how his articulation and development of them relates to the rest of his proposals about medical ethics and meaningful reform therein. So, for example, Garcia says this:

What privileges the Magisterium's teaching is that the Holy Spirit guides her, leading her in a certain direction, toward a certain destination. This suggests that the Holy Spirit's influence will be more evident in the conclusion of a piece of moral reasoning, than it is in the reasoning itself. The point of that guidance is to keep the substance of the Church's teaching free from error, not to keep its thinking cogent. Providing rational defense for what the Spirit guides the Church to teach is not a part of her magisterial mission, even as it was not a part of Christ's.

With all due respect, I don't understand the above separation between conclusions and reasoning. At the least, it suggests that the Spirit of Truth would be unconcerned about invalid inferences and unsound argumentation as long as the bottom line was correct. And while it is true that Christ wasn't a philosopher, he certainly was a lover of Truth, as even the most minimalist trinitarian theology would attest. Moreover, he surely was a teacher who enjoyed at least some modest success. Aquinas says that all truth comes from God (ST I.16.6) and more specifically through the Word of God (I.34.3) who must also be reckoned the principal teacher of all (I.117.1.ad 1). Pope and bishops continue this teaching ministry. In the New Testament, see I Timothy 3:2 and Titus 1:9. In the documents of Vatican II, see *Lumen Gentium*, §25, which labels the pope "supreme shepherd and teacher of all the faithful" and §12 of *Christus Dominus* (The Decree Concerning the Pastoral Office of Bishops) says that "the duty of teaching" is "conspicuous among the principal duties of bishops."

But teachers shirk their duty when they promulgate conclusions apart from persuasive arguments (construed broadly). In the absence of such rationale and in the presence of coercion to adhere to what one cannot bring oneself to accept, authority becomes authoritarian. (See the fine essay by Fr. Richard McCormick, "Authority and Leadership: The Moral Challenge," *America*, July 20, 1996, pp. 12-17. On p. 13, McCormick writes, "We submit to authority in the hope that it will become leadership. Authoritarianism is authority that has ceased to struggle to become leadership.") Bishop Kenneth Untener of Saginaw explains that if this happens, the perception is that "the teaching church has committed a teacher's cardinal sin: it has become more concerned about itself than about truth." (Bishop Kenneth Untener, "'Humanae Vitae': What Has it Done to Us?" *Commonweal*, June 18, 1993, p. 12.)

The Catholic corrective which Garcia speaks of with hope obviously cannot operate if the Church withdraws 'sect-like' from the culture's wider controversies and embraces the irrelevance attendant upon such withdrawal (as the second horn of MacIntyre's dilemma suggests). Garcia himself clearly implies a public role for Catholic teaching and witness in the health care field so that "Perhaps the 'ethicists' will learn and eventually follow." The problem I see with that in light of the other things he's said is that the Church will never get a seat at the table if its authority is perceived as authoritarian, if coercion replaces persuasion, and monologue (however enlightened) replaces dialogue (however impaired). Then I think there is little reason to be hopeful that the darkness of this time will not long abide and painfully so.

The Church will surely be a more effective conversation partner if it is seen to model within itself the virtues of careful listening, mutual respect, and productive dialogue. One may well admit that the Church is an institution *sui generis,* but that in itself does not negate the benefits (accruing both to the Church's Magisterium and the wider community) of diversity or the advantages of openness to the witness of unfolding human experience that Garcia had defended earlier in his lecture. I believe, then, that he doesn't exhaust the alternatives when he writes:

> How much should authority count for? I will say only that this is the question of who is more likely to be right: (a) one's own limited knowledge and fallible reasoning, subject as it is to prejudices, self-delusion, and temptations to see oneself in the best light, or (b) the teaching office of the Church, where fallible humans act, but under the

guidance of the Holy Spirit? (Garcia admits on the next page that this may be a "simplistic" rendering, but also says that he doubts "that the further complications that completeness requires really change the central point.")

Allow me, in closing, to make one point about (a) and one about (b).

In the section of his lecture entitled "Beyond the New *Freedom* and *Dignity*," Garcia very persuasively describes the moral corrosion accumulated through misplaced notions of autonomy and dignity. There he develops John Paul II's concerns in 1993's *Veritatis Splendor* about the modern secular absolutization of autonomy and contrasts it with the "genuine moral autonomy" that the pope identifies with participating in the law from God (participated theonomy). He quotes John Paul's statement that our "free obedience to God's law effectively implies that human reason and human will participate in God's wisdom and providence." (Garcia quoting *Veritatis Splendor*, §32.) These are lofty words, but the confidence Garcia has in this notion of freedom and the participation it implies in the source of all truth seems mysteriously to evaporate when applied to the non-mitred in the very next section. In contrast, the *Catechism of the Catholic Church* says, "When he listens to his conscience, the prudent man can hear God speaking" (§1777); and Vatican II says in §16 of *Gaudium et Spes*, "Conscience is the most secret core and sanctuary of a man. There he is alone with God, whose voice echoes in his depths." Indeed, it is true that fallible humans with mitres act under the guidance of the Holy Spirit, but not to add that they too may be subject to prejudices, delusions, and temptations to earthly power is to give a very ahistorical presentation of the Church and to forget all too soon the corrective benefits of diversity and pluralism that Garcia had earlier elevated.

Finally, as Fr. Richard McCormick has persuasively argued, to affirm allegiance to the teaching office of the Church leaves completely undetermined how that office should exercise its authority, to whom it should listen, whose experience it might heed, how it should include the wisdom of competent lay people, what place it should make for corrective critical response to papal formulations, and so on. (See Fr. Richard McCormick, "The Shape of Moral Evasion in Catholicism," *America*, October 1, 1998, pp. 183-188 (especially pp. 186-187).) Therefore, we may not have to choose *either* individual conscience *or* magisterial authority. As the Catholic vision for so many other things has historically been a both/and, so too may it be here.

I think Garcia himself gives an example of this productive, corrective dialogue when he discusses personhood. He is careful in that discussion not to link personhood with any particular abilities or capacities (like rationality or freedom). Such would simply be to play Singer's own game again while simultaneously attempting to mount a critique of it. Instead, Garcia renders the preciousness of human nature in its innate penchant to develop capacities for thought and autonomous action. But he also acknowledges that these capacities may be blocked by organic or social obstacles. Therefore, and in itself, "The capacity for such reasoned, freely-chosen obedience is not a part of human nature." But not everyone in the tradition has been this careful. I take it that Garcia is directly disagreeing with Pope John XXIII, who wrote in *Pacem in Terris,* "Any human society, if it is to be well-ordered and productive, must lay down as a foundation this principle, namely, that every human being is a person, that is, *human nature is endowed with intelligence and free will.*" [italics mine] (Pope John XXIII, *Pacem in Terris*, §9.) It is certainly a question worth further exploration whether the western theological tradition has been too quick to identify personhood and creation in the image of God with rational capacities. Again, this plays right into Singer's hands and is related to so much that Garcia wants to criticize. Such criticisms do the Magisterium and all the People of God a service.

The Church is a pilgrim people (*Lumen Gentium*, §§48 & 50), and pilgrims learn as they go. Traditions are shadows ever lengthening and, for the discerning eye of the observer, they afford old things to be put in new perspective and novel lessons learned about what we thought we already knew. In this regard, Bishop Untener develops a wonderful analogy of the mutual dependence of mapmakers and explorers. Both need each other: the mapmakers need the explorers so that those who actually walk the terrain may help the mapmakers refine the precision of their sketches by furnishing additional data gathered through their wanderings; and the explorers need the mapmakers to guide their travels, to have some bigger sense of how the tectonic plates of human experience assemble, and to be warned of dangers hidden in shadows or lurking over the horizon. (Untener, *op. cit.*, pp. 12-13.) If the Church models this kind of pluralistic dialogue, then with the promises of Christ and under the guidance of the Holy Spirit, the dusk marked by Minerva's Owl need not be feared, for daylight has been faithfully spent and provisions made for the journey ahead.

THE CRISIS IN MEDICINE: PROFESSIONAL LIFE IN THE AGE OF MANAGED CARE

Edmund Pellegrino

It is a special privilege to deliver the Clarke Family Lecture a second time. It bespeaks a degree of confidence I will find it difficult to justify. The difficulties not withstanding I am grateful for the invitation.

As was the case last time, I asked David Solomon to suggest a topic he thought might be appropriate and might fit comfortably into the general outline of this year's conference. David said, "What I think physicians are worried about is the question – is it possible to be an ethical physician in the present climate of managed care?"

I was gratified because it is the question I am most frequently asked by conscientious physicians all over our country whenever I speak about professional ethics, i.e. about the obligations and duties of physicians to their patients. I hear it also from nurses and other health professionals who together with physicians feel overwhelmed by the demands of a system of care whose aims are economic and political primarily rather than ethical.

Confusion about the answer to David's questions is the source of demoralization and early retirement on the part of our most morally sensitive physicians and unseemly vindictiveness on the part of the less morally sensitive. Yet, if we think about what it is, and who it is, that we are, there can only be one answer. We must remain faithful to our moral purpose or lose any claim to moral credibility or to the title of "physician" or "nurse." If we capitulate, accommodate or compromise, then we become the technicians, bureaucrats and proletarians the health care "industry" wants us to be.

My worries are less for what these mean for the practice or social standing of the profession than what it does to the persons we are committed to serve – those who need our knowledge and skills, and who need it as patients and persons not as insured lives, consumers, or purchasers of just another commodity called health care. I address my remarks therefore to physicians, nurses and other health professionals. Theirs is an especially demanding call whose moral dimensions can never fit the rubric of a mere occupation.

I will use medicine as my paradigm case for several reasons: I know it best and I am still close enough clinically to speak from experience of the way practice has changed. I shall be critical of my own profession. I have learned that nurses do not look kindly on physicians who moralize about nursing. I do not, however, think nurses will object if I suggest that they face the same question of moral integrity, that the ethical issues they face fundamentally are the same, and that nurses in their own way must answer David's question in the affirmative. Indeed, all of us who claim to be "healers" must confront the ethical challenges of that claim. Allowing therefore for the differences in our roles, I believe that what I say is relevant analogically for nursing and the other health professions.

For more than a quarter of a century medical ethics has been the focus of powerful forces for change. It has been and continues to be reshaped by the rise of participatory democracy, in the consumer mentality, in civil rights and patient's rights movements, in the distrust of all authority and institutions, in the decline in religious belief, and in the critical surveillance of every precept of the traditional Hippocratic Ethic. To this has been added the bureaucratization, institutionalization, and commercialization of all the professions.

The most serious consequence of all of this has been the shift from physician authority to patient autonomy and from freedom to make clinical decisions at the bedside to decision making within a framework of restrictions imposed by managed care organizations. When I gave the first Clarke Family lecture managed care was in its incipiency. Today it is the single most powerful force in restructuring medical care and practice. For economists, policy makers, and politicians this is what medicine has needed for a long time; for conscientious physicians, whose patients become sick enough to actually need its services, managed care, as it now exists, is a present and growing threat to humane, considerate, and compassionate care of the sick.

Managed care goes, unerringly, to the heart of medical ethics, to the gold standard of that ethic – the primacy of patient welfare and the obligation of the physician to act for the patient's welfare. Managed care forces a re-definition of who and what physicians, patients, and health care ought to be. It redefines the kind of society we want to be and how we want to treat the vulnerable persons among us – the sick, the poor, the very young, and the very old. Managed care exposes undercurrents of social and ethical unrest that have been latent for many years. The boldness of its challenges to professional ethics makes clear the degree of our confusion about our identity. It forces us physicians to decide whether we define ourselves as physicians by economic or ethical criteria.

This afternoon I would like to approach David Solomon's question as a question of moral identity since how we identify ourselves will determine the way we answer this question. I will argue that managed care is not intrinsically evil but that the way it is practiced today is morally inadmissable. I will argue that managed care poses unacceptable conflicts in the physician's ethical obligations which place ethics and economics into conflict with each other when they should be complementary. By examining the impact of managed care as currently practiced on the moral imperatives of the physician-patient relationship it will become clear that physicians have no choice but to recover the ethical primacy of patient welfare or desist from claiming to be an ethical enterprise or even a profession.

Such a conclusion does not preclude the design of systems of managed care that satisfy ethical requirements nor does it excuse physicians from their societal responsibilities for the optimum use of health care resources. A reorientation of systems of managed care around the centrality of the ethics of medicine with economics as the science of means whereby the ethical ends are best achieved is therefore necessary.

SOME DEFINITIONS

Managed can be defined under three categories: (1) *de facto* rationing, (2) systematized rationing, and (3) implicit/explicit. *De facto* rationing is really not rationing. It is an unplanned, fortuitous distribution of services based on accidental factors like ability to pay, social or educational status, geographical location. There has always been *de facto* rationing but this does not, as some erroneously argue, justify systematic rationing.

Systematized rationing is the organized systematic conscious planing to accomplish a specific end – a distribution of resources according to some specified principle such as quality care, the good of patients, cost containment, profit, competitive edge, etc. Managed care today is systematized, not *de facto*, rationing.

Systematized care can be implicit or explicit. In today's managed care system, implicit rationing makes the physician the rationing agent by assigning him or his organization x dollars for patients for z period of time to be used as he sees fit, with penalties for exceeding x and rewards for conserving it. Explicit rationing, on the other hand, is a system in which some organization external to the physician decides what services and under what conditions the physician may employ by pre- or post authorization

Managed care is, per se, a morally neutral concept. Its moral status depends upon the ends it presumes to serve, the means whereby it achieves them, and the priorities it follows in achieving its ends. From the traditional ethical point of view the ultimate determinant of moral probity is the degree to which the system serves the needs of the one who is ill. Any other end, such as cost containment, profit, efficiency, productivity, or redistribution of wealth, unless it directly serves the welfare of the patient presenting himself, is open to ethical challenge. This principle will be developed further as we examine the ethical dilemmas of managed care at the bedside.

Managed care comes in various forms, some are morally acceptable, some morally dubious, and some morally reprehensible on this standard.   Clearly a managed care system that has improvement of the quality of care as its end is commendable; one whose ends is cost containment alone is morally dubious; one that has profit as its end is morally suspect since profit as a driving force eventually displaces compassion.

The ethical problems attending managed care as it is organized today center on the fact that almost all varieties are converging on the profit motive.   This is a response to the commodification of health care in the current economic climate of commercialization of every aspect of life and to the current fascination with competition and with the market place as the arena for all service transactions. As a result, patients become clients or consumers; physicians are providers or stakeholders; health care is an industry and an investment opportunity; and health care executives demand the inflated salaries and golden parachutes of corporate executives.

The corporate ethos displaces traditional professional ethics. Productivity, efficiency, competitive product lines, competitive edge, mergers, and profit margins dominate the discourse. Subscribers are sought not among the sick – they are too costly – but among the young, the wealthy and the well who pay the premiums and do not use the resources of the plan. Meanwhile the physician becomes a hireling, a tool of corporate interests, not the advocate for the good of the patient. Ethics is piously affirmed because, after all, it is good for business.

No one can object to productivity, efficiency, or lowered costs if they are effected to improve the quality of care. Indeed, on the traditional ethical model they are morally obligatory. So is the avoidance of unnecessary care. Whenever managed care effects these changes for the express purpose of improving care, it gains moral stature. That is why, as a concept, managed care is not intrinsically unethical.   As a teacher, investigator, and practitioner I have expended considerable energy in pointing to the evils of unnecessary care urging diagnostic and therapeutic parsimony, i.e. ordering only what will demonstrably improve our diagnostic and prognostic accuracy and our therapeutic outcomes.

Guarding against unnecessary care constitutes the morally obligatory gatekeeper role, one consistent with the best traditions in medical ethics. It is the gatekeeper role in managed care which is objectionable since its aim is to reduce costs or increase profits with patient care only a secondary consideration. Clinical guidelines, cost benefit, cost effectiveness, and outcome studies are therefore not unethical. They have been encouraged by managed care for economic reasons, but when they serve the improvement of the quality of care they meet the test of moral probity very well. Certainly, they should not be abandoned because of the moral defects of managed care as it exists today.

MANAGED CARE VERSUS PATIENT CARE

Notably absent in the national debate over the Clinton Administration's proposed health care reform was its impact on those the system was purported to serve. Of course, all the participants – the government, the insurance industry, and even the professions – piously invoked the welfare of patients as their motive. But even a cursory scrutiny of their arguments quickly uncovered the underlying motives of self-interest – not always even enlightened. Now that we have had some experience with the system that emerged from that debate it is important to examine the ethical conflicts inherent in managed care at the bedside.

First is the erosion of the trust relationship. To be sure in the past all physicians were not equally trustworthy that is why the world's literature abounds in satirical portraits of venal physicians. But the majority of physicians could be trusted to respect the first principle of medical ethics to act for the welling being of the sick person. Physicians and patients at least were allies in the modern insurance era.

From the patient's point of view this has changed. The physician as a hireling of the "plan" is clearly in a position of divided loyalty. Patients constantly wonder, and even ask, whether the denial of care is because it is unnecessary or because its denial means a bonus for the doctor and a profit for the plan. In many a patient's eyes *primum non nocere* has given place to *primum non expendere*. The risk of under treatment is a reality especially with respect to the aged, the infant, and those handicapped mentally whose lives fail the quality tests of a youth and fitness entranced society.

The distrust is further enhanced by the fact that the managed care industry, under the federal Employees Retirement Insurance Act (ERISA) is protected from liability for wrongful acts. The Medical Director of an HMO claims not to be making medical decisions but simply a decision about benefits eligibility whenever he second guesses the attending physician. How long this spurious defense can last in the face of litigation is problematic at this time.

Second is the so called "hassle factor" – the inconvenience, stress, anxiety, impersonality, rebukes, and disputes patients encounter when they seek care. Added to the vulnerability, dependence and anxieties any illness entails, patients experience the hassle factor as peculiar category of unusual punishment. This says nothing of the loss of time, confusion, and dismay of having gone to the wrong hospital, MRI facility, or laboratory because of changing contractual arrangements between "providers" all based on who provides the lower cost.

Third, there is the much despised "gag" rule which forbids a conscientious physician from revealing his disagreement with the allowed treatment, hospital, or specialist the plan approves and insists upon. Patients need to know about their doctor's financial arrangements, at least in so far as fiscal rewards and penalties go. All the conflicts of interest present during the fee for service era are magnified when the physician is a double or triple agent. When the physician is also owner of the managed care organization or a shareholder, directly or indirectly, then the patient has no advocate to rely upon against the system when the patient has a complaint.

Fourth, there is the much vaunted but illusory "freedom" of the patient as a consumer to choose the kind of plan he wants and how much he wants to spend on health care. The fact is that the employer chooses the plan not the employee and this choice can change with little notice when a cheaper one comes along making continuity of care by one's preferred physician doubtful or impossible of attainment. In any case even the illusion of freedom vanishes when one is acutely ill. Then if one has made the wrong choice – an inadequate plan, one with limited coverage or chosen no plan at all – what is the physician to do? To be consistent, devotees of the free market ethos would have to say that patients must suffer the consequences of their wrong choices. Yet few would go so far as to suggest that we refuse to treat those who neglected their health and bet on freedom from illness in trade for other things they might have wanted. No matter what the social attitude might be the physician is impelled to treat and society is impelled to cover the expense in some way.

Very few people, however well-educated, physicians, administrators and economists included, possess the clairvoyance to foresee every medical eventuality. Few, if any, can choose the precise plan that will protect them against every catastrophic illness. The idea of the free individual freely making his choices, taking the risks he wants to take, and living with the consequences of his choices simply collapses in the face of illness. A health care system built on this fiction flies in the fact of the reality of each person's inevitable fragility and finitude.

A fifth moral conflict in managed care centers on the ineradicable fact of physician complicity. Understandably, physicians may feel compelled – by the need to protect legitimate self interests or those of their families – to compromise professional integrity and to accommodate to the pressure of managed care. Some compromises may be legitimate, others inexcusable. It all depends upon the degree of betrayal of trust and beneficence they entail.

What is certain is that – at least at the present time – everything that happens or is omitted in patient care is ordered by the physician. Even in this day of team care, the physician is the final common pathway and the final guardian of what happens medically to the patient. For any serious departure from the best standard of care the physician is an accomplice. This is true even in a system of managed care which deliberately pits the physician's self interest against the patient's. The law recognizes this fact of complicity and the special fiduciary relationship between doctor and patient. The physician is held responsible for providing the standard of care. He is not excused because managed care policy violates that standard. Economic considerations can no more eradicate legal responsibility than they can eradicate ethical responsibility.   The full weight of the recognition of this moral and legal complicity has yet to impress itself on physicians, patients, or the public. As the managed care system finds itself increasingly squeezed between rising costs, falling profits, and the ethical demands of patient care more corners will be cut. The current ERISA protection against liability will be weakened or eliminated.

At some point physicians, as a body, will be forced to protest and to refuse to participate in certain practices. Not to do so is to become corrupted by the system. Many are already "gaming" the system – adjusting disease categories and severity to fit what is authorized by the plan. Good as the intention may be – to help the patient – such practices cannot be justified. Neither can another corrupting move, namely unionization, be justified in the name of protecting the patient. A physician's union would only provide further evidence of our defection from the role as advocate of the patient's welfare.

A sixth and final ethical conflict is the temptation to be "practical" – to set ethics aside as fine ideal but not a viable option in today's crisis. On this view, the problems I have been enumerating are temporary – the price we must pay until the kinks in the system are straightened out. This argument resembles in kind, if not in severity, the argument I often heard from my friends who saw hope in the Soviet system. My friends were well-intentioned colleagues who assured me that the atrocities of totalitarianism were abuses and temporary phenomena before the dawning of the new economic utopia. It is well to remember too that one of the first acts of the

Presidium of the Soviet state was to subvert the Hippocratic Oath to the purposes of Communist ideology. Medical ethics can be subverted to economics and commerce just as it has, in times past, been subverted to politics.

THE PROPER ROLE OF ECONOMICS

None of what I have said to this point should be taken as a denial of the legitimate role economics can and does play in medicine and medical care. The problem is not the proper use of economics but the inversion of the priority ethics should take over economics. Economics is a science of means, concerned with how best to use our resources – physical, human, and fiscal to achieve certain goals. It provides scientific data about the state of our economy as a whole and as a manifestation of human behavior. As such it can teach, measure, and devise optimum systems for achieving whatever goals we set.

Economics has no special competence in deciding what goals we ought to set and what kind of society we ought to be. It certainly cannot tell us what constitutes a good society in the moral sense. Its studies, deliberations, and data are crucial in designing a health care system but only after we have decided whether health care is a commodity, a legal right, a privilege, or a moral obligation of a good society. Economics under the constraint of ethics is indispensable for any workable and just health care system. Economics can enter into decisions at the bedside under certain specified conditions. Mentally competent patients may validly refuse treatments they deem too expensive given their life plans or those they may have for their families. Likewise competent patients may execute living wills or appoint durable powers of attorney whom they empower to make decision about costs of care or its discontinuation when they cannot make decisions for themselves.

Correspondingly physicians are obliged, when two treatments are of comparable effectiveness, to use the less expensive treatment. What is not defensible – though many disagree on this point – is to use cost alone as a criterion for withholding or withdrawing effective or beneficial treatment from mentally incompetent persons – the demented, the very old, the infant, or the retarded. The physician is, and should remain, the advocate for his patient. The physician must not become the agent of personal or social policy in protecting the resources of society. In such cases decisions should be based on the clinician's best estimate of the relationship between effectiveness and benefit on the one hand and the burdens of treatment on the other. This will keep the intrusion of the physician's biases and prejudices or his estimate of the patient's quality of life to a minimum.

COST CONTAINMENT – THE PHYSICIAN AND THE PROFESSION

It would be a serious misreading of my intention to interpret what I have said thus far as a plea for social and economic license on the part of physicians. This is far from the case. The physician's role is a vital one on at least four levels: (1) at the bedside, (2) as an expert in the science of medicine, (3) as a member of a moral community, and (4) as a citizen.

At the bedside, as I already mentioned, the physician is obliged to use the cheaper of two treatments or tests when they are equally effective. Even more important is the elimination of truly unnecessary care, i.e. care that is ineffective, non-beneficial, or freighted with burdens disproportionate to its effectiveness and benefit. Sadly, even before managed care, excessive treatment, and with it the consummation of vast sums, often resulted in unnecessary and even harmful care.

The first step, therefore, for the individual physician – and the profession as a whole – is to begin with themselves and, as a moral obligation, to practice rational, scientific medicine and to enforce standards of professional competence on this ground. This is not the place to dilate on our failures in this respect in the past. No matter what managed care plans may ordain, individual physicians cannot excuse over or under treatment on grounds of the policies or practices of their managed care employers.

Likewise to retain ethical integrity individual physicians must continue to be patient advocates. They must refuse the goal of rationer at the bedside and defend the patient against the erroneous or capricious decisions of the managed care medical director when there is evidence of potential harm to the patient.

As I will indicate in a moment, I do not expect individual physicians to carry the full weight of reform or protest by themselves. Their obligations to resist or to say no are directly related to the degree of harm they can foresee for their patients. Every disagreement with the health plan or its medical director is not an excuse for ethical self-righteousness. Nor can anyone prescribe for another physician how much he must risk in personal loss or harm to protect his patient in a given situation.

At the second level of obligations, there is the duty as an informed expert to provide sound, objective, and disinterested advice to policy makers on the clinical foundations for policy or guideline recommendations. Physicians relate to public or community policy bodies as experts to courts of law. Without sound expert input health care policy cannot be rational or scientifically sound. For his part the clinician must be sure that his advice is up to date, that it takes opposing views into account, and that it is as free of self-interest as possible in an imperfect world.

At the third level, the physician acts as a member of a moral community which is what a profession is in fact. Physicians are united by a common ethical ideal, the ethic of the trust relationship with patients in which the welfare of the patient is the primary ethical imperative. Medical professional associations exist as agencies for collective expression of the ethics of physicians. The purpose of professional associations, therefore, is not the welfare of physicians but of patients. Professional associations, thus, are obliged to act as a body whenever the health care system is inimical to patient welfare. As a moral community this means doctors, collectively, must strive for a just health care system and must educate policy makers in the character of such a system.

Finally at the fourth level, physicians are citizens like everyone else and as such they are expected to participate in the process of democratic government. In that capacity, physicians are free to express their own beliefs about economics, business practices, the rights of patients or physicians, and to vote for a system that meets their criteria for justice. These may be different from those espoused by the professional organization but they must be ethically justified all the same.

Physicians who act conscientiously at these four levels of societal purpose can best meet their obligations to safeguard societal resources and advance the good of all patients. This is far better, ethically and societally as well, than their acting as the rationer of health care or turning away from the ethics of individual patients to something called "social ethics." We will all be better protected if the individual physician is bound by his fidelity to the agent before him and if rationing and allocation decisions are made by some public mechanism. This assures the patient that the doctor remains the patient's advocate and friend and is not a double or triple agent.

BEYOND TODAY'S MANAGED CARE

It is uncertain at this time whether managed care as it exists today – energized by the ethos of the market place – can, will, or should survive. If I were to venture a guess, I would predict its self-destruction for several reasons. First, as the insured population ages, those who are now healthy and profitable will become ill, chronically ill eventually, and their care costly. Costs will rise, profits will drop, and the investment opportunity will be deflated. Second, one can anticipate increasing public protest, especially from the educated middle class who are vocal and influential. Legislative controls of HMOs will be demanded. Third, in one way or another the current protection from liability under ERISA will be challenged; malpractice and personal injury suits will multiply and juries will award large damages. In the end, the public will demand a reformed system.

Unfortunately, when the entrepreneurs who now sustain managed care corporations leave the field for better financial returns, they will leave very little behind. They have virtually destroyed the voluntary community hospital system as well as the *pro bono* activity of the profession. It is hard to envision what will fill the vacuum.

There is one bright prospect in this gloomy prognosis. This is the opportunity to devise a managed care system driven by ethical imperatives. Here the goal of managed care will be the quality of patient care with productivity, efficiency, and competence directed to the end of patient care and not the end of profit. Rationing will need to be an element but it, too, will need to satisfy certain ethical disiderata, for example, to be ethically justified rationing would: (1) have to be dictated by a true economic emergency, one in which it can be shown that health care expenditures are in fact compromising other societal goods; (2) require that measures other than rationing should be exhausted before rationing, e.g. reduction of administrative costs (now estimated as 25%), paring down of executive salaries, removal of profits, price reductions when amortization of new equipment (like the MRI) is accomplished; (3) demand that other discretionary expenditures should be examined critically to see whether the claim that we are spending too much on health is taken for granted. The amount of money spent in the United States on alcohol, tobacco, sports, entertainment, and a host of pursuits and pleasures is staggering. No one can expect vast shifts of these monies to health care but one can certainly ask what kind of people are we choosing to be? After all our budgets reveal what we value better than does our rhetoric.

If these three preliminary steps are taken, rationing health care could be ethically entertained. But to be ethically implemented another set of criteria must be satisfied: (1) the allocation and access policies must have been arrived at by some democratic method which allows for informed consent on the part of the populace. Mechanisms which make expression of opinion and which make appropriate means for assuring response to these opinions need to be elaborated. The principle of distribution which gives the "rationale" for rationing should be clear and freely disclosed to public surveillance. (2) The physician must not be the rationer for reasons developed earlier in this essay. Rationing thus must be explicit and not implicit. (3) Society must see provision of health care to all its citizens as a moral obligation of a good society.

CONCLUSION

Within such a system, driven by ethical and not economic imperatives, physicians can and must be ethical, patients will be protected, societal needs will be addressed, and there will be no questions about the integrity of physicians, nurses, and other health professionals.

Physicians today increasingly ask how it is possible to be ethically responsive in a world dominated by the ethos of managed care. That ethos, as managed care is operated today, is antithetical to the traditional ethic of medicine. The fault is not in the managed care concept but in the way that concept is implemented in today's commercialized and market driven health care.

Physicians must recognize the points at which managed care conflicts with professional ethics and must strive to alleviate or eliminate those conflicts. Without recognizing who and what they are, physicians cannot prevent themselves from being transformed into proletarians, technocrats, and bureaucratic functionaries with special skills in a system not of their making.

Managed care can be ethically inspired under certain conditions and, if those conditions are met, physicians can maintain professional integrity and patients can be served as fellow humans in need of helping and healing and not as beneficiaries of an insurance apparatus – necessary as sources of income.

Response to
THE CRISIS IN MEDICINE: PROFESSIONAL LIFE IN THE AGE OF MANAGED CARE

Kevin McDonnell

Speaking with customary vigor, Ed Pellegrino struck a nerve with the physicians who had the privilege of hearing him present his paper. It is a reflection on a timeless issue in medicine (and all professions) – how can physicians wholeheartedly serve their patients while drawing their income from medical practice? Is there not an irresolvable conflict of interest between physicians and their patients? Have modern financial arrangements, managed care in particular, finally revealed the depth of that conflict? Pellegrino responds that managed care, especially financially managed care, presents a critical challenge to the contemporary physician. Ever optimistic, he concludes that medicine can rise to the challenge by drawing on the moral community of physicians. By way of commentary, I agree with Ed Pellegrino's conclusion but suggest that the community of physicians will only regain its moral strength and meet this challenge if physicians are salaried.

Plato put the issue clearly in the first book of his *Republic*. His character Thrasymachus, arguing that those in authority invariably act in their own self-interest, challenges Socrates. For example, Thrasymachus claims that the shepherd fattens his sheep not for their good but for the shepherd's own lunch. Invoking the example of medicine, Socrates replies, "The true doctor concerns himself with the patient's interest and not his own. The true doctor is like a ruler whose subject is the human body; he is not a mere money maker"(342d). The entire *Republic* may be read as a lengthy response to the accusation of Thrasymachus. Ed Pellegrino's paper is, fortunately, a briefer restatement of the issue and a response to one way this issue presents itself to modern medicine.

For most of the history of medicine, fee for service structured the financial relation between physicians and patients. This system rewarded physicians financially for providing more services, some of them perhaps only marginally beneficial to their patients. And it handsomely rewarded the unscrupulous in the medical profession who provided completely unnecessary services.

The fee for service system has extensive side effects, both positive and negative. For one, it stimulates advances in medical practice and research. Since new services generate increased fees, there are very tangible rewards for developing treatments and technologies. Pharmaceutical companies advance this argument in support of their prices – high prices support the research required for the developments of new drugs and treatments. The fee for service system also encourages patients and physicians to look at medical care as a consumer good because it fits the model of other items in the marketplace. A consumer society assumes that the more goods or service individuals have, the better off they are. Forgetting for the moment that patients are those who are sick or at least threatened with disease, patients sometimes think of themselves as consumers and believe that the more medical care they receive, the better off they are. They take the slogan "You get what you pay for" to apply equally to the plumber, the auto company, and the doctor. As insurance became an ever larger part of medical care, consumers had the luxury of buying something without concern about or even awareness of price. The inevitable result was a huge increase in the cost of medical care.

Managed care is an assemblage of systems to control the costs that fee for service medicine generated. When Ed Pellegrino spoke, the major concern about managed care was the huge salaries and stock market bonuses accruing to executives of managed care companies. At present, those concerns have been replaced by such issues as the bankruptcy of managed care corporations, the dramatic decline in their stock prices, and the financial crisis of those physicians who assumed some of the financial risks typically borne by insurance companies. By the time you read Dr. Pellegrino's paper and this comment, the symptomatic issue will almost certainly be different. Nevertheless, while the symptoms may differ, the underlying disease is the same one correctly diagnosed by Ed Pellegrino who defines managed care as "any system of care consciously organized to influence the clinical behavior of health professionals in the direction of some specified end." As Plato and Pellegrino argue, the end of medicine is not an open-ended "some specified;" the end of medicine must be nothing other than healing the patient.

Medicine has always needed to provide for the support of its practitioners. Pellegrino forthrightly acknowledges that physicians have all too often taken advantage of their superior knowledge and social position to advance their financial interests at the expense of patients. Still, in a fee for service environment, these moral failures belonged simply to individuals. Moral failure was unsystematic; it was not a feature of the system. When managed care organizes medicine around a financial goal, it imposes a systematic immorality. It misdirects medical care toward an end, goal, or purpose to which it is not by nature suited. As Plato argues in the *Republic*, government devoted to the benefit of the governors rather than the governed is tyranny. If medicine's goal becomes money making, then patients will be tyrannized. Ironically, in managed care systems operating in fancy buildings with expensive equipment, physicians are also tyrannized. Such systems are run for the advantage of investors and their managers who are, as investors, solely interested in making money.

Because fee for service is not really a system but a ramshackle collection of arrangements, whatever moral problems exist in those arrangements can be addressed by dealing with individual physicians. One by one, physicians must be steeped in the ethic of medicine that demands unswerving devotion to the benefit of the patient. The processes of selecting those for medical training, inculcating the requisite professional virtues, and sustaining those virtues through long careers is a daunting task that inevitably will be dotted with failure. Such arrangements appeal for the treatment that Pellegrino advances in his several books on virtue ethics and, in my view, no one has contributed more than Ed Pellegrino to inspiring professional virtues among physicians.

Since system is so essential to managed care, however, medical ethics must expand its scope beyond examining only bedside issues to exploring issues in the systems of medical care. Insurance and social policies now structure much that happens or does not happen at the bedside. Physicians need to examine not only their individual consciences but also the social structures in which they work to insure that their clinical activities are wholeheartedly devoted to the benefit of their patients. There are two parts to this task. The first is the negative one of eliminating the destructive facets of managed care. The second is establishing social structures that promote the basic goal of medicine.

Ed Pellegrino is well known for his scathing critique of some clearly evil structures of managed care. He mentions several in his paper, notably capricious decision making by distant authorities and a loss of freedom for both physicians and patients.

In discussing the capricious decisions of the case managers employed by managed care organization, Pellegrino notes that we need to examine the whole picture. (He then promptly gives in to the clinician's temptation to give two or three outrageous examples from his own experience.) It seems to me, however, that the issue is not so much capricious decisions but systematically mis-constructed decisions. Managed care is, in many ways, a reaction to the caprices of individual physicians ordering tests, treatments, medications, and hospitalization in patterns that are not generally beneficial for patients. Beyond ineffective and inefficient medicine, managed care is designed to eliminate the conflicts caused by physicians ordering or charging for tests because of their financial interest in doing the test or ordering the procedure. Many managed care organizations were formed in part to provide care according to the best professional standards. They encouraged professional education and set standards for tests and the prescription formulary designed to enhance patient care.

Financially-driven managed care changed all that. The focus shifted from clinical quality as established by peer physicians to the financial health of the managed care organization. What appears capricious to the practicing physician may appear totally rational to the managed care accountant. As Pellegrino notes, cost containment, *primum non expendere*, is the driving force in financially managed care. Since managed care is a system, it cannot appeal merely to the self restraint of physicians; it must have a systematic way to control costs. It therefore generates utilization reviews, financial hold-backs, and other devices designed to restrain what are taken to be, and sometimes are, the capricious decisions of physicians.

The second destructive feature of managed care is its attempts to limit patient and physician choice. Patients' choices are limited by the gatekeeper role that managed care organizations assign to primary care physicians. The impetus for establishing gatekeepers was to prevent patients from referring themselves to specialists for care that primary care doctors could appropriately and more cheaply provide. Lack of access to preferred physicians has become one of patients' most persistent complaints about managed care.

Physicians, on the other hand, are concerned with gag rules and other restrictions on their ability to recommend the treatments that they believe are in the best interests of their patients. Having accepted the limitation on their professional authority that patient autonomy requires, physicians resent the authoritative impositions of insurance plans or HMOs. After many physicians turned away from the paternalism of old-fashioned medicine, they now find that power wielded by some remote financial entity.

Currently, both patients and physicians are becoming successful in rolling back the restrictions that managed care has placed on their choices. Physicians have persuaded legislatures to outlaw "gag rules" that restrict them from informing patients of all the choices available. Congress is considering versions of a patients' bill of rights that would enable patients to appeal the treatment-limiting decisions of managed care organizations. Customer demand has also forced many managed care organizations to pay for the services of alternative practitioners and not fully validated medical treatments. All these measures rob financially managed care of its crucial rationale – cost control. The restrictions on care to which Ed Pellegrino rightly objects are rapidly being swept away.

The task of developing a positive way to insure that medicine retains its focus on the goal of healing is far more elusive. Medical insurance premiums and drug prices currently are increasing. In this 2000 election year, political leaders are again floating plans for health care reform. Since price increases are the principal stimulus for reform, the proposals will almost certainly be financial in focus and, therefore, will not direct medicine back to its proper aim.

Dealing with the proper aim of medicine requires remembering that most physician and nursing services are devoted to sickness care. Health care, on the other hand, is often a legitimate consumer good, consisting of such things as good nutrition, effective exercise, and sound personal hygiene. Consumers can shop for health products because they enter the marketplace with strength and vigor, wielding resources such as *Consumer Reports,* nutritional labels, and medical school newsletters. In contrast, the clinical encounter generally provides sickness care. People come to physicians when they lack strength and vigor, when they are at a special disadvantage. (The marketing of health care, designed to put a positive face on everything, has disguised this important reality.) While some physician visits lie outside this description – minoxidil was once available only by prescription – the weakness of patients is a distinguishing feature of the clinical encounter. The professional codes of physicians and nurses, requirements of competence, confidentiality, and beneficence, are required to protect the vulnerable. In such an encounter, it is not enough to give information or warn of dangers; patients are vulnerable and need support. They lack the power and strength to be good consumers.

The possibility of insurance demonstrates the validity of the distinction between health care and sickness care. (Like "life" insurance, the product is often misnamed "health" insurance.) One can only buy insurance against undesirable events: sickness, death, accidents, etc. We save for consumer goods; we insure against losses that are out of our control.

The positive solution to the problems of managed care has to come from a reawakened recognition that professionals, whether doctors, lawyers, or teachers, undertake a profession because of the vulnerability of their patients, clients, or students. Because of the weakness of the people they help, society has validated the professions, giving them powers not allowed to ordinary participants in the marketplace. Teachers have tenure to insure their freedom to express controversial views because society has judged that it needs such views to flourish. Physicians control access to powerful drugs because preventing their abuse is in society's interest. Society grants physicians their licenses to protect the vulnerable ill against substandard care.

Society well-compensates the professions for their service to the vulnerable. It allows these professions extensive power to supervise and control their members, to establish educational and other standards that pose substantial barriers to the entry of competition, and it grants each a monopoly on the provision of its services. This enormous power is justified because human weakness is one principal motivation for establishing society, and even those of us who are financially secure are not safe against the assault of illness and death.

In the last several decades, American physicians have used their power as a profession for ends both good and bad. American physicians are among the richest of the richest people in the world. However, as they have done so, physicians have increasingly lost control of their own practices. Physicians responded so warmly to Ed Pellegrino's paper because, in appealing to traditional professionalism, it promises the return of professional control. No amount of juggling or restructuring of the present managed care systems is going to accomplish this goal. Physicians will regain professional control only when their rewards are no longer primarily financial. I do not think that serious reform of health care is possible unless it includes changes to the way physicians are paid.

Each year in my medical ethics course I ask students to name a single reform they would make to improve the structure of American medical care. Reflecting on Ed Pellegrino's paper forced me to answer this question myself. My answer: physicians should be paid a salary or a fixed sum per patient (capitation) free of financial risk.

While this proposal may seem startling or threatening to many physicians, there is nothing in it that is not already in place in some parts of American medicine. The proposal does not ask that physicians receive less than they presently earn. The important element is removing financial risk. Various strategies to assess and manipulate risk have driven much of the dramatic increase in the cost of medical care in the past 25 years. Physicians should simply remove themselves as far as possible from this manipulation.

If physicians are salaried, they will be working, almost certainly in groups, for large organizations: hospitals, insurance companies or even government agencies. As salaried employees, they will bond more closely to each other and have a strong incentive to control their working conditions. Their incentives will be professional control rather than financial profit.

In effect, physicians will work in a system akin to that of college professors. They would live on good salaries, negotiate wages and working conditions, and, most important, establish almost complete control over their primary working environment. They will have considerable say in the selection of new colleagues and the conditions of their attaining full professional status. They will work in an environment which can reward well-coordinated care with the mutual respect that accompanies shared efforts. (Obviously, this is a grossly idealized picture of academic life.)

Rather than countering objections to the proposal, let me mention two major shifts that such arrangements might produce.

First, they would shift the external incentive of medical practice from money to honor. This is at least one step up the scale of rewards that Plato outlines in the *Republic*. As professional control increases, the incentive will be the respect of one's peers, those with whom one works closely to attain a common goal. Since their honor is at stake in the quality of care provided by both colleague physicians and the medical institutions for which they work, physicians will have a justification and incentive to demand structural changes in medicine that will benefit patients.

Second, and most important, such a shift in physicians' reward system would enable them to refocus their attention on the primary goal of medicine. Healing the sick and helping the vulnerable is the intrinsic goal of medicine. No person or profession can sustain itself if it does not focus on its intrinsic goals. Money is important; physicians no less than others are entitled to recompense for their work. Honor is essential; people cannot sustain themselves and their work without the respect of their fellows. But most important in human flourishing is sustaining oneself with the inherent joys of what one is doing. When physicians can again focus on taking care of patients, the joy will return to the practice of medicine.

Refocusing physicians toward the goal of medicine requires that they escape from the tyranny of money. Ironically, the money that brings freedom in the market, the freedom to buy and sell as one pleases, has robbed physicians of their professional control. At the conclusion of his *Republic*, Plato pictured the way his ideal city might decay into tyranny. The rule of wealth was midway down that slippery slope, one step before social chaos that only tyranny could control. The redirection of the energies of the rulers away from their proper goal of regulating the state started the ideal city down that slope. Socrates advances the metaphor cited at the beginning of this essay that the physician is the ruler of the body in a way similar to the way the ruler rules the state. Without just rule directed to the benefit of those ruled, medicine may slide down Plato's slippery slope, whizzing through a phase of chaos to end in tyranny.

PRACTICING PATIENCE: HOW CHRISTIANS SHOULD BE SICK

Stanley Hauerwas

(Portions of this lecture appeared in *Christians among the Virtues: Theological Conversations with Ancient and Modern Ethics*, Stanley M. Hauerwas and Charles Pinches, University of Notre Dame Press, 1997.)

This is a memorable occasion for me. It's wonderful to be back among people who are dear to me and have changed my life forever. I don't come back to South Bend very often, but it floods me with emotion when I do. And so I am honored to give this lecture and doubly honored by the friends who claim me here. Actually, I mean, it's wonderful to be back with Solomon. David taught me to read Trollope for which I will be forever grateful. I remember once I was talking to David and I said, "Have you read them all?" And he said, "No, no, you've got to save three or four for those really black periods in your life. You know he only wrote forty-seven." – a true Trollopean.

I   THE GOD THAT FAILED: THE PATHOS OF MEDICINE IN MODERNITY

In 1979 Alasdair MacIntyre wrote in response to articles on theology and medical ethics in a special issue of the *Journal of Medicine and Philosophy*:

> What ought we to expect from contemporary theologians in the area of medical ethics: First – and without this everything else is uninteresting – we ought to expect a clear

statement of what difference it makes to be a Jew or a
Christian or a Moslem, rather than a secular thinker, in
morality generally.   Second . . . we need to hear a
theological critique of secular morality and culture. Third,
we want to be told what bearing what has been said under
the first two headings has on the specific problems which
arise for modern medicine. ("Theology, Ethics, and the
Ethics of Medicine and Health Care: Comments on Papers
by Novak, Mouw, Roach, Cahill, and Hartt," *Journal of
Medicine and Philosophy*, 4 (1979), p. 435.)

That issue of the *Journal* had been planned and edited by James
Gustafson and myself in the hope that theology might reassert its
voice in matters having to do with medicine and with medical ethics.
Subsequent developments have made clear that that issue of the
Journal did little to convince anyone that theology had or has
anything distinctively important to say about these matters. Our
failure in that respect, I think, has everything to do with our inability
to meet the kind of expectations that MacIntyre delineates for
theologians.

Such expectations ask us to emphasize the differences, but
theologians, particularly in this time called modernity, have largely
attempted to play down the differences. Indeed, it has been the task
of theology in recent times to suggest that Christians pretty much
believe what anyone would believe on reflection. The call for
theology to be a "public" discourse, for example, has been the
attempt to show that theological convictions do in fact measure up to
the standards of truthfulness generally recognized in liberal
democratic societies. Only if theology meets those standards can
Christians enter the public arena without apology. (For an article that
nicely describes these developments, as well as suggesting some of
the beginnings of dissenting positions, see Scott Giles and Jeffrey
Greenman, "Recent Work on Religion and Bioethics: A Review
Article," *Biolaw: A Legal and Ethical Reporter on Medicine, Health
Care, and Bioengineering*, II, 7-8 (July-August, 1994), pp. 151-160.)

This strategy has been particularly apparent in religious thinkers who specialize in medical ethics. If Christians, or other religious communities, were characterized by practices or convictions that would make a difference for how medicine was practiced and understood, then Christian ethical reflection would be marginalized. Allegedly, medicine represents an objective, or at least neutral, set of practices that can be used by anyone irrespective of their peculiar personal situation or beliefs. So any attempt to show that theology might make a difference is perceived, morally and politically, as an act of aggression.

I have been identified as one who has emphasized the "differences." Accordingly, I am sometimes described – usually by people who think it's a good idea to have an American flag at a university – as a "sectarian, fideistic tribalist" – a set of attributions in which I take great pleasure. The danger in emphasizing the differences, of course, is that for the Christian, difference can never be an end in itself. If we let our distinctiveness become an end in itself, then we might be tempted to describe "the world" in blacker terms than is warranted.

My first title for this paper may have exemplified that temptation: "The God That Failed: The Pathos of Modern Medicine." After some reflection, however, I decided that no one needs another attack on the characteristically Promethean presumptions of modern medicine. A much more urgent and potentially constructive requirement is to remind ourselves – that is, we who bear the name "Christian" – how we should be patients and, accordingly, how that might shape the kind of medical care that we receive. In other words, one of the things I'm really interested in is changing the focus of the debate. Everyone talks about the "docs." I want to talk about us patients. What kind of patients should create a corresponding medicine? Yet to do that I need to provide, in accordance with MacIntyre's second expectation, a theological critique, or at least an account, of the secular morality and culture that currently shapes medicine and medical ethics. As a way to do that, I am going to say a bit about my original proposed title.

The title, "The God That Failed," originally was used for a book of essays by former communists describing how they became communists and why and how they lost their faith in communism. (*The God That Failed*, edited with an Introduction by Richard Crossman. (New York: Harper and Row, 1963).) The book was first published in 1949. It contains essays by Arthur Koestler, Ignazio Silone, Richard Wright, Andre Gide, Louis Fisher, and Stephen Spender.   Arthur Koestler, one of the essayists, notes that communism, like all true faiths, "involves a revolt against the believer's social environment, and the projection into the future of an ideal derived from the remote past. All utopias are fed from the sources of mythology; the social engineer's blueprints are merely revised editions of the ancient text." (*Ibid.*, p. 16.) For many today, medicine is construed analogously to a Koestler-like understanding of communism – that is, the medical utopian presumption that illness could be cured or at least controlled by medicine is increasingly questioned. You can see that in the development of AIDS. AIDS just shouldn't be there. We knew that if we could deal with cancer and heart failure, we'd be on our way. No new illnesses. Then AIDS comes along . . . that's not in the cards. We are now soon to experience the rise of a whole new set of infectious diseases which our antibiotics have rendered all the more powerful. This is not good news for the American public. Medicine represents another utopia, another god, that has failed.

Like most gods that fail, moreover, medicine is now seen not as a mode of liberation, but as a legitimating ideology which allows some people to control others in the name of liberation. Moreover, like most effective forms of control, the power that medicine exercises over our lives is not perceived as oppressive exactly because the very nature of such power stems from and is secured by its invisibility. In this regard, medicine is but another supervisory strategy so characteristic of modern political regimes. Insofar as we desire what medicine teaches us to desire, we willingly shape our lives to be good medical subjects. The very understanding of our bodies, our "biology," produces and reproduces us to be good servants of the current regime of medicine. For a wonderful set of essays that question the understanding of the body prevalent in modern medicine see *Troubled Bodies: Critical Perspectives on Postmodernism, Medical Ethics, and the Body*, edited by Paul Komesaroff (Durham: Duke University Press, 1995). In his introduction, Komersaroff observes, "The infiltration of the categories of medicine into the way we think about pregnancy and childbirth, menopause, sexual relationships and caring for a sick relative, for example – or, for that matter, merely eating, exercising or just lying in the sun – may profoundly transform the quality of these experiences. In these cases, medical modes of thought introduce into previously unproblematic life experiences evaluative criteria that are formulated in purposive-rational terms. That is, they are presented as purely technical values." (p. 3.) Take for example the notion that we think of our bodies now as a collection of organs. Who does that serve? That's not science. You do not even have to read Foucault to understand that. That we now understand ourselves as having bad kidneys serves those who want to take care of bad kidneys.

The rise of medical ethics in the last twenty-five years is but part of this system of control. Just as princes once surrounded themselves with priests in order to legitimate their power to rule, so physicians now employ, for purposes of legitimizing their own authority and prestige, that strange creature only modernity could produce, the "ethicist." The stress on patient autonomy so characteristic of modern ethics may seem to belie such a legitimating function, but ironically the stress on autonomy turns out to produce the kind of ahistorical accounts of moral agency that most effectively hide from us the power of medicine to shape our lives. Nothing so profoundly betrays the accommodation which contemporary "ethics" has made imperative than the former's penchant for devising rules and guidelines that ostensibly help us resolve hard decisions about life and death. What is lost by concentrating on such "decisions," however, are the forces and structures that make us think that it is incumbent on us to make such choices. For an extraordinary account of how "ethics" has served to legitimate the presumptions of modern medicine, see Gerald McKenny's forthcoming book, *To Relieve the Human Condition: Bioethics and the Technological Utopianism of Modern Medicine* (Albany: State University of New York Press). McKenny observes, "A moral discourse which related the health of the body as well as its mortality and its susceptibility to illness and suffering to broader conceptions of a morally worthy life was succeeded by a moral discourse characterized by efforts to eliminate suffering and expand human choice and thereby overcome the human subjections to natural necessity or fate. The result is that standard bioethics moves within the orbit of the technological utopianism of what I call the Baconian project and its agenda and content are designed to resolve certain issues and problems that arise within that project." McKenny identifies the "Baconian project" with the attempt to eliminate suffering and to expand the realm of human choice through technology.

I can help you feel this out. I teach seminarians. Most people coming to seminary today are not kids anymore. They are usually failed businessmen and they are people who are just tired of being lawyers. They say something like, "I'm just really not into Christology this year. I'm really into relating. I'd like to take some more clinical pastoral education." And we say, "Right, go do that – we are all wounded healers. I mean ministry is relating; that's good." Now a kid can go to medical school today and say, "I'm just really not into anatomy this year. I'm really into relating. I'd like to take some more courses in psychiatry." The medical school faculty says, "Well, who in the hell are you kid? Screw off. Take anatomy or ship out." Now what accounts for that difference? Is it that medical education is so much more morally serious than divinity school education? You're the difference and the reason is very simple. No one believes that an inadequately trained priest might damage his or her salvation since no thinks anything is at stake in salvation. But you do think that an inadequately trained doctor can hurt you. Now I'll tell you what salvation is. When I talk to lay audiences, that is the people who are not associated with medicine,

I ask them how they want to die. And it's very clear. They all want to die quickly in their sleep, painlessly, and without being a burden. They don't want to be a burden because they don't trust their children. They want to die painlessly and in their sleep because, when they die, they don't want to have to know they're dying. They ask doctors to keep them alive to the point that when they die they don't have to know that they're dying and then no one can blame doctors for keeping us alive to no point. It's a wonderful double game. At one time, in the middle ages, what people feared was a sudden death, because what they feared was God. When you fear God, you need to confess your sins. You need to reconcile with your neighbors and so on. You don't want to face God with sin on your soul and you can do something about that. We no longer fear God. We fear death. And that's the reason why medicine is the only priest-craft around that's still interesting, because medicine is about helping us face death without having to come to terms with death.

When I teach seminarians, I try to help them gain a sense of the past power of the church over people's lives by asking them to think how it feels to experience the amazingly technical, administrative, and bureaucratic complexity of a major medical center. Most of us – that is, those of us who are unfortunate enough to find ourselves patients in such centers – feel deeply out of control. Our feeling of powerlessness creates in most of us a corresponding sense that we must somehow please those who are "caring" for us because, otherwise, we fear we may be hurt. Moreover, the hierarchical politics of such medical centers are usually enough to make the description "Byzantine" inadequate. Indeed, if there is anything to the analogy between medicine and Christianity as a social and political power, then some of the current reaction against medicine can be interpreted as the only kind of reformation that makes sense in modernity. The church, after all, is far too weak an institution to make revolt worthwhile. Calling medicine into question, however, is a much more interesting and engaging proposition.

Yet I think the comparison of communism and medicine as instances of "gods that failed" is quite misleading, or at least insufficient to meet MacIntyre's expectation for a theological critique of secular morality and culture. Such an account is inadequate because it overestimates the intensity and pervasiveness of the revolt against medicine. There is, as well, not that much dissent against the current mode of medical ethics. At least to this point such "revolts" have had little effect, since those who raise such questions can be easily dismissed as medical oddities or romantic advocates of moral irrationalism. Medicine is not a god who has failed because revolts against it are so effortlessly deflated, absorbed, or repudiated. That characterization of medicine is morally insufficient.

My point, quite simply, is that medicine is not the god that failed. What has failed is the kind of medicine produced by modernity, which I think is in deep trouble, not because of its pretensions, but because of the role which medicine necessarily has come to play in liberal social orders. That role, quite simply, was and is to bandage the wounds of societies constructed on the premise that God does not exist. Colin Gunton is to be commended for his attempt to read modernity in this fashion. See his, *The One, the Three, and the Many: God, Creation, and the Culture of Modernity* (Cambridge: Cambridge University Press, 1993). I am, in general, quite sympathetic to Gunton's account, though I might have a different reading of who have been and currently are friends and enemies. John Milbank's *Theology and Social Theory* (Oxford: Basil Blackwell, 1990) provides an important contrast to Gunton. Gunton suggests that Milbank is insufficiently trinitarian and, as a result, fails to see that "modernity" did not begin with nominalism and the Reformation, but is rooted earlier (p. 55). I confess that I am not learned enough to enter into such debates, but the hard problem with which both Gunton and Milbank are struggling is how to narrate the "secular" theologically. The great temptation is that secular modes of discourse are now so powerful that theological claims no longer seem to do any work – thus we fail to supply what MacIntyre says we must, that is, a *theological* critique of secular culture and morality.

Few have accomplished this task better than Cardinal Newman. According to Robert Pattison, Newman regarded what most people take as the character of liberalism, that is, a movement for individual rights, free markets, and material progress, as but the trappings of liberalism. For Newman, liberalism's political program was but a symptom of the heretical belief that shaped its basic principles. Liberalism was only a modern version of the Socinianism of the Reformation and that but a version of that Arian heresy of the fourth century. According to Newman, what offended the Arians about Nicaea and Constantinople was not that the Church declared the Son to be "the same in nature" as the Father, but that anything at all was declared about God. The Arians denied our knowledge of God in Christ and, as a result, became the first liberals. In other words, part of what it means to be human is to be capable of being trained in measuring the adequation of truth. However, in the face of the limits of language and our inability to express the truth fully within its parameters, truth must finally be constructed as a contest of wills. Pattison, a liberal, admires Newman because "he was the last good mind in which the dogmatic principle still excited all the ideological excitement of seventeenth-century controversy. As a result, he denominated ancient theological errors and modern social theories indifferently by the interchangeable names Arianism, Socinianism, Hoadlyism, and liberalism. Newman is the missing link between the belief of the old world and the ideology of the new. As he seemed absurd to his brother, so must he to us; his absurdity is inseparable from his message, which is that those things that the worldly mind of the modern era considers ridiculous – namely, the orthodox assertion that belief has a real object, that truth is abiding, and that words can dogmatically state truth – are in fact sublime realities." (*The Great Dissent: John Henry Newman and the Liberal Heresy* (Oxford: Oxford University Press, 1991), p. 143.) In other words, the problem, as John Paul II knows very well, is atheism. Such social orders, which we rightly call liberal, take as their central problem how to secure cooperation between self-interested individuals who have nothing in common other than their desire to survive.

Cooperation is secured by bargains being struck that will presumably secure the best outcomes possible for each individual. (Obviously the account of such bargains varies from Hobbes, to Locke, to Rousseau, and in our own day, to Rawls and Nozick. Such differences matter, but all I am concerned with is to articulate how medicine works in social orders so conceived. The current enthusiasm for rational choice methodologies in the social sciences is a wonderful confirmation of bargaining as the central metaphor for social organization today. For a good critique of the inability of rational choice methods to deliver what they promise, at least in political science, see Donald P. Green and Ian Shapiro, *The Pathologies of Rational Choice Theory: A Critique of Applications in Political Science* (New Haven, CT: Yale University Press, 1994).)

My way of putting this . . . and it's important that it's my way of putting it, because you cannot let the enemy have your terms . . . the project of modernity is to produce people who believe that they should have no story except the story they chose when they had no story. They call that freedom. David and I know better since we are Texans. It would never have occurred to us to choose it. It was destiny – gift. The Jews know it too. Jews and Texans are the only people left who can come to terms with this. But there is a deep difficulty embedded in cultures of modernity that want to produce such people. Notre Dame is built upon this presumption. You take lower class Catholic kids and put them through a liberal arts education and they learn that they should buy Van Gogh prints and not tigers on velvet. And therefore, they think they have become free. What they have become is tasteful consumers. Therefore, they are less likely and less able to resist the powers that are bearing down on them. Buying tigers on black velvet can be a very deep form of resistance. And part of the problem is that such societies make freedom fate. Who told you the story that you should have no story except the story you chose when you had no story? Who told you that? Why did that become your story?

Liberal societies presuppose the only thing people have in common is their fear of death, despite the fact that they share no common understanding of death. So liberalism is that cluster of theories about society that are based on the presumption that we must finally each die alone. Our fear of such a death becomes a source of cooperation. But in liberal society, our cooperation itself reveals the crucial modern presumption that there is nothing quite important enough in our lives that we should risk dying for it. (This paragraph is a slight rewording of a footnote from my *Naming the Silences: God, Medicine, and Suffering* (Grand Rapids: Eerdmans, 1990), p. 123.) I have reproduced it here since I think it the heart of the argument of that book, though few have recognized the importance I attribute to this point. That is, of course, not the fault of my readers, since I was in truth trying to disguise the main argument of that book. *Naming the Silences* is allegedly a book about the suffering and death of children, and I hope it is at least that. But I also wanted to make the case that medicine has become the theodical project of modernity, part of whose task is to save liberalism. That is why I claimed that the book was really an exercise in political theory. I am not here simply trying to articulate in a straightforward fashion what I attempted to do indirectly in that book. *Naming the Silences* has recently been reprinted by Eerdmans under the title *God, Medicine, and Suffering*. Eerdmans thought my original title was hurting the sales of the book. So much for being subtle.)

That's the reason why Americans are dying to have something worth dying for. And that's the reason Americans have become such effective killers. Oh, give us the Gulf war! What a wonderful thing! We get to show we are ready to sacrifice . . . at least Iraqis. And if you don't believe what I was saying about modernity, let me point out the great mystery passage from *Casey*, namely, "At the heart of liberty is the right to define one's own concept of existence, of meaning, of the universe, and of the mystery of human life." How extraordinary! You're a creature. You're going to die. That's the bottom line.

But in liberal societies our cooperation itself reveals the crucial modern presumption that there's nothing quite important enough in our lives, that we should risk dying for. Will Willimon and I wrote a little book called "Resident Aliens" in which one of the passages that made people the most angry, and there were many of them, was, "The greatest enemy of Christianity today is not atheism." What's destroying Christians today is not atheism. If only we could produce some interesting unbelievers. But since we are not particularly interested in producing believers anymore, we have a lot of trouble producing interesting unbelievers. "The greatest enemy of Christianity is sentimentality. The deepest form of sentimentality is people's presumption that they can have children in such a manner that the children do not have to suffer for their convictions." So we wind up bringing up children to make up their own minds. Give me a break! It's not serious. You just drive people crazy.

Yet, at the same time, we all know we must die. Even more telling, we know that the way we die reflects the forms of cooperation, which often take the form of competition, created to hide our own deaths from ourselves and from one another. In such social orders, medicine becomes the insurance policy to give us a sense that none of us will have to come to terms with the reality of our death.

Nowhere is this better seen than in the transformation of the traditional medical imperative, "Do no harm," which has as a corollary, "When in doubt, do not act." It has now become incumbent on physicians to act, for, if they do not, their patients will lose hope or believe the physician to be incompetent. The imperative to act, moreover, drives medical research to discover ever new modes of intervention in order that the physician's power to affect our lives might be enhanced and extended. Of course, the more medical intervention we have, the greater the possibility of making mistakes. To avoid error, physicians become increasingly specialized in the hope that by knowing more and more about less and less they will be prone to commit fewer errors. Which, of course, ironically results in more error, precisely because the patient happens to be more than the sum of his or her parts; but, unfortunately, he or she is increasingly cared for by a medicine that is something less than the sum of its specializations.

It is crucial to note, however, that no one can be blamed for this state of affairs. I often observe that, if you really want to know who the American people are, all you have to do is look at whom they elect to Congress – a sobering judgment. In like manner, I assume that we get exactly the kind of medicine and corresponding medical care that we deserve – again, a sobering judgment. Medicine but exemplifies a secular social order shaped by mechanistic economic and political arrangements that, in turn, reflect the metaphysical presumption that our existence has no purpose other than the arbitrary purposes we create and impose.

The pathos of medicine is that its practice was formed by quite a different set of presuppositions. For example, at least some physicians still presume that they are to care for a patient even though they cannot cure or even alleviate, to any significant extent, the patient's malady. I am acutely aware that this puts the issue too simply, since part of the power of modern medicine is constituted by its power to name "illness" that should then be subject to medical intervention. I have dealt with such questions in my *Suffering Presence: Theological Reflections on Medicine, the Mentally Handicapped and the Church* (Notre Dame: University of Notre Dame Press, 1986), but discussion of these questions seems rightly to me to be unending. Medical care, moreover, is still governed by the presumption that a patient is to be cared for in a manner independent of and precinding from all other considerations concerning the worth of the patient to the wider society. Our pathos as physicians and patients is that we no longer are constituted by practices that make such presuppositions intelligible, let alone coherent. This is one of the reasons, I suspect, that medicine has seemed such a fertile ground for theological reflection, since, at least, some of the practices of medicine continue to constitute a space that allows certain theological claims to retain a semblance of intelligibility and persuasiveness.

II   THE CHRISTIAN VIRTUE OF PATIENCE

No practice signals medicine's ambiguous presence in modernity better than the presumption that the subject of the physician's art is called "a patient." I am well aware that this is being changed to "customer," but nonetheless, we still have cultural lags. I like cultural lags. Cultural lags are very important and you can make something of them. We Methodists even still say that we believe in the Trinity. Now that's a cultural lag that you can make something of. Now that I am back among the Methodists, I have discovered that we have a conviction. It's that God is nice and that we ought to be nice too. We ought to be nice since we are a sanctificationist people. So you can do something with cultural lags.

We are, of course, the most impatient of patients, an observation that should not be surprising if the analysis I have given to this point is even close to being right. Yet the very fact that we are still called patients provides an opportunity for reflection on what difference it might make for how we, as Christians, come to know ourselves as patients who are truly patient. By exploring what it means for the Christian to embody the virtue of patience, I hope at least to suggest how we might begin to make some headway toward addressing MacIntyre's expectation that the theologian should say what difference it makes to be a Christian, as well as suggesting what that difference might mean for the specific problems arising from the modern practice of medicine.

There are at least two unusual aspects to this way of proceeding that should be highlighted at the beginning. The first has to do with the retrieval of the virtues for modern ethics and, the second, the centrality of one particular virtue for the practice of modern medicine. Emphasizing the importance of the virtues for how one thinks about ethics, and in particular medical ethics, has only recently begun. A welcome exception is *Virtue and Medicine: Explorations in the Character of Medicine*, edited by Earl E. Shelp (Dordrecht: D. Reidel Publishing Company, 1985). Karen Lebacqz's essay "The Virtuous Patient" (pp. 275-288) is particularly relevant for what I am trying to do in this essay. Lebacqz argues that three virtues – fortitude, prudence, and hope – are central to the task of being a patient. My only difficulty with her account is knowing from whence such virtues come. William May has also developed the importance of the virtues in his "The Virtues in a Professional Setting" in *Medicine and Moral Reasoning*, edited by K.W.M. Tulford, Grant Gillet, and Janet Martin Soskice (Cambridge: Cambridge University Press, 1994), pp. 75-90. For an overview of recent work in medical ethics on the importance of virtue see my article, "Virtue and Character," in the new edition of the *Encyclopedia of Bioethics*. There are many reasons why the virtues have been neglected in modern Western ethics, but perhaps the most significant factor in their recovery is their unavoidability if one wishes to provide any coherent account of the tradition in which one is standing. Alasdair MacIntyre's *After Virtue* (Notre Dame: University of Notre Dame Press, 1984) is, of course, the best account not only of why the virtues have been ignored in modernity but of why the virtues must be unavoidably located within tradition-shaped practices if they are to make any sense. What is particularly important for my purposes is to show how the absence of a thick account of the virtues makes any consideration of the virtues or a virtue in medicine far too abstract. In other words, the great problem with becoming a patient is that too often the first time we are forced to exercise patience is when we become sick, and that is probably the worst time to begin to be patient. It's hard enough knowing how to be patient when you are well, let alone when you become ill. So, if we are to understand the inescapable importance of patience as a virtue, we cannot begin by considering the patient in the context of medicine – which may well mean that I will test your patience even as I must ask you to bear with me as I explore how Christians have understood patience as an integral virtue to the Christian life.

The second unusual aspect of my approach is the identification of patience as a significant virtue. If the virtues in general have been ignored in recent moral reflection, the virtue of patience has even been less prominent, which creates the problem of knowing how to begin to think about patience, since we have such a dearth of examples. Happily, however, patience has played a prominent role in Christian accounts of the moral life, and I propose to begin where those accounts begin – namely, with God.

I was first made aware of the significance of patience as a virtue by struggling with John Howard Yoder's account of non-violence as embodied in Christ's cross. Yoder observes that apparent complicity with evil, which the nonresistant stance allegedly involves, has always been a stumbling block to nonpacificists. In response, Yoder points out "that this attitude, leaving evil to be evil, leaving the sinner free to separate himself from God and sin against man, is part of the nature of *agape* itself, as revealed already in creation. If the cutting phrase of Peguy, '*complice, c'est pire que coupable*,' were true, then God Himself must needs be the guilty one for making man free and again for letting His innocent Son be killed. The modern tendency to equate involvement with guilt should have to apply *par excellence*, if it were valid at all, to the implication of the all-powerful God in the sin of His creatures. God's love for men begins right at the point where He permits sin against Himself and against man, without crushing the rebel under his own rebellion. The word for this is divine *patience*, not complicity." (See *The Original Revolution* (Scottdale, PA: Herald Press, 1971), pp. 64-65.) Drawing on Yoder, I argued in *The Peaceable Kingdom: A Primer in Christian Ethics* (Notre Dame: University of Notre Dame Press, 1983), that hope and patience are central Christian virtues (pp. 102-106). I have continued to find ways to display that contention in my subsequent work, though as far as I can tell, without much success. For one of my favorite attempts to try to remind us of the importance of patience, see the last chapter of *Christian Existence Today: Essays on Church, World, and Living In Between* (Durham: Labyrinth Press, 1988), pp. 253-266. The title of the chapter is "Taking Time For Peace: The Moral Significance of the Trivial."

Cyprian, for example, begins his "On the Good of Patience" by observing that philosophers also claim to pursue the virtue of patience, but "their patience is as false as is their wisdom." For how can anyone be either wise or patient unless he knows the wisdom and patience of God? In contrast, Cyprian says, that Christians:

> [A]re philosophers not in words but in deeds; we exhibit our wisdom not by our dress, but by truth; we know virtues by their practice rather than through boasting of them; we do not speak great things but we live them. Therefore, as servants and worshipers of God, let us show by spiritual homage the patience that we learn from heavenly teachings. For that virtue we have in common with God. In Him patience has its beginning, and from Him as its source it takes its splendor and dignity. The origin and greatness of patience proceeds from God its Author. The quality that is dear to God ought to be loved by man. (Cyprian, *De Bono Patientia*: *A Translation with an Introduction and Commentary*, by Sister M. George Edward Conway, S.S.J. (Washington, DC: The Catholic University Press of American, 1957), p. 65.)

Cyprian's account of patience closely parallels Tertullian's earlier treatise, "On Patience." The latter can be found in Volume III of *The Ante-Nicene Fathers* (Grand Rapids: Eerdmans, 1989), pp. 707-717.

Augustine drew on both Tertullian and Cyprian for his "On Patience," which can be found in *A Library of Fathers of the Holy Catholic Church, Anterior to the Division of the East and West*, translated by Members of the English Church (Oxford: John Henry Parker Press, 1937), pp. 542-562. Sister Conway provides a very helpful comparison of these three treatments of patience. Augustine is careful to explain that just as God is jealous without any darkening of spirit, so He is patient without "thought of passion." (p. 544.)

According to Cyprian, God's patience is clearly shown by the way he endures profane temples, replete with earthly images and idolatrous rites meant to insult God's majesty and honor. Yet nowhere is God's patience more clearly exemplified than in the life of Christ. Tertullian likewise observes that the patience of God made it possible for him to be conceived in a mother's womb, await a time for birth, delay growing up, and even when grown up to be less than eager to receive recognition, having himself been baptized by his own servant. Throughout his ministry, Jesus cared for the ungrateful, and even refrained from pointing out the betrayer who was part of his own company. Tertullian says, "Moreover, while He is being betrayed, while He is being led up 'as a sheep for a victim,' [for] 'so He no more opens His mouth than a lamb under the power of the shearer,' He to whom, had He willed it, legions of angels would at one word have presented themselves from the heavens, approved not the avenging sword of even one disciple." (Tertullian, p. 708.)

Tertullian and Cyprian alike make much of Matthew 5: 43-48, since the refusal to return evil for evil is the very character of God and, accordingly, through imitation, the way the sons and daughters of God are made perfect. As Tertullian says, "In this principal precept the universal discipline of patience is succinctly comprised, since evil-doing is not conceded even when it is deserved." (*Ibid.*, p. 711. Cyprian's reflections on Matthew are found on pages 68-69.) Such patience is not only in the mind, but in the body, for according to Tertullian, "[J]ust as Christ exhibited it in his body so do we. By the affliction of the flesh, a victim is able to appease the Lord by means of the sacrifice of humiliation." (Tertullian, p. 715.) Now don't miss the fact that you find that profoundly offensive. None of you are going to pray the prayer of the Middle Ages, "Thank you for giving me this sickness that I may take on Christ's cross." Tertullian continues, "By making a libation to the Lord of sordid raiment, together with scantiness of food, content with simple diet and the pure drink of water in conjoining fasts *to all this*; this *bodily* patience adds a grace to our prayers for good, a strength to our prayers against evil; this opens the ears of Christ *our* God, dissipates severity, elicits clemency." (*Ibid.*) Thus, that which springs from a virtue of the mind is perfected in the flesh, and, finally, by the patience of the flesh, does battle under persecution. (Cyprian observes that the Christian should not hasten to revenge the pain of persecution, since vengeance is the Lord's. "Therefore, even the martyrs as they cry out and as they hasten to their punishment in the intensity of their suffering are still ordered to wait and to show patience until the appointed time is fulfilled and the number of martyrs is complete." p. 89.)

I have to tell you that I first began to think about patience primarily in relationship to pacifism. The deepest challenge to those of us committed to non-violence is that we stand and watch the innocent suffer for our convictions. The just war people have to do the same thing. It's not like there is some special case for us. And so it is a deep problem for Christian life that you have to be patient while watching the innocent suffer for your convictions.

Suicide is, accordingly, out of the question. Job is the great exemplar in this regard, resisting his wife's suggestion that he should curse God and die. Augustine calls upon those who would kill themselves under persecution to look to "this man," meaning both Job and Christ. Like true martyrs who neither seek death nor invite it prematurely, they ought to bear all patiently rather than "to dare death impatiently." According to Augustine, all that can be said to those who have killed themselves under persecution is, "Woe unto them which have lost patience!" (Augustine, pp. 550-551.)

Augustine, following Tertullian and Cyprian, maintains that only that patience which is shaped by Christ is true patience. As Augustine says, "properly speaking those are patient who would rather bear evils without inflicting them, than inflict them without bearing them. As for those who bear evils that they may inflict evil, their patience is neither marvelous nor praiseworthy, for it is not patience at all; we may marvel at their hardness of heart, but we must refuse to call them patient." (Augustine, p. 544.) Aquinas uses this quote to counter the claim that patience is not a virtue, since it can sometimes be found in wicked men. (See *Summa Theologiae*, translated by Fathers of the English Dominican Province (Chicago: Encyclopedia Britannica, 1952), II-II, 136, 1, 2.) Such patience cannot come from "the strength of the human will," but rather must come as a gift of the Holy Spirit. (Augustine, p. 551.) The name of that gift is, of course, charity. Augustine says of this charity:

[W]ithout which in us there cannot be true patience, because in good men it is the love of God which endureth all things, in bad men the lust of the world. But this love is in us by the Holy Spirit which was given us. Whence, of Whom cometh in us love, of Him cometh patience. But the lust of the world, when it patiently bears the burdens of any manner of calamity, boasts of the strength of its own will, like as of the stupor of disease, not robustness of health. This boasting is insane: it is not the language of patience, but of dotage. A will like this in that degree seems more patient of bitter ills, in which it is more greedy of temporal good things, because more empty of eternal.(Augustine, pp. 557-558.)

Augustine, like all Christian theologians, makes constant appeals to scripture in support of this argument – I Corinthians 13:4 being, of course, the central text. Charity must form patience, but it is equally the case that charity needs patience. In a remarkable passage, Cyprian says,

Charity is the bond of brotherhood, the foundation of peace, the steadfastness and firmness of unity; it is greater than both hope and faith; it excels both good works and suffering for the faith; and, as an eternal virtue, it will abide with us forever in the kingdom of heaven. Take patience away from it, and thus forsaken, it will not last; take away the substance of enduring and tolerating, and it attempts to last with no roots or strength. Accordingly, the apostle, when he was speaking about charity, joined forbearance and patience to it, saying: Charity is magnanimous, charity is kind, charity does not envy, is not puffed up, is not provoked, thinks no evil, loves all things, believes all things, hopes all things, endures all things. By this he showed that charity can persevere steadfastly because it has learned how to endure all things. And in another place he says, "bearing with one another in love, taking every care to preserve the unity of the Spirit in the union of peace." He proved that neither unity nor peace can be preserved unless brothers cherish one another with mutual forbearance and preserve the bond of unity with patience as intermediary." (p. 81.)

Augustine knows that most of us become patient because we lust after the world.

Aquinas, like Tertullian, Cyprian, and Augustine, maintains that true patience is that which comes from God. Like them, he is aware that many people seem to display patience without the gift of the spirit, but the problem with construing patience as a "natural virtue" is that it is not shaped by the appropriate sadness and joy constitutive of Christian patience. For Aquinas, a true understanding of our place as creatures must include an insuperable sadness and dejection about our condition. Christ's suffering on the cross exemplifies the sorrow that must be present in every Christian's life. I am indebted to Lee Yearley's wonderful account of Aquinas's view of patience in his *Mencius and Aquinas: Theories of Virtue and Conceptions of Courage* (Albany: State University of New York Press, 1990), pp. 136-143. Crucial for understanding Aquinas's views is the significance of his account of the passions, and in particular, sadness as a passion. See *Summa Theologiae*, I-II, 35-39. Yearley, quite rightly, observes that Aquinas thinks his understanding of the place of sadness in the Christian life is the crucial difference between Stoicism and Christianity. The Christian cannot seek to be free of sadness for without the appropriate sadness we lack the ability to be joyful. Christians must "be saddened by their own frailty, by the suffering present in the world, and by their inability to change either fundamentally." (Yearley, p. 137.)

Josef Pieper, however, rightly notes that Thomas's account of patience does not entail passivity. Patience is a necessary component of fortitude, which, as Pieper observes, seems incongruous for many people because for them patience has,

Come to mean an indiscriminate, self-immolating, crabbed, joyless, and spineless submission to whatever evil is met with or worse, deliberately sought out. Patience, however, is something quite other than indiscriminate acceptance of any and every evil: "The patient man is not the one who does not flee from evil, but the one who does not allow himself to be made inordinately sorrowful thereof." To be patient means to preserve cheerfulness and serenity of mind in spite of injuries that result from the realization of the good. Patience does not imply the exclusion of energetic, forceful activity, but simply explicitly and solely the exclusion of sadness and confusion of heart. Patience keeps man from the danger that his spirit may be broken by grief and lose its greatness. Patience, therefore, is not the tear-veiled mirror of a 'broken' life (as one might easily assume in the face of what is frequently presented and praised under this name), but the radiant embodiment of ultimate integrity. In the words of Hildegard of Bingen, patience is "the pillar which nothing can soften." And Thomas, following Holy Scripture (Luke 21:19), summarizes with superb precision: "Through patience man possesses his soul." (*The Four Cardinal Virtues* (Notre Dame: University of Notre Dame Press, 1966), p. 129.)

From Aquinas's perspective, the problem is how to prevent sadness, which we appropriately feel, from becoming depression, despair, or apathy. Aquinas says, "Patience is to ensure that we do not abandon virtue's good through dejection of this kind." (*Summa Theologiae*, II-II, 136, 4, 2.) Yearley highlights this wonderful passage:

Patience makes us capable of being rightly saddened without succumbing to the temptation to give up hope. A patience-formed sadness produces joy because each is the effect of charity. Such a joy, "[M]akes us delight in the divine good as shared by us . . . [yet joy] can be impeded by something contrary to it, (so that) our joy can be mingled with sadness, in the sense that we grieve over what opposes this participation in the divine good in ourselves, or in our neighbors, whom we love as ourselves. (*Summa Theologiae*, II-II, 28,2.)

I have used Yearley's translation of this passage. Crucial for sustaining such joy in the midst of sadness is the kind of materialism required in the Christian belief in the Incarnation and Resurrection. Our belief in the bodily Resurrection – that is, that the Resurrection is not so much a throwing off of our human flesh but rather an exchanging of our present body for a new body so that we may dwell in a new heaven and a new earth, means that Christians hope that "all manner of things shall be well" can never be a facile optimism that evades the reality of pain. As Dr. Jim Fodor observed to me:

Simply to encourage people to see things differently, while leaving things as they are, is to reinforce their slavery, the reinforcement of which is all the more insidious precisely because it is disguised as a proclamation of the truth to set us free. Christianity, in other words, is not merely a way of 'regarding,' 'looking at,' or 'interpreting' reality. Christianity is not a 'theory' but a way of life, a way of discipleship. And discipleship is concrete, specific; it occurs – or fails to occur – in particular practices and patterns of engagements, relationships, suffering, and worship. Thus the importance of the practice of 'bodily patience' for guarding against the tendency, all too common among many modern Christians, to affirm 'the primacy of the spiritual' to the neglect of the material conditions of redemption. The practical, material display of Christian virtue necessary for patience is in finding a gift from God and not something we cultivate willfully or from our own strength, apart from God's help. In fact, patience is often something we reluctantly accept, if at all, and then only after a long and painful struggle to acknowledge our creaturely limits and the sense in which most things in our life remain out of control.

Lee Yearley rightly suggests that Aquinas's account of patience combines two different, even apparently paradoxical, attitudes. Christians must judge our earthly life according to the standard evident in God's goodness. Yet Christians must also adhere to the future good of possible union with God and the present good evident in God's manifestations in the world and in people's lives. Neither side of such an attitude can be lost. We must persist in such sadness, yet that very sadness must not be allowed to overwhelm the pursuit of the good, the accurate recognition of its forms, and a correct belief about the world's ultimate character. "This attitude is distinctive enough that it can arise, Aquinas thinks, only from the theological virtues. Charity's friendship with God is most crucial, but the attitude manifest in patience also rests on faith and displays the mean between presumption and despair that appears in hope." (Yearley, p. 139.)

Christian patience, like all the virtues that come from charity, is a gift. There are, of course, semblances of the virtues. Patience in particular is frequently confused with the virtues not formed by charity. For example, there is a kind of tempered optimism in which people "either rest too confidently on their past experiences of overcoming dejection or manifest a phlegmatic or unreflective disposition at inappropriate times. Their optimism, then, reflects a flawed hope that is close to dullness or presumption. It displays an untempered attitude that expresses itself in the naive belief that all will turn out for the best." (*Ibid.*) That's Stoicism; that's not Christianity. Yearley notes that Aquinas did not examine the semblances of patience in the systematic manner in which he explored the semblances of courage. Yet given patience's close relation to endurance, the crucial aspect of courage, Yearley rightly uses the semblances of courage to suggest analogies for how Aquinas might have understood the semblances of patience.

Though the comparisons of the semblances of patience (and courage and other virtues) with true patience are usually negative, it is a mistake to assume that positive comparisons are not also a possibility. Since we are God's good creatures, we should expect to find in those who are not Christians indications of God's patience. The problem, then, is not that non-Christians fail to exhibit any of the virtues, but that they do and because they do they are just as likely to display them in ways that may be either destructive and/or constructive. The Christian advantage is to be part of God's people, which makes us vulnerable to the judgments of others who have acquired the wisdom necessary to understand the interrelation of the virtues. That's why it's so important, as Aquinas understands, that you have to have passion for sadness. You don't want to deny it. You cannot deny it. You cannot have *apatheia*. The Christian has no such wan hope, sustained as we are by a patience that looks to our misfortunes, even the misfortune of our illness and death, as part of our service to one another as God's people.

III   CHRISTIAN PATIENCE AND BEING A PATIENT

Those who believe there is no God or those who believe that God does not matter have no time for such patience. Our lives are constituted by what Albert Borgmann characterizes as a kind of addiction to hyperactivity. Believing, as we do, that we live in a world of infinite possibilities, we find ourselves constantly striving, restless for what we are not sure. (Albert Borgmann, *Crossing the Postmodern Divide* (Chicago: University of Chicago Press, 1992), pp. 97-102.) We call our restlessness freedom, but too often such freedom seems more like fate, especially when we get exactly what we strive after only to discover that it does not satisfy – thus the peculiar combination in modern life that seems to conjoin an attitude of metaphysical indeterminism with Stoic fatalism.

As Christians, of course, we should not be surprised to discover that our world is constituted by impatience. Tertullian ascribed to the devil the creation of impatience, since the devil could not endure the patience God exemplified in creation. According to Tertullian, the devil passed to Eve that same impatience when, through his speech, he "breathed on her a spirit infected with impatience: so certain is it that she would have never sinned at all, if she had honored the divine edict by maintaining her patience to the end." (Tertullian, p. 710.)   Gerald J. Schiffhorst, in a similar fashion, argues that in *Paradise Lost* Milton "relies on patience to express the Christian's proper response to the divine will while ironically revealing the anti-heroism of Satan, whose blind impatience reverses what Milton called the 'better fortitude' of patience.   Satan's struggle to fight God is undercut by the 'pleasing sorcery' of a false heroism whereas Adam learns to arm himself with patience 'to overcome by suffering' what God will unfold.   The centrality of 'patience as the truest fortitude' (*Samson Agonistes*, 654) in revealing this fundamental contrast demonstrates the importance of the virtue in the poem" ("Satan's False Heroism in *Paradise Lost* as a Perversion of Patience," *Christianity and Literature*, 38, 2 (Winter, 1984), p. 13).   Schiffhorst provides a very helpful contrast of Christian patience with Stoic indifference by noting the difference between the Christian understanding of providence and the Stoic idea of fortune.   He notes that "this basic Christian-pagan distinction helps us recall that Christ's victory over death was a victory over Fortune, and so the virtuous Christian can have everlasting life by imitating Christ's perfect patience.   As Miles Coverdale says in his important Elizabethan treatise on patience, 'The   impatient man complains against God and ascribes prosperity to his own wisdom, blaming blind Fortune for adversity.   Without ascribing dispassionate Stoic virtues to Satan, we can nevertheless say that his false heroism is rooted in a stubborn pride and that he exhibits all the passions of the impatient man: wrath, despair, grief, and envy.'" (pp. 14-15.)   For a wonderful collection of essays on patience, see Gerald J.   Schiffhorst, ed.   *The Triumph of Patience: Medieval and Renaissance Studies* (Orlando: University Presses of Florida, 1978). Particularly interesting is Elizabeth Kirk's essay entitled, "'Who

Suffreth More Than God?': Narrative Redefinition of Patience in *Patience* and *Piers Plowman*," pp. 88-105. She not only provides a wonderful commentary on the medieval poet of the *Pearl*, but ends with a delightful quote from Chaucer's Parson that she thinks contains everything written large in *Patience* and *Piers Plowman*:

> Patience, that is another remedie agayns Ire, is a vewtu that suffreth swetely every mannes goodness, and is nat wroth for noon harm that is doon to hyn . . . This vertu maketh a man lyk to God, and maketh hym Goddes owene deere child, as seith Crist. This vertu disconfiteth thyn enemy. And therfore seith the wise man, If thow wolt vengukysse thyn enemy, lerne to suffre . . . And understond wel that obedience is parfit, whan that a man dooth gladly and hastily, with good herte entirely, al that he should do. (p. 102.)

She passed her impatience on to Adam, which in turn produced impatient sons. The very impatience that "had immersed Adam and Eve in death, taught their son, too, to begin with murder." (Tertullian, p.710.) As a pacifist, I find Tertullian's suggestion that our violence lies in our impatience as intriguing as it is persuasive. That murder was the fruit of impatience, as Cain impatiently refused his God-given obligation to his brother.

Yet surely medical care has been one of God's gifts which is our prerogative to use as a hedge against the impatience of the world. To care for one another when we cannot cure is surely one of the many ways we serve one another patiently. It makes no sense to be committed to alleviating the other's pain in a manner that makes all other considerations irrelevant if we have not been made to be patient people. Yet it is surely the case that the powers of impatience have breathed on the practice of modern medicine and, accordingly, led it to promise more than it can or should deliver. In the frustration of being unable to meet impatient expectations, we are threatened with a medicine that kills in the name of relieving suffering. That's how you have to read Kevorkian. Once medicine promises to keep us alive, then it must put us to death. Otherwise medicine is not being compassionate, which is the surest sign of why compassion is indeed a distressful virtue when it is separated from the truth of the cross. Compassion will just drive you crazy. You will do the most inhumane things in the name of love.

Christians are, of course, as implicated in this strange reversal as our non-Christian neighbors. But these issues are far too serious to play, "Who is to blame?" The challenge is rather whether Christians have any contribution to make that would help us discover the proper limits of our care of one another through the office of medicine. It is not the Christian's task to suggest new and better theories about medical care, though some Christians engaged in that care may have some contributions to make. Rather, if Christians have anything to offer, it is to be patients who embody the virtue of Christian patience.

To be patient when we are sick requires first that we learn how to practice patience when we are not sick. God has given us ample resources for recovering the practice of patience. First and foremost, we have been given our bodies which will not let us do whatever we think we should be able to do. I am acutely aware, as anyone must be after the work of Foucault, that appeals to the "body" are anything but unproblematic. Recent historical work helps us better understand why Paul could think that nothing was more "spiritual" than the body or that the body as the peculiarly "spiritual" has great potential for helping us rethink the relation of Christian practices and the practice of medicine. I have in mind such works as Peter Brown's, *The Body and Society: Men, Women and Sexual Renunciation in Early Christianity* (Boston: Faber, 1988) and my colleague, Dale Martin's, wonderful book, *The Corinthian Body* (New Haven: Yale University Press, forthcoming). Particularly important is a better understanding of the "therapy of desire" characteristic of Christian practice in contrast to the assumptions of Galen and the other Hellenistic philosophic schools. For example, we need a Christian account parallel to Nussbaum's *The Therapy of*

Desire. Brown's book is obviously a good beginning, but one has the feeling that we are just beginning to understand better what Augustine and Aquinas understood far better than we about the nature of the passions. I am indebted to Mr. Thomas Harvey, a graduate student at Duke, for a paper in which he explored how Augustine provided an alternative to Galen's understanding of the body. We are our bodies and, as such, we are creatures destined to die. The trick is to learn to love the great good things my body makes possible without hating my body, if for no other reason than that the death of my body is also my death. To practice the patience of the body is to be put on the way to holiness as we learn that we are not our own creations.

Secondly, we have been given one another. To learn to live with the unavoidability of the other is to learn to be patient. Such patience comes not just from our inability to have the other do our will, but more profoundly is constituted by the love that the presence of the other can and does create in us. For our loves, like our bodies, contain our deaths. Such love, if it is not to be fearful of its loss, must be patient. Patience names the time required for the constitution of the story that we must be able to tell together, the story that in fact constitutes our love.

I am aware that the emphasis on patience as the virtue essential to the doctor-patient relationship may appear particularly perverse, since it seems to make the patient even more powerless. There is rightly an asymmetry between the doctor and patient inasmuch as the physician has authority that the patient does not or should not have. Once, however, it is understood that medicine names an activity in which doctor and patient are jointly involved, I think how patience works in such a relationship not so much as to increase the possibilities of abuse of power but to decrease the possibility of such misuse. Crucial in this respect is how Christian patience requires the Church for its display. Without the kind of friendship, dependency, trust, and mutual nurturing imbedded in the worship of God, patience always risks the possibility of becoming malformed. That is why I suggested in *Suffering Presence* that institutionalized medicine requires a church for sustaining the kind of presence that physicians, nurses, and others in medical settings provide. The hospital, I suspect, is the best exemplification of the kind of care the Church should make possible and sustain. Dr. Jim Fodor suggested to me that it would be fascinating to compare the ways people come under the care of either the Church or the hospital.

People do not "choose" to be sick, but they often "choose" the hospital as the place they should receive care. How the necessity of the choice to go to the hospital is made is surely one of the significant issues before us.

Thirdly, we have been given time and space for the acquisition of habits that come from worthy activities such as growing food, building shelters, spinning cloth, writing poems, playing baseball. Such activities not only take time but create time by forcing us to take first one step and then another. Moreover, these activities must be passed on to future generations through tradition-constituted practices and stories. Patience constitutes our ability to tell such stories well so that we and our children may be rightly entertained. One of the institutions that embodies that patience is called "University." How do we justify what we are doing here, right now, in the face of so much hunger? How do you justify Notre Dame in the face of so much injustice, if you don't think the university is the place where we pass on, from one generation to the other, the wisdom garnered, hard won, in patience, as a people learning to live together.

These resources, these practices of patience – and there are others – are not simply "there," but are shaped by the narrative of God's patient care of the world. This is but another way of insisting, with Aquinas, that it is impossible to have patience without charity – that is, without friendship with God. Put simply, our very ability to take the time to enjoy God's world, when we are well as when we are sick, depends on our recognition that this is God's world.

Yet, when we are sick, talk of joy seems too much a gesture of false courage. Still, Aquinas maintained that the sadness occasioned by our own and another's illness is not to be denied. The acknowledgment of such sadness is part of the Christian gift for the sustaining the ill and those who care for the ill. To be a patient who has been formed by the virtue of patience, however, is to be a patient who does not believe that life is an end in itself. Indeed, a patient formed by patience knows that the enemy is neither illness nor the death that it intimates, but the enemy is all that would tempt us to be impatient or fatalistic in the face of our "bad luck." I put quotes around this phrase to indicate its everyday usage but also to mark my unease with the phrase. Luck is a Stoic, not a Christian, notion that implies fortune that is blind. Christians do not believe the world is constituted or determined by fortune since we believe we are under God's providential care. These matters are too large for treatment here, but, for at least some of my thoughts on such matters, see my "Can Aristotle Be a Liberal: Nussbaum on Luck," *Soundings* 72, 4 (Winter 1989) pp. 675-691.

If we as Christians could be such patient patients – and there is every reason to think that we can – I suspect that we might well have a witness to make to our non-Christian neighbor. We might even have something to say, not only about the kind of people who should be called to be physicians and nurses, but about the kind of training they should receive as well. To do that, we would have to take the risk of being different. But then that is no great risk for a people who, because they have learned to be patient, believe that they have all the time in the world for such worthy work.

(I am indebted to Dr. Jim Fodor, Mr. Scott Saye, and Dr. Katherine Miles Wallace for their critique of this essay, as well as for their suggestions for how it might be improved.)

Response to
PRACTICING PATIENCE:
HOW CHRISTIANS SHOULD
BE SICK

Michael J. Baxter

IN MEMORY OF AN IMPATIENT PATIENT

My father had a stroke in August 1976 at the age of fifty-eight. It put him in the hospital for about a month and left him with the right side of his face partially paralyzed and drooping. "Why didn't you tell me about my face?" he asked as he looked at himself in the bedroom mirror for the first time in four weeks. "It's not that bad," I assured him, "it'll straighten out." It did straighten out eventually, but that trip home from the hospital marked his entry on to a path of declining health that he was never able to get off for the next sixteen years.

Up to that point, my father had been active, vital. He was a big man, a six-foot-four, 285-pound bear of a man. He worked for the State of New York for forty years, first, in the Public Works Department as a draftsman, then in the Education Department as a cost analyst for the state museum being put in downtown Albany. But he did not live to work. He worked to live. Like many of his generation, he returned from overseas to start a family with his war bride. He bought a lot outside of Albany and contracted for a house that he himself finished building when the contractor went bankrupt. He and his friends poured the concrete for the cellar floor. He and my mother's father hauled in railroad ties to construct a split-level back yard that was big enough for a large patio and screen house on the upper level and for baseball, football or horseshoes on the lower level. It was the best place in the neighborhood for me and my sister and our friends to play hide-and-go-seek at night. It took an hour and a half to mow, another hour to clip the hedges. My father worked in the yard on Saturdays before settling in to watch the Yankees or the Giants on T.V. He and my mother had people over to the house just about every weekend, neighborhood friends on Fridays or Saturdays, or my mother's family on many Sundays. They had hamburgers, hotdogs, steaks (when they could afford it), and clams on special occasions cooked in the big steamer stored in the tool shed out back. The beer was always flowing. They knew how to throw a party. And my father was always at the center of it. When Jay Hulihan, Bill Cookfair or one of his other friends would walk up to the back porch, they'd often shout out, "Where's Big Jack?" That's what people called him. "Big Jack."

In spite of his vitality, my father had health problems for most of his life, mainly having to do with his legs. He was hit by a piece of shrapnel during the war and spent several months in a military hospital in Italy before returning to the front lines. His injury brought him a purple heart and a limp that got more pronounced as the years went by, especially when he worked in the yard all day. But his real problem emerged in his thirties after a friend next door noticed that he was thirsty all the time and needed to pee a lot. It turned out he had diabetes, a disease that even then was quite manageable. Thus every morning while growing up I would witness what at that time was a diabetic's prescribed ritual. My mother would use tongs to dip a hypodermic needle into boiling water and set it on the counter to cool. Then my father would use it to draw the insulin (80 UPH) out of a little, refrigerated glass bottle, plunge it into the fleshy part of his upper arm, inject the insulin, then pull the needle out fast and quickly wipe his arm with a cotton swab soaked in alcohol. It was a simple, two-minute routine but without it he would "have a reaction," as my mother would somberly remind my sister and me. I remember two reactions. The first, when I was in grade school, left him stretched out on the living room floor with my mother spoon feeding him frozen orange juice concentrate straight from the can. He went into the VA hospital and I remember being hoisted up outside his window and talking to him while he wore a surgical mask. The second episode occurred some years later while he and I were shopping in Woolworths. He suddenly grabbed a handful of Hershey bars and headed past the cash registers and right out the door, all the while leaning heavy on my shoulder, using it as a moving hand rail. Once we made it to the car, he sat in front of the steering wheel stuffing the candy bars into his mouth. After he came out of it, he turned and ordered me, "now, don't go telling your mother." She knew his eyesight was worsening and he was experiencing numbness in his hands and feet and he didn't want to get her all worked up. Besides, he didn't want to contend with a dietary regime that would exclude some of the things he loved most in this world, like peanuts, potato pancakes and a nightly six pack of beer. He was not one to alter his lifestyle.

With time, his medical problems caught up to him. At the end of my freshman year in high school, we moved out of the house and yard of my childhood into a one-story ranch house. My mother liked this house better than the other one, but the more pressing reason was that, as she'd put it, "your father couldn't take the stairs." The yard was also more manageable. For a while, his patterns did not change much. He took on more responsibility at work. He coached my Pop Warner football team and came to all my high school games. He shouted his way through my wrestling matches and gloated when I won. He drove with my mother several times to visit me at Allegheny College in Meadville, Pennsylvania. The two of them flew with another couple to visit their son in California. But these trips took their toll on his legs, leaving him moaning in bed for a day or two afterwards. Looking back, I think he had a sense of living on borrowed time. I feel this most poignantly when I recall the summer between my junior and senior years in college when my roommate Eddie came to stay at our house for three weeks. For Eddie and me, it was three weeks of partying: me going to work as a lifeguard at the local pool around ten in the morning, Eddie coming to join me in the afternoon, then the two of us going out and coming back in the middle of the night to cook eggs in the kitchen. But we would always come back to the house before going out and drink beers with my father and have a lot of laughs. He let us know that he could "still keep up with you guys." For those three weeks he did. But on the day my father dropped Eddie off at the Thruway exit so he could hitchhike home – that was the day my sister walked up to me while I was up in the lifeguard chair and told me, "We gotta go to the hospital. Dad had a stroke."

Not long after my father went into the hospital, the people working for him told us that he had been having blackouts of some sort for months. The doctors surmised that these were "mini strokes." He never returned to work; he was "forced to retire" as people put it. The following January, they threw a banquet for him and gave him a gold watch for his forty years of service to the State. From then on, his life was centered at home. It was not the kind of retirement he had been looking forward to. No trips to Buffalo to see his cousin Jess. No drives across country in a Winnebago. He had a hard enough time driving around Delmar and into Albany. His eyes got worse due to the diabetes, so much so that his family and friends started commenting on how dangerous he was on the road. For several years, he barely made it through the eye exam to renew his license, one time with the help of a friend of mine who cued him as to the letters located on the bottom line of the chart. We all got a kick out of it when he and Bruce told the story, but he knew his driving days were numbered. The next year he turned in his license voluntarily.

In the early years after the stroke, my father did not vigorously pursue the regime of recovery that the doctors and physical therapists prescribed. He had limited mobility in his left leg. His left arm was cold to the touch. His massive torso was getting weak and flabby. But the biggest obstacle was his emotional state. At first he was weepy and sad, a common response among stroke patients. After that, he became angry. Then he became depressed. Throughout it all he was afraid, deathly afraid, not so much of another stroke but of the diabetes. He knew what the future holds for a diabetic who lives long enough to endure it: diminished vision, loss of circulation in the hands and feet, infection, and eventually amputation. He endured them all. He could no longer read and had to resort to books-on-tape (provided by the State for the legally blind). He could barely see the TV screen. And his feet were fitted for special shoes designed to prevent blisters, a diabetic's nightmare because of the likely onset of infection. This nightmare befell him in the summer of 1984. With admirable persistence and the help of a newly developed technique, the doctors in the VA contained the infection for the better part of a year. But after a half dozen trips into the hospital, my father came home in the summer of 1985 with most of his right foot gone, leaving him with what he called "my stump." It was still possible for him to walk with a prosthesis, but only with tremendous difficulty and always with the danger of another blister developing. So he had to rely on what he'd always dreaded relying on: a wheelchair.

It would be wrong to characterize these years as total darkness for him. After all, he saw a lifelong dream come true with the birth of his grandson in 1984. Although he was unable to attend my ordination in 1985, he and my mother made it out to Phoenix the next year to see the house of hospitality I helped start. He still got around town with the help of his friends and plenty of people came to see him. And my mother was there to take care of him, although she wasn't about to quit her job as a manager of a women's clothing store to put up with his cussing and shouting and his moods; "I'd go out of my mind," she'd hiss, whether or not he was in the room. He was surrounded by family and friends, but at the same time, his surroundings were shrinking. Most days he moved from his bed to the kitchen to his reclining chair in the living room to the back deck during nice weather, and no further. Eventually he would sleep at night by kicking back in his chair until the morning sun poured through the living room window. In my visits home, I would often stay up with him and we'd catch up on gossip, reminisce, and he'd bring me up to date of his illness, of this alien within. That was when he would say he wanted to die, but he'd usually express his death wish less explicitly. "I'm ready to go." Or, taking a line of Fred

Sanford's (Red Foxx) in the TV show "Sanford and Son," he'd look up, clutch his heart, and say in bad ghetto slang, "I's waitin' for da' big one."

The big one came in December 1987. Again I got the news from my sister, this time just before going out to say Sunday morning Mass in Phoenix. That night, I was at his bedside listening to the monitors and watching the ventilator pump oxygen in and out of his lungs. He had had a massive coronary, leaving him with a "floppy heart." The two things keeping him alive were the ventilator and the high powered heart drugs that were being administered intravenously. When he came to a day later, he gestured with his hands that he wanted the ventilator out. When they took it out, he made it clear that he wanted the heart drugs discontinued as well. After talking it over and swallowing hard, we agreed. Over the course of twelve hours starting Friday evening, my father would be weaned off the heart drugs. His hospital room that Friday afternoon was the scene of a procession of a dozen or more family and friends coming to say good-bye. In-laws he had known for half a century came out of the room weeping. One old friend, Steve Yelich, a former parole officer for the Corrections Department who looked every bit the part, left shaking his head and muttering tearfully, "I can't believe this is it." Another friend, Kay Hulihan, couldn't bring herself to come in. Then my mother and sister said good-night while I stayed in the room, ready to call them at home when the time came. We talked a long while that night. He said he was happy Kathy and I had turned out well and expressed confidence that we would take care of our mother. He was more peaceful than I had seen him in years. As he faded in and out, my eyes went back and forth between his face and the monitors. At one point, he coughed and the monitors spiked. "I lost my breath," he whispered. "Later tonight," I thought, "you'll lose it and won't get it back." It was like watching him move toward the edge of a cliff. I passed the hours reading psalms while he slept, and eventually fell asleep myself. The next morning, when we met with the doctor on duty for the weekend, he told us that my father would probably die sometime that day. The morning after that, he told us the same thing. On Monday morning, the attending physician admitted that there had been a misdiagnosis. Us: "What do you mean, Doc?" Him: "Looks like his heart is stronger than we thought." As we left, my mother, feeling both relief and exasperation, announced that she was going down to the cafeteria. My sister and I were punchy. In the elevator on the way up to the floor I asked her, "How are we going to break it to Dad? He's going to be okay."

We joked about it quite a bit afterward. And Steve Yelich told my father that he wasn't getting any more tearful farewells. My father died four and a half years later, his worst years by far. He did make it out to Buffalo one last time. And he and my mother made it to their fiftieth wedding anniversary, an event 150 people gathered to celebrate. But medically speaking, it was all downhill. A few weeks after the anniversary party, he went back into the VA Hospital, this time for what was a multi-system shutdown: weak heart, high blood pressure, kidney failure, and so on. During his last few days, he was vomiting up a dark, granular substance that the medical staff called "coffee grounds." One afternoon, when they were transferring him from gurney to bed, his body gave out. My mother, who had been at the hospital since early morning, was out having lunch. My sister, who had just been in to see him and left to come back later, was on her way home. I was grading papers in Durham, North Carolina. Once again, my sister was the one to call me, this time to tell me he had died. That was on May 7, 1992.

I have recounted the life and times of Big Jack because I think it has something to say in response to Hauerwas's call for Christians to be "patient patients." Amid all his health problems and all his trips in and out of hospitals, he was anything but that. He didn't usually do what the doctors told him. He didn't usually listen to my mother and the rest of us when we pleaded with him to take care of himself. He ate and drank what he wanted to, when he wanted to; and when he couldn't eat and drink what he wanted to, he got away with what he could. On good days, he was pleasant and fun to be around but never without sarcasm. On bad days, he was self-pitying and bitter. At any time, he could erupt into yelling and shouting. One time, my sister warned him that she wouldn't bring his grandson over to the house anymore if he didn't knock it off. He was hard on his many doctors, nurses, and therapists. He was, to put it mildly, an impatient patient.

This is not to say that we should follow my father's lead of being an impatient patient. We should watch what we eat, drink in moderation, and do what the medical staff tells us to do unless the directive is obviously misguided. Good health is a gift from God and we should do what we can to preserve it. In his own way my father imparted this wisdom on me when he urged me numerous times in my young adulthood to "stay in shape." But however faithfully I fulfill his last will and testament, I am still vulnerable to the kind of trials and tribulations to which he was subjected during the final sixteen years of his life. I have had to go in and out of hospitals only two times, once for pneumonia and once for a broken nose. This second time was complicated by the fact that in fixing my nose the doctor mistakenly severed the artery behind my left eye which then had to be repaired with another surgery, which, in turn, left me with double vision. He refused to acknowledge any mistake on his part, owing, I suppose, to the possibility of a lawsuit. As I lay in my hospital bed the night after the second surgery, a close friend of mine, Michael Garvey (to whom Hauerwas gives honorable mention for wearing a tie to his talk), made light of my ordeal by scribbling on the nurse's chalk board in my room, "Patient Angry." A much needed bit of comic relief. But I also look back on those words as a reminder of how bad a patient I will probably be when I go in for something worse, of how susceptible I am to the passions and demons that undermine our ability to embody the virtue of patience. Hauerwas is certainly right to remind us that our ability to be patient patients hinges on our ability to be patient in the ordinary circumstances of everyday life. But we also need to be reminded that however virtuous we are in the ordinary circumstances of life, when those circumstances change for the worse and we are forced to deal with a stroke or a heart attack or some other medical catastrophe, we may also have to face far less edifying and admirable parts of ourselves. We scarcely know ourselves, and we may never know ourselves unless or until we confront what the Greeks called "The Furies."

A modern version of this Greek worldview is articulated to me every so often by Steve Yelich's second son, Glen, who used to bring the books-on-tape to my father. A few years back Glen was jogging around the fields at the high school where he works as a counselor and psychologist when he was struck down by a seizure that the doctors still haven't been able to explain. He lost his long-term memory almost entirely (he didn't even remember that my father had died) and has been able to regain it only after a monumental effort in mentally reconstructing his past, and then only partially. He looks at his seizure as an instance of bad luck, one of the countless tragic events that occur each day in a universe governed by nothing more than chance. Always ready to engage in a debate, he challenges me to prove otherwise, to explain why it is that God, if He exists, would single out some people for disaster and others for good fortune. Trained by Hauerwas, I steer away from proposing logical solutions to this problem and take up the Wittgensteinian tack of argument through exemplification, appealing to the examples of people Glen and I both know: Bill Cookfair, a good friend of his father and mine who became Catholic in 1980 while dying of pancreatic cancer; Joan Cookfair, his wife and widow who raised four kids on her own, has always gone to Mass several times a week, and remains to this day a staunch advocate of (as she would put it) "the Faith"; Joe and Julie Cannizzarro, whose son Patrick came down with kidney disease ten years ago, who for the past two years have had to deal with Joe's colon cancer, who both work full time, and whose faith helps them to play the hand that's been dealt to them, though they embrace it without any pretension. Trained in modern psychology, Glen's response is roughly the same: "if it helps them to deal with it, more power to 'em." At some point, we'll start talking about old times and leave our ongoing debate where we always leave it, batted back and forth between the Faith and the Furies.

In my litany of people whose faith has helped them to endure medical illness, I do not include my father. A non-churchgoer who always maintained that a person's religion is a private matter between him and God, his belief was located somewhere between my traditional Christianity and Glenn's modern skepticism, but closer to Glenn's. Over the years, I would try indirectly to impart to him at least something of the vision reflected in Hauerwas's paper; how we should fear God more than death; how we should always strive to integrate the acquired virtues more fully into our lives and always pray for the infused virtues so that those virtues would be perfected; how we should shun impatience and rest assured with the knowledge that sickness is a legacy of the Fall that is being overcome by the victory of the New Adam, Christ. I wanted him to know the beauty and inspiration of the patristic vision that Hauerwas so helpfully articulates. But at one point or another, he would say, as he often said in response to my theological talking and writing, "words are cheap." Some theologians would fail to appreciate such a response, but Hauerwas is not one of them. If he has taught us anything over the years, it is that in the face of the cross, words are cheap. So I expect that Hauerwas would not disagree with what I saying about the difficulties in being a patient patient. Still, it bears repeating, as a way of remembering a reality that many of us forget: for some people who are sick over the course of many years, whose lives are consumed by the suffering signified in the cross, it is often difficult to see anything *but* the cross, and that this can try one's patience. It is a reality that any one of us may come to know first-hand.

And yet, in the face of such a reality, it is important to remember another reality: that the cross signifies not only suffering, but also God's mercy, and that this fruit of Christ's passion comes to us in the form of works of mercy. Works of mercy such as when Glenn sat with my father listening to his books. Or when my mother helped him through the thirty-minute ordeal of going to the bathroom. Or when my sister would sit with him out on the back deck, or when all of us when we buried him four days after he died. Works of mercy that he himself brought to many others too, which were surely on people's minds as we drove him to the cemetery adjacent to the school which he attended from seventh to twelfth grades and laid him to rest in a grave only a hundred yards from the baseball diamond where he played as a kid. What I thought of that morning in May was the many times that my father brought me to that same diamond when I was a kid and patiently taught me how to throw and catch and hit a baseball. It was a glimpse of the patience by which all of us, after wavering throughout our lives between patience and impatience, will be brought into the presence of God.

DEALING WITH DEATH

John T. Noonan, Jr.

(This lecture later appeared in *The Notre Dame Journal of Law, Ethics & Public Policy*, V. 12, Issue 2 (1998), pp. 387-400.)

Well, thank you for such a kind and generous introduction. It is always a pleasure to be here at Notre Dame and I always enjoy being in this particular conference room which is so well suited for discussion. I hope that there may be questions and comments after my formal presentation, and I'd be glad to engage in such discussion following it.

Both our professions, the medical and the legal, deal with death – not all the time, but enough of the time that awareness of death lurks in our subconscious as it lurks in the subconscious of ministers of the Gospel. This afternoon I shall speak to you about how assistance to die provided by a physician has been addressed by judges. I shall do so concretely in terms of *Compassion in Dying v. State of Washington*, the case with which I am most familiar by virtue of having decided it on appeal. I shall go on to sketch the larger contexts – moral, cultural, and religious – that are relevant to consideration of the issues raised. I hope to outline for you the central legal factors and at the same time convince you that the legal factors need to be set in larger contexts.

To begin with the case: I first encountered *Compassion in Dying* in the Fall of 1994 when by a random selection process it was assigned to me to preside at argument in Seattle over the State's appeal from a judgment of the district court. The district court had passed judgment on a Washington statute entitled "Promoting a suicide attempt." The entire state statute reads as follows:

(1) A person is guilty of promoting a suicide attempt when he knowingly causes or aids another person to attempt suicide.

(2) Promoting a suicide is a Class C felony. (Wash. Rev. Code § 9A.36.060 (1994))

The district court held the statute to violate the Constitution of the United States on two grounds. First, the Supreme Court in *Planned Parenthood v. Casey* had announced an extraordinary new autonomy centered on "the right to define one's own concept of existence, of meaning, of the universe, and of the mystery of human life." (505 U.S. 833, 851 (1992).) Conceivably, such a right could have been linked to freedom of religion; but the Court made no attempt to so link and limit what was announced in such encompassing and absolute terms. This announced right, this liberty interest, was read by the district judge as "highly instructive and almost prescriptive" in indicating that there was a constitutional liberty for terminally ill persons to decide whether or not to end their lives. (*Compassion in Dying v. Washington*, 850 F. Supp. 1454, 1459 (W.D. Wash. 1994).)

To this decoding of what is derisively called the "mystery passage" of *Casey*, the district court added a thought taken from the *Cruzan* case, decided by the Supreme Court in 1990. *Cruzan*, as you may recall, was the case in which the parents of Nancy Cruzan, in a coma from an automobile crash, sought a court order directing the withdrawal of their daughter's artificial feeding and hydration equipment. The state court of Missouri held there was not clear and convincing evidence of Nancy's own desire to have life-sustaining treatment withdrawn and the state refused to authorize its withdrawal. The Supreme Court affirmed the state decision, but in passing acknowledged the common law right not to be touched against one's will and almost as the corollary of that right "a constitutionally protected liberty interest in refusing unwanted medical treatment." (*Cruzan v. Director, Missouri Dept. of Health*, 497 U.S. 261, 278 (1990).) If a competent adult could terminate a life support system, then – so the district court reasoned – a competent adult could ask a physician's help in ending life. What difference would there be between disconnecting the life-sustaining tubes and injecting a fatal dose of poison? (*Compassion in Dying*, 850 F. Supp. at 1467.)

Hearing the argument on appeal, I was first struck by the abstractness of the case. The name plaintiff, Compassion in Dying, was a nonprofit, whose avowed purpose was to assist persons described by it as "competent" and "terminally ill" to hasten their deaths by providing them information, counseling, and emotional support but not by administering fatal medication. Three individuals were plaintiffs in their own right, their identities cloaked by an order permitting them to litigate under pseudonyms. They were now deceased. Jane Roe had been a sixty-nine year old physician, suffering from cancer; she had been bedridden for seven months at the time the suit was brought and died before judgment was entered by the district court. John Doe had been a forty-four year old artist, who was partially blind at the time of suit and was also suffering from AIDS; he had been advised that his disease was incurable; he died prior to judgment. James Poe had been a sixty-nine year old patient suffering from chronic pulmonary disease; he was connected to an oxygen tank. He died after judgment and just prior to the hearing of the appeal. (See *Compassion in Dying v. Washington*, 49 F.3d 586, 588 (9th Cir. 1995).)

Four physicians also joined the suit asserting their own rights and those of their patients. Harold Glucksberg had specialized in the care of cancer patients since 1985 and was a clinical assistant professor at the University of Washington School of Medicine. According to his sworn declaration, he "occasionally" encountered patients whom he believed he should assist in terminating their lives, but did not because of the statute; he referred to two such patients, both deceased. Abigail Halpern was the medical director of Uptown Family Practice in Seattle and served as a clinical faculty member at the University of Washington School of Medicine. In her practice, according to her sworn declaration, she "occasionally" treated patients, dying of cancer or AIDS, whose death she believed she should hasten but did not because of the statute; she referred to one such patient, now deceased. Thomas A. Preston was chief of cardiology at Pacific Medical Center in Seattle and Professor of Medicine at the University of Washington School of Medicine. According to his sworn declaration, he "occasionally" treated patients whose death he believed he should hasten but did not on account of the statute; he referred to one such patient, now deceased. Peter Shalit was in private practice in Seattle and the medical director of the Seattle Gay Clinic; he was a clinical instructor at the University of Washington School of Medicine. According to his sworn declaration, he "occasionally" treated patients whose death he believed he should hasten but did not on account of the statute; he referred to one such patient, now deceased. (*Id*. at 589.)

The case as presented seemed to me to be a hypothetical. A hypothetical, as we use the term in law schools, means a plausible set of facts that might need decision but does not yet present an actual controversy. The name plaintiff, "Compassion in Dying," had a good name – who would not want compassion in dying? – but no discernible interest in the issue as its purpose was not to promote suicide by any physical act. All the patient-plaintiffs were dead. Only the physicians remained. But the physicians were not asserting the interest of any actual patient, only the interest of some hypothetical persons they might have occasion to treat.

There was the additional problem of whom the district court's judgment covered. According to elementary principles of law, the judgment in favor of the dead plaintiffs was a nullity. (*Id*. at 593.) Did the physicians and their hypothetical future patients represent a class? According to the Federal Rules of Civil Procedure, certification that a class exists is required to sustain a class action. (Federal Rules of Civil Procedure, Rule 23.) No class was certified. There was good reason why no certification had been attempted: it would have required the plaintiffs and the court to say who the terminally ill were.

It was suggested in argument that a definition of the terminally ill could be supplied from the Washington statute governing the refusal of life-sustaining treatment, a statute which does define "terminal condition." (Wash. Rev. Code § 70.122.020 (9).) There were three difficulties: "Terminal condition" and "terminally ill" were different terms. The examples given by the plaintiffs showed considerable variation as to whom they considered the terminally ill to be and there was wide disagreement in the definition of the terminally ill among the states in this country. Life itself is a terminal condition, unless terminal condition is otherwise defined by a specific statute. A terminal illness can vary from a sickness causing death in days or weeks, to cancer, which Dr. Glucksberg noted is "very slow" in its deadly impact, to a heart condition which Dr. Preston noted can be relieved by a transplant, to AIDS, which Dr. Shalit declared is fatal once contracted but can run its course over years. One could only guess which definition of terminally ill would satisfy the constitutional criteria laid down by the district court. Consequently, an amorphous class of beneficiaries had been created in this non-class action; and the district court had mandated the state to reform its law against the promotion of suicide to safeguard the constitutional rights of persons whom the district court had not identified. (See *Compassion in Dying*, 79 F.3d at 839.)

In the end, for these and six other reasons you will find set out in 49 F.3d 586, our panel, 2 to 1, reversed the district court. We, in turn, were reversed, 8 to 3, by our own court sitting *en banc*, (79 F.3d 790 (1996)) which in turn, on June 26, 1997, was reversed by the Supreme Court of the United States, 9-0. (*Washington v. Glucksberg*, 117 S. Ct. 2258 (1997)) Like all professionals, the judges found it hard to agree on a difficult question. Fourteen judges had upheld the law, nine had held it bad; but of course the last word belonged to the Supreme Court. By the time the case had reached this tribunal, the winningly-named plaintiff, Compassion in Dying, had disappeared, and the lead name was Dr. Glucksberg's. The Supreme Court did not pause to ask who the plaintiffs were, who the terminally ill were, or who had actually secured the judgment of the district court. A companion case, *Vacco v. Quill*, was also before the court. Here a three-judge panel of the Second Circuit had held unconstitutional the New York statute that classified aiding a suicide as a species of manslaughter. (*Quill v. Vacco*, 80 F.3d 716 (2d Cir. 1996) (N.Y. Penal Law § 125.15 held unconstitutional).) This decision, too, was reversed. (*Vacco v. Quill*, 117 S. Ct. 2293 (1997).)

The state of the law after *Glucksberg* and *Vacco* may be summarized succinctly as follows: The liberty guaranteed by the Fourteenth Amendment and protected from violation by the states does not include the right of competent, terminally ill adults to hasten their deaths by obtaining medication prescribed by their doctors with the intent to kill them. (*Washington v. Glucksberg*, 117 S. Ct. at 2275.) In Chief Justice Rehnquist's opinion in *Vacco,* a distinction was accepted between prescribing lethal medication and "aggressive palliative care," which would both mitigate pain and hasten death. (*Vacco v. Quill*, 117 S. Ct. at 2298-2299.) The distinction was said to rest on the intention of the physician. In Chief Justice Rehnquist's opinion in *Glucksberg*, *Cruzan* was distinguished as responding to the long-standing common law tradition that one can refuse to be touched; therefore one could refuse to be treated. (*Washington v. Glucksberg*, 117 S. Ct. at 2270.) *Planned Parenthood v. Casey* was explained away as not establishing a general right to autonomy in "any and all important, intimate, and personal decisions." (*Ibid.* at 2271.) In addition, a remarkable concession was made by justices who hitherto had opposed *Roe v. Wade*, justices who had hitherto been the champions of the right to life, Chief Justice Rehnquist and Justices Scalia and Thomas. These three justices agreed that the abortion liberty was a fundamental, traditional liberty. (*Ibid.* at 2267.) The concession was a high price, presumably paid for Justice Kennedy's vote for the Chief Justice's opinion.

Five justices – Breyer, Ginsburg, O'Connor, Souter and Stevens – also spoke through separate opinions. Justice O'Connor, explicitly joined by Justices Breyer and Ginsburg, said she did not address whether a competent person who was "experiencing great pain," that is, uncontrollable physical pain, had a constitutional interest in controlling the circumstances of death. (*Ibid.* at 2303 (O'Connor, J., concurring); cf. 2311 (Breyer, J., concurring).)

Justices Stevens and Souter indicated a similar openness to a "particularized" case. (See *ibid.* at 2290 (Souter, J., concurring); *ibid.* 2309 (Stevens, J. concurring). See the commentary of M. Cathleen Kaveny, "Assisted Suicide, the Supreme Court, and the Constitutive Function of the Law," *Hastings Center Report* 27, No. 5 (1997) 31-32.) Five justices, in short, appeared to view the constitutionality of statutes banning assisted suicide as open to challenge if the challenge is narrow and focused on a patient suffering without medical relief.

Looking back at this course of three years of litigation, one thinks that the role that the medical profession should have in bringing about death would appear to be normally one for that profession to decide and for the legislature that licenses and regulates that profession to approve. As you are aware, the American Medical Association disapproves of doctors killing their patients, even with a patient's consent; the legislature of Washington, like most legislatures, had concurred in this judgment and had made such medical practice criminal. These judgments appear to be quintessentially professional and legislative. How do judges acquire the superior status to scoff at the professionals' reasoning and to mock the legislative judgment and declare the law violative of a fundamental liberty?

I entered on the consideration of this case with some reluctance because it asked me to empathize, to a degree, with someone wanting to put himself or herself to death and with a doctor wanting to help effectuate this desire. I knew neither desire from my own experience. Like every other living being I did not and do not know what death entails – what follows on the cessation of physical life. So how judge sensibly of a desire to bring about this condition that is cloaked in mystery?

From observing my colleagues, I have no doubt that some particular personal characteristics, such as age and health and the death of close relatives, influenced the judges who actually took up such a question. Inevitably, the judges' own experience of life played a part. But there were also larger, more public variables at work. I list them as moral, cultural, and religious, and I look at those favoring the result ultimately reached.

MORALS

Law and morals are intermixed. Every legal position, every judgment of a court, every enactment of a legislature incorporates some position on the human good, that is, on what is moral. Analytically, however, law and morals can be separated, and the moral positions embodied in the law can be examined for their soundness. Having set out what the law now is and may become after *Cruzan, Glucksberg,* and *Vacco,* I will look at three moral positions reflected in the law. I think none of them are easy to arrive at. I think none of them beyond debate; but, let me say what I think they are.

The first is that it is morally proper to administer medication with the intention of alleviating pain even though you as the physician know that medication will also impair vital functions and hasten death. Traditionally, this practice has been defended under the rubric of double effect: you are doing a single act with two effects, one good and one bad, and the good effect is proportionate to the bad effect, and your intention is focused on the good effect. The analysis is based on Thomas Aquinas's example of self-defense: you strike the aggressor threatening your life; your intention is self-defense; your blow has the effect of preserving your life and taking his; your action is good. (Thomas Aquinas, *Summa Theologiae,* 2-2, 64, 7.) To the traditional terminology it is objected that when you foresee exactly what the bad effect of your double-effect act will be, you cannot disclaim responsibility for the bad effect by claiming that you only meant to accomplish the good effect. (See *Quill v. Vacco,* 90 F.3d at 729; Note, "Physician-Assisted Suicide and the Right to Die with Assistance," 105 *Harv. L. Rev.* 2021, 2028-31 (1992).) In plain English, you have both defended yourself and killed another in the case of self-defense. You have relieved pain and killed the patient in the case of lethal medication. In each case you are responsible for a death. But in each case your action was justified. You have a right to defend yourself. You have a right to relieve pain. You are not doing bad things and trying to justify them by good ends – a morality that is elastic. You are, rather, acting in a world where you cannot control all the consequences. If you are justified in seeking the good effect, the bad effect, not disproportionate to the good effect, will not make your action evil. This analysis supports the position, although not the terminology, of Chief Justice Rehnquist.

The *Catechism of the Catholic Church* also supports Justice Rehnquist's terminology and his focus on intention. Theologians – at least a reputable number of them – insist that a human being can distinguish between the effect intended and the effect foreseen, and to be without sin you must intend only the good effect, such as the preservation of your life in self-defense and the alleviation of pain in lethal medication. (See *Catechism of the Catholic Church* (1994) 491.) This emphasis on intention may be rationalized in terms of intention forming individual character or in terms of the intentions of physicians forming the character of their profession: no one wants a profession whose character is formed collectively by the intention to kill. The emphasis on intention may also be explained, perhaps better explained, in terms of being what is subject to God's judgment.

Modern American law does make a distinction between intention, defined as purpose, and knowledge of what one's action is "practically certain" to bring about; but the distinction often makes no difference to criminal liability. (Wayne La Fave and Austin W. Scott, Jr., *Criminal Law* (2nd ed. 1986), sec. 3.5.) For example, in *Regina v. Hancock*, House of Lords, 1986, the defendants – strikers patrolling a bridge and watching for strikebreakers on the road below – pushed a forty-six pound block off the bridge, killing a strikebreaker in an oncoming taxi. The defense was that the strikers were merely trying to put a barrier in the road. The House of Lords held if the defendants appreciated that their act was highly likely to cause death, the jury could infer their intent to kill. In other words, foreknowledge of the likely result is a normal basis for attributing intention to the one causing the result. John Finnis seems to me to agree, defining murder as "killing with intent to kill" or "the doing without lawful justification or excuse an act which one is sure will kill." (Finnis, "Intention and Side Effects" in Frey and Morris, eds., *Liability and Responsibility: Essays in Law and Morals*, 49.) Rather than rely on the terminology of the criminal law, I would draw attention to our common sense response to the difference between intention and foreknowledge of a certain result. For example, we wear a comfortable pair of old shoes. We know that wearing them we will wear them out. We foresee that this will happen. Our intent, however, is not to wear them out, although that is what will surely happen. Or take a more romantic situation. Cyrano tells Roxanne that he will kill himself if she marries François. It is clear that Cyrano means this, but she goes ahead and marries François. Cyrano carries out his threat. Roxanne did not intend to kill Cyrano, even though she knew he was a man of his word. Or take a collective example: we all drive our automobiles, knowing that as a consequence fifty thousand persons will be killed this year. We know the deaths will happen. We foresee the deaths. We do not intend them. No one thinks we are collectively murderers. We intend the good of driving our cars; we accept, with regret, the foreseen consequences. Intuitively, practically, as a matter of fact, we accept the distinction between intending and foreseeing, but it is not an easy distinction.

The second moral position to be considered here is the one undergirding *Cruzan* – the right to refuse treatment. As stated in *Cruzan,* the right may be argumentatively construed as the right to kill yourself by starvation or dehydration. (For a vigorous critique of such an interpretation, see M. Cathleen Kaveny, "Assisted Suicide, Euthanasia, and The Law," 58 *Theological Studies* 129-131 (1997).) So stated, it is offensive to common morality. It is also contradicted by Chief Justice Rehnquist's declaration in *Glucksberg* that there is no constitutional right to suicide. (*Washington v. Glucksberg*, 117 S. Ct. at 2270.) Accordingly, to even pose a plausible position, *Cruzan* must be recast to find at its heart the view that no one has an obligation to preserve life by extraordinary means. One gets back to the ordinary-extraordinary distinction. That proposition does require examination.

The proposition is open to at least three objections. First, if nature is our norm, does not the natural drive of self-preservation make no distinction between the ordinary and the extraordinary? If you are on the Titanic, you will grasp anything to stay afloat. Secondly, as what is ordinary is constantly changing with technological developments, the distinction between ordinary and extraordinary is unstable. A glass to hold water and a fork to eat food with might have been extraordinary once. Third, there are extraordinary things like a rare drug and there are ordinary things like food and water delivered by unusual methods; the ordinary-extraordinary distinction blurs these categories. It might be that one would naturally refuse to try a rare drug, but one does not naturally refuse food and water. These are the objections summarily stated and I'll attempt my own answer to them.

The answer to the first objection appears to be that an average or mediocre human nature, not an heroic one, should be taken as the norm, and mediocre human nature will seek only average remedies or means of survival. The answer to the second objection is that the categories of ordinary and extraordinary will change over time, but for a given period they are stable. The answer to the third objection is that the lines could be drawn differently, but a line that treats the complicated delivery of food and water as extraordinary is not unreasonable. In the end, as some modern moralists have concluded, it is the patient himself or herself who must decide what is extraordinary. (Kaveny, "Assisted Suicide" at 141; cf. Paul Ramsey *The Patient as Person* (1970) 131.) In sum, the ordinary-extraordinary distinction is not written in stone, but is fairly flexible and as flexible passes moral muster. *Cruzan's* dictum on the right to refuse medical treatment is salvageable if this position is adopted. In the background is the common sense position that one is not called to remedy all the evils of the world of which one becomes aware. One, in short, is not called to the morality of Don Quixote. If one is not called to remedy all evils, one may – even in the case of one's own body – draw a line where extraordinary efforts are not required. You are not called to a superhuman effort to save even your own life. The morality is not mediocre but that of common humanity.

The third moral position to be examined is the one foreshadowed as a possibility for the law by the openness of a majority of the justices in *Glucksberg* to a narrow challenge to the law on assisted suicide. By implication, they might hold assisted suicide to stop intolerable pain is good. That cases of untreatable pain occur – "compelling, heartwrenching cases," as Yale Kamisar calls them – appears to be a datum. (Yale Kamisar, "Physician-Assisted Suicide: The Problems Presented by the Compelling, Heartwrenching Case" (1998) 4.) They are the kinds of cases effectively presented by journalists sympathetic to legalized euthanasia. How frequent these cases are is a matter of dispute. Timothy Quill and Robert Brody, physician-advocates of physician-assisted suicide, put them at 2 percent in their experience of dying patients. (Timothy E. Quill and Robert Brody, "You Promised Me I Wouldn't Die Like This," 155 *Arch. Intern. Med.* 1250, 1251 (1995).) The New York Task Force on Life and the Law simply said that the cases were "extremely rare." (*When Death Is Sought: Assisted Suicide And Euthanasia In The Medical Context* (1994) 40.) I assume that there are no reliable statistics. It may be true, as Dr. Ira Byock in his book *Dying Well* observes from experience, that the pain of dying is never wholly physical, and "comfort is always possible." ((1997) 214-215.) Nonetheless, I think we must confront the possibility that, in some cases, physical pain can be assuaged only by life-threatening medication.

The principal argument, it seems to me, for permitting assisted killing here is this: you agree that it is proper to relieve pain medically even though one effect of the medication is to hasten death. Here is simply a case where instant pain relief is required; the dosage will relieve the patient totally while killing him. Surely the speediness of the solution should not make a moral difference.

From a religious perspective, the speed does make a difference in its complete arrogation to the doctor of the decision of God. I shall return to this objection but not consider it further at this point. The main objection is that it is wrong to frame any law on the basis of rare examples. "Hard cases make bad law" – a legal truism that holds as well for moral rules. If the hard case is focused on, the easy, ordinary case is overlooked. The majority of dying persons – the poor, the emotionally disturbed and the handicapped – would be injured by a rule facilitating assisted suicide. (*When Death Is Sought*, 100 and 129.) A law or rule should be made for the majority of cases.

The reply to this response is, why not set a norm for the majority but also create a well-marked exception for the unusual case? And the counter-reply here is that, at least where there is legislation and also some public pressure, the predictable tendency will be to push the exception so that it swallows the rule. If only *moral* rules and exceptions are at issue, the reliance is on conscience to keep the distinction between norm and exception clear, and it can be argued that conscience should be trusted. If that is done, then the objection that the exception will swallow the rule fails as a moral objection, leaving only an objection that seems to me to be focused on religious faith and to be considered further under that heading.

CULTURE

I turn from moral analysis to the cultural. Mixed as the moral and the cultural are, they are analytically distant. I start with the author whose corpus, next to the Bible, probably most shaped our literary universe: Shakespeare. In *Othello*, there is a suicide, unassisted, presented as the emotional sword stroke of a man who, as he says, does not know where to go. No one, I think, reads *Othello* as a play about suicide. In *Hamlet*, the famous "To be or not to be" speech contemplates suicide – unassisted suicide, *quietus*, accomplished, as Hamlet puts it, by one's own "bare bodkin" or dagger. But Hamlet quickly thinks that the mystery of what lies beyond death, "the undiscovered country," is sufficient deterrent. (III, 1, 79.) The prince has already acknowledged that "the Everlasting has set his canon 'gainst self-slaughter." (I, 2, 131-132.) In *King Lear*, the king is reduced to a state where suicide would seem to be a desirable option; the pain is entirely psychological but it is overwhelming, intolerable. Lear has been broken. Yet suicide is not attempted by the king. Rather, it is his friend Gloucester who, having lost his eyes and his son Edgar, is tempted to it. Blind, Gloucester meets Edgar (not in fact dead). Edgar disguises himself and pretends to assist his father in his suicide attempt. Believing he has been led to the brink of a cliff in Dover, Gloucester leaps, only to fall on the ground. Not realizing yet that he's been deceived, he is nonetheless repentant and declares:

> You ever-gentle gods, take my breath from me,
> Let not my worser spirit take me again
> To die before you please.   (IV, 6, 221-223.)

The attempted suicide, foiled rather than assisted by Edgar, and Gloucester's reaction to the failure stand as a small illustration of what is the great theme of *Lear*. It is given to Edgar to restate it in Act V.

> Men must endure
> Their going hence even as their coming hither.
> Ripeness is all. (V, 3, 9-11.)

That is the theme that resonates in our culture. In the face of the greatest adversity, it is not for a human being to determine when he dies. Like birth, death is the decision of a Higher Power; and it is the Higher Power who says what ripeness is.

Let me turn to a different sort of cultural icon, Henry James's *The Wings of The Dove*. As you know if you've seen the recent movie, it involves a kind of love triangle; but if you remember the book, it is also the story of the interaction of a London physician with the dying heroine, Milly Theale. The physician is Sir Luke Strett, regarded as "the greatest of medical lights." Conscious that she may be seriously ill, Milly consults him. He treats her not as an object, not as a collection of symptoms, but as a person. "But what does he say?" Kate Croy asks Milly. Millie answers, "That I'm not to worry about anything in the world and that if I'll be a good girl and do exactly what he tells me, he'll take care of me for ever and ever." (p. 195.)

Milly has indeed a mortal illness. Unable to cure her, Sir Luke does care for her until the end with absolute devotion, tact, and fidelity. He cannot prevent her death. He does not accelerate it. His ministrations are set off against the manipulations of Kate. It is this contrast that the movie has lost by lopping off Sir Luke, as the movie, like Kate, looks only to the bottom line. *The Wings of the Dove*, James's novel, is as much about how the dying should be treated as it is about dying gracefully. Assisted suicide is implicitly rejected. It is no accident that its physician bears the name of the author of the third Gospel.

R E L I G I O N

Culture and religion are no more sharply distinct than law and morals or morals and culture. Every culture has a religion at its center. Our culture reflects our Jewish and Christian roots. At the same time, our religion is affected by our culture. But there is no doubt that, for Jews and Christians, the first text of religion is scriptural. It is illuminating for a Christian to observe how death is treated in the Gospels.

Killing enters the Gospels only four times. The first time, almost at the outset of Matthew, is the killing of the baby boys of Bethlehem. (Matthew 2:16-18.) We are not told the number, though Matthew calls it a "massacre." It is a terrible foreshadowing of the propensity of power to make victims of the most helpless.

The second time is the execution of John the Baptist. He is a prisoner because he has told a powerful man that the woman the man is with is not the man's wife. It is not a welcome message. John is put to death because the woman wants this troublemaker eliminated. (Matthew 14:3-12.) Again the episode presages the reaction of the mighty to the Christian message.

Near the end of the Gospel of Matthew, as the Passion begins, a suicide occurs: Judas, characterized as "the betrayer," hangs himself. (Matthew 27:5.) It has been argued that, in the Judaism of that day, a suicide could be a sign of repentance. (David Daube, "Judas," 82 *California Law Review* 95 (1994).) In the context of Matthew, Judas's act does not appear to be penitent or praiseworthy. In Acts, Luke is even more scornful: Judas "falling headlong, burst open in the belly;" an act of suicide is not mentioned but may be assumed to have been known to Luke's readers. (Acts 1:18-19.)

The fourth killing is that of Jesus. Jesus is presented as risking this death, indeed as knowing that this particular kind of death will be inflicted on him. The suffering that accompanies the dying is clear, and the Gospels' treatment of the whole sequence culminating in the death emphasizes the suffering. Together, these events constitute the Passion of Our Lord. (Matthew 26:1-27:56) In Christian theology, the death and the accompanying suffering are redemptive.

As the following of Christ and the taking up of the Cross are presented to Christians as what should be done, suffering and death cannot have a wholly negative value for Christians. Not only is death inescapable, not only is some suffering inescapable, the follower of Jesus in undergoing them imitates him. In Christian theology, the follower's suffering and death are also redemptive. In the light of this theology, in the light of the Passion of Our Lord, a Christian cannot make the elimination of suffering a good trumping all other goods. Christian belief therefore provides a basis for the Christian to reject suicide and assisted suicide.

Like all human beings, Christians must shun suffering as an evil and shun death as the ultimate evil, effecting the separation of the soul from its natural setting and depriving the body of its form. The example of Jesus and the participation in the redemptive process will not alter these truths, but will confer on the believer a sense that these evils have a purpose, that they are not meaningless torture. Redemption – why it is needed, how it takes place – is a mystery; but for the believer it is also a reality in which he or she can play a part.

Close to self-contradiction, the Christian paradox of redemption parallels a second paradox: the believer, believing that to die is the necessary step for union with God, must not take the step voluntarily, must not accelerate the end of life on earth. Paradise must be postponed. Why? If one is firm in one's belief, death is the gateway to unearthly happiness. Why should the happiness be put off and misery endured on earth?

The answer – we all know it – is that our lives are not our own. God is the creator, who has brought us into being here and who will determine when we leave. Older theology spoke of God's dominion over us as though we were His property. Pope John Paul II, followed by the new *Catechism of the Catholic Church*, has emphasized that we are created with a special relation to God, who is our sole end; it is that relation which makes each life sacred. (p. 486.) We cannot lay violent hands on the life of another human being or on our own. Our "going hence" is as much in His will as is our "coming hither." We can, for just reason, risk the termination of our lives. We can even take measures to alleviate unbearable suffering that have the effect of hastening death. We can even assent to the respirator's being turned off, the intravenous drops being discontinued, the ending of the sustaining of our life by extraordinary efforts. Assent of this kind does not create a precedent permitting everyone to determine the manner and hour of their death.

Acknowledging the sovereignty of God, accepting the mystery of Redemption, following in the footsteps of Jesus, the Christian physician will do all that can be done to postpone the natural evil of death and its accompanying suffering; will not usurp the Creator's choice of the moment for the soul to leave the body; and will work to sustain the faith, hope and love of the believer who in suffering identifies with Jesus.

Response to
DEALING WITH DEATH

David Solomon

John Noonan's paper is written against the background of a tumultuous three year period in American constitutional and cultural history when it appeared for a moment that the courts of this country would take it in their own hands to discover (or perhaps declare) a constitutional right to physician assisted suicide. The results of such a decision on the part of the courts would have surely been as culturally significant – and as unpalatable to many – as has been the Roe v. Wade decision in 1973 that utterly transformed the legal landscape of abortion. The court's possible intervention to craft such a constitutional right first received wide public attention in the spring of 1996 when two different federal appellate courts produced majority opinions finding such a constitutional right. It was strange enough that two courts should discover such a right at almost exactly the same time, but even more strangely the courts provided quite different arguments for the right, construed it in quite different ways and launched their opinions from opposite sides of the country. The Second Circuit on the East coast based its decision on attacking the moral significance of the traditional distinction between killing and of letting die. (*Quill v. Vacco*, 80 F.3d 716 (2d Cir. 1996) (N.Y. Penal Law § 125.15 held unconstitutional).) The Ninth Circuit on the West coast based its decision on broad considerations of autonomy and liberty. (*Compassion in Dying v. Washington*, 49 F.3d 586, 588 (9th Cir. 1995).) When these opinions were announced, many felt certain that it was all but inevitable that the Supreme Court in due course would affirm the outcome (especially since it had been given two different powerful arguments from which to choose).

In the year after these appellate decisions were announced, the public discussion of the morality and legality of physician assisted suicide was carried on enthusiastically. There were unprecedented numbers of concurring and dissenting briefs written and the discussion in the press, both high and low, was almost overwhelming in its extent and its passion. Among the many remarkable pieces written about these matters in the year after the *Vacco* and *Compassion in Dying* decisions was Ronald Dworkin's *The Philosophers' Brief*. (The *Brief* was filed as an *amicus* brief in *Vacco* and *Compassion in Dying* and was printed in *The New York Review of Books* in the spring of 1997.) In it, Dworkin presumed to speak on behalf of all philosophers (otherwise why the definite and not the indefinite article) in announcing that philosophers had reached conclusions in their airy academic hang-outs that made it mandatory that the Supreme Court affirm these decisions, and do so quickly and overwhelmingly. The religious, cultural and moral disagreements about the issues involved were deep, with traditional Christian groups, led by the Catholic Church, main stream medical organizations like the American Medical Association and groups concerned for the well-being of the disabled leading the opposition to the recognition of such a constitutional right, while secular academics and traditionally liberal public interest groups supported such a right.

Ronald Dworkin and those philosophers he represented so ably (the brief was cosigned by Thomas Nagel, Robert Nozick, John Rawls, Thomas Scanlan, and Judith Jarvis Thomson) were surely surprised, along with many others, when the Supreme Court handed down its decision in June, 1997 and overturned both decisions in unanimous votes, 9-0. (*Washington v. Glucksberg*, 117 S. Ct. 2258 (1997) and *Vacco v. Quill*, 117 S. Ct. 2293 (1997).) Whether progress was postponed or a bullet dodged is, of course, still disputed.

In the aftermath of the failure of this attempt to render physician-assisted suicide legal by judicial means, it was widely predicted (even by many of those at the conference where Judge Noonan first presented this paper) that many states would put in place legislatively that right to physician assisted suicide that the Supreme Court had refused to put in place judicially. This seemed especially likely since five of the justices who concurred in the unanimous decisions wrote separately and expressed some sympathy for a constitutional case that would find a more finely-honed and less sweeping right to physician assisted suicide. State legislatures seemed ideally suited to craft legislation that could define a more narrowly circumscribed right. Such a right appeared to have popular support and every chance of being enacted into law.

Once again, however, pundits on this issue have been surprised. In the eleven years since the Supreme Court so overwhelmingly failed to find a constitutional right to physician assisted suicide, only Oregon has found a legislative route to legalization. Although many states have taken up the issue either in the legislature on through voter referenda, only in Oregon is physician assisted suicide presently legal. Even there, a lengthy court fight was necessary to sustain this legislation, and even though it is now legal there, it has been much less used than its supporters expected and it is still the object of constant attack by its opponents. (Timothy E. Quill, M.D., "Legal Regulation of Physician-Assisted Death – The Latest Report Cards," *New England Journal of Medicine* 356:1911-1913 (2007).)

Judge John Noonan is in an ideal position, of course, to comment on this particularly exciting stretch of constitutional and cultural history. It does not, of course, begin with the two appellate decisions discussed above but stretches further back to the earlier *Cruzan* and *Casey* decisions and other court decisions instrumental in shaping the judicial discussion of these matters. (*Cruzan v. Director, Missouri Dept. of Health*, 497 U.S. 261, 278 (1990) and *Planned Parenthood v. Casey* (505 U.S. 833, 851 (1992).) Judge Noonan played a prominent part in the legal proceedings as the lead judge in the original ninth circuit panel that, by a 2-1 vote, overturned the district court decision finding a constitutional right. His panel's decision, in turn, was overturned by the entire 9th circuit sitting *en banc*. (*Compassion in Dying v. Washington*, 49 F.3d 586, 588 (9th Cir. 1995).) Apart from his particular involvement in this case, however, his position as one of the premier Catholic intellectuals of his generation, as well as his scholarly work on the history of Catholic legal and moral thought, make his comments on these matters particularly important. He had been a prominent opponent of the revolutionary changes in our approach to abortion law in the 1970's and it should not be surprising that he would have equally strong views on the judicial route to the legalization of physician assisted suicide.

In this paper, Judge Noonan both gives an account of the main outlines of the judicial battles that raged over these matters in the years 1996-1997, and also explores the broader moral, cultural and religious issues that are implicated in what at first might seem to be dreary and dusty jurisprudential matters. On the first matter, his account of the judicial controversies, I will have little to say. He was clearly shocked, as were many of us, that the courts presumed in *Cruzan* and *Casey* to intervene so dramatically in matters surely best left to other seats of public authority. Noonan favors giving the medical profession a larger role in dealing with these matters. As he says, "Looking back at this course of three years of litigation, one thinks that the role that the medical profession should have in bringing about death would appear to be normally one for that profession to decide and for the legislature that licenses and regulates that profession to approve." And speaking ever more critically of the interventionist judiciary in these cases, he says, "How do judges acquire the superior status to scoff at the professionals' reasoning and to mock the legislative judgment and declare the law violative of a fundamental liberty?" Although Noonan leaves this a mere rhetorical question, there is no doubt that he believes that the answer does the court no credit.

The most important part of Noonan's piece, however, is its comprehensive review of a broad range of considerations – he divides them into moral, cultural and religious – that he takes to provide the background for the court's decision. One cannot help but notice how wide-ranging these considerations are. This may not seem surprising given the broad cultural significance of the move to legitimize physician assisted suicide, but it flies in the face of one commonly accepted view of the role of judges in reviewing the constitutionality of disputed legislation. It is sometimes suggested that judges, as befits the blindfold Lady Justice wears in the statues that frequently represent her in judicial settings, must be blind to considerations other than narrow considerations of constitutional language and judicial precedent when making appellate decisions. Noonan, to the contrary, suggests that not only is this broad set of considerations relevant to the matter at issue, but that even the personal experience of some of the judges could have been determinative of their decisions. As he says, "From observing my colleagues, I have no doubt that some particular personal characteristics, such as age, and health and the death of close relatives, influenced the judges who actually took up such a question."

The broader considerations discussed by Noonan that influenced the judicial decision bear two marks: first, there are "public variables at work" in the decision and, second, they are factors "favoring the result ultimately reached." While it would have been impossible for Noonan to discuss the private and personal characteristics of the judges that might have borne on their decisions, one might wish that he had found room in his paper not only for the views on those public variables that favored the courts final decision, but also those that opposed it. Perhaps he believes that those views have been sufficiently aired in the work of Dworkin and others who wrote so prolifically in support of a judicial decision discerning a constitutional right to physician assisted suicide. In the remainder of the paper, I will discuss briefly the moral views that Noonan takes to be embodied in the law concerning end of life medical treatment. His brief discussions are models of philosophical reflection, and I will pay them the usual respect we pay serious philosophy by raising objections to them.

There are three moral positions that Noonan takes to be "reflected in the law." First, the view that it is permissible for physicians to use medical means to treat suffering even when they are aware that the use of such means might hasten death. This position, as Noonan notes, is simply an application of the traditional doctrine of double effect in the context of treating dying patients. Double effect requires us to regard in radically different ways the moral significance of intended consequences of our actions and those consequences that are merely foreseen, but not intended. While Noonan admits that the distinction between the intended and the merely foreseen is "not an easy distinction," he believes that most persons accept it intuitively and practically. His brilliant discussion of a number of examples where ordinary people quite clearly presuppose the distinction in their thought and action provides a powerful argument that it is indeed widely accepted in ordinary life.

The critics of this distinction, however, do not dispute that it is presupposed in many contexts of ordinary life. They argue rather that, by presupposing it, persons are led to act in ways that are either inconsistent or arbitrary. (See James Rachels, "Killing and Letting Die," *New England Journal of Medicine*, 292:78-80 (1975).) The most formidable critics of the traditional doctrine of double effect do not deny that it is a fixture in "folk" thinking about the moral quality of action, but rather claim that folk thinking embodies fundamental mistakes and needs to be changed. In order to counter these critics, Noonan would have to resort to arguments of a quite different character than he provides here. While I am confident that such arguments are to be had – and that the traditional doctrine of double effect can be sustained – the arguments Noonan gives here will be inadequate as a response to these opponents.

The second moral view embodied in the law is the view that patients have the right to refuse extraordinary medical treatment. As Judge Noonan well knows, the distinction between ordinary and extraordinary medical care has become increasingly difficult to draw with any precision in our age of high-tech medicine where almost every medical procedure would seem by the standards of even the recent past quite extraordinary. He recognizes that in order to preserve the usefulness of this distinction the criteria for the extraordinary cannot be fixed and timeless, but must change over time. While a dose of penicillin might have been extraordinary in 1942, it is hardly that today. Many would argue that even cardiac by-pass surgery is no longer an extraordinary procedure. The danger of admitting that the standard for extraordinary care is not fixed is that this admission might open the door to the view that anything goes with regard to what counts as extraordinary. Noonan is aware of this danger and counters with his claim that while the criteria for the extraordinary may not be fixed over time, nevertheless "for a given period they are stable." This, alas, simply replaces the problem of the fuzziness of the notion of the extraordinary with the problem of the fuzziness of the extent of the "given period." Exactly when did penicillin become ordinary? Not surprisingly, Noonan is driven to the position that "it is the patient himself or herself who must decide what is extraordinary." While this view might seem edifying and respectful of patient autonomy, it is difficult to see how it can sustain the moral position that Noonan set out to defend. The distinction between ordinary medical care and extraordinary was introduced to attempt to set some reasonable limits to the kinds of medical treatment that a patient may refuse in life or death decisions. If the criteria for what counts as extraordinary are to be set by patients themselves, it is difficult to see how this could set limits in any meaningful sense. It is as though motorists could be convicted of speeding only if they were going faster than their own personal standard of highway safety would allow. Not only would few speeders be convicted in such a world, but the whole idea of speeding violations would lose its sense and the institutional practice of writing tickets for speeding drivers would surely disappear.

The third moral view embodied in the law is in many ways the most complicated of the three to unravel. While the first moral view allows that it is permissible, in accord with the principle of double effect, to administer pain-relieving drugs with the intention of relieving suffering even when one foresees that the drugs may shorten life, the third view queries how we should behave toward patients when pain is severe and untreatable. May we not in the case of persistent, severe and untreatable pain take steps with the patient's consent to end life directly? Indeed, is this not the only humane action to take in such a case? If one gives an affirmative answer to these questions, one will be committed to the view that assisted suicide to stop intolerable pain is good. The five justices who assented to the Supreme Court decision but wrote separately from the majority opinion by Justice Rehnquist all found this line of reasoning quite compelling. They indicated that if a case were presented to the Court that focused on this consideration alone, they might be willing to affirm a right to physician assisted suicide in cases of this sort.

Judge Noonan nevertheless does not think that this line of reasoning can be decisive in a legal context. His reason for rejecting it is based on the fact that the cases where pain is severe, persistent and untreatable are rare ones and making these cases the focus of legislation concerning medical treatment at the end of life leads to bad law. His complete response to this argument is worth quoting at length: "The main objection is that it is wrong to frame any law on the basis of rare examples. 'Hard cases make bad law' – a legal truism that holds as well for moral rules. If the hard case is focused on, the easy, ordinary case is overlooked. The majority of dying persons – the poor, the emotionally disturbed and the handicapped – would be injured by a rule facilitating assisted suicide. A law or rule should be made for the majority of cases." While he agrees that it might be possible to write a restrictive law for the majority of cases and "create a well-marked exception for the unusual case," in the context of the law where legislation and public pressure are factors in shaping the rule and exception, "the predictable tendency will be to push the exception so that it swallows the rule." He fears then, that while we might strive to make a narrow exception to the prohibition of physician assisted suicide for the case of untreatable pain, given the political realities of legislative and marketing pressures in contemporary culture, the exception would be inevitably expanded.

He does not say, but might have, that this is precisely what happened in the expansion of the class of abortion rights. It is quite clear that the Supreme Court did not anticipate at the time they crafted the Roe v. Wade decision that within five years of that decision there would be one and a half million abortions in this country each year. Nor did most commentators on the decision at the time it was published expect that the decision would create a strong pro-choice lobby that would effectively oppose any attempt to set even the most narrowly focused restrictions on the legal right to abortion. Hardly anyone could have anticipated that the principles laid down in Roe would be used a quarter of a century later to oppose even the prohibition of such inhumane practices as partial-birth abortion.

There is an interesting tension in Judge Noonan's treatment of this third view, however. While he thinks that in the legal context it would be unwise to create a law which generally prohibits physician assisted suicide while making an exception for the case of untreatable pain, he argues that things are different in the moral context. As he says, "If only *moral* rules and exceptions are at issue, the reliance is on conscience to keep the distinction between norm and exception clear, and it can be argued that conscience should be trusted. If that is done, then the objection that the exception will swallow the rule fails as a moral objection, leaving only an objection that seems to me to be focused on religious faith and to be considered further under that heading." The most natural reading of this passage would suggest that Judge Noonan finds a moral argument for allowing an exception to the moral rule against physician assisted suicide convincing while he rejects the argument for such an exception in the legal case. A complete discussion of the issues here would lead us into territory that we can't explore on this occasion, but it is worth noting that if Judge Noonan is correct that there are powerful and persuasive arguments for allowing exceptions to the *moral* rule against physician assisted suicide while there are equally compelling arguments for not allowing such an exception in the *legal* case, he sets up a tension between the moral and legal that is likely to make orderly public discussion of the issue of physician assisted suicide very difficult indeed.   If he is right, conscientious and reasonable citizens will find moral grounds for performing actions that they will have equally powerful legal reasons for prohibiting.

Judge Noonan writes as a Christian, however, and as he makes clear in the final section of his paper, Christians will have reasons of their own for rejecting any exceptions to the prohibition of physician assisted suicide. Christians know "that our lives are not our own. God is the creator, who has brought us into being here and who will determine when we leave. . . . We cannot lay violent hands on the life of another human being or on our own." While Judge Noonan writes eloquently about the views shared by Christians on this matter, his discussion of the nature of Christian approaches makes the public policy problem concerning physician assisted suicide even more difficult.   He has already argued that secular moral approaches to physician assisted suicide are likely to conflict with the most reasonable approach to legal regulation to this issue. He now argues that Christian approaches to this issue will necessarily also conflict with secular moral approaches.

We can be grateful to Judge Noonan for not only clarifying incisively the interwoven cultural, moral and religious threads in the current debate about medical treatment at the end of life, but for also providing a profound explanation of why this contemporary debate has so persistently resisted resolution. We can also be grateful that someone like Judge Noonan, with his comprehensive grasp of the background issues on this matter, is in a position on the Ninth Circuit Appelate Court to pass judgment on our legislative efforts to respond to this issue.

DEATH AND DIGNITY
"APART AND NOT A PART"

Gilbert Meilaender

(This lecture appears in *Religious Commitment, Personal
Narrative, and Healthcare Ethics,* edited by David Smith
(Westminister: John Knox Press, 2000.)

Thank you very much, David. I am pleased to be here and I am
honored to give this lecture that has been given by so many
distinguished people. I am a little disconcerted that so many of them
should be here today to hear me, but I'll do my best on this rather
morbid topic that I have chosen. Let me say just a word, first, about
where I'm headed so that you'll be able to hang with me. Roughly
what I shall do will fall into three parts. First, I'll get the theoretical
part over with at the outset. It will reflect on the sense in which we
should or should not think of death as an enemy. So that will be the
first issue that I take up. Then I shall turn to a couple stories about
dying patients in order to play them off against that more theoretical
discussion. And finally, I shall try to pull the threads together at the
end and draw some conclusions. You can see what you think of that.
But, in short, I am not, except in some tangential ways, going to be
aiming directly at the hot button issues. I'm not directly talking about
euthanasia or physician assisted suicide or currently topical policy
issues. I'm talking about something a little more fundamental out of
which we come at those other issues. So that's where I'm headed.

Dietrich Bonhoeffer wrote from prison:

We are paying more attention to dying than to death. We
are more concerned to get over the act of dying than to over
come death. Socrates mastered the art of dying; Christ
overcame death as "the last enemy" (I Cor. 15:2 6). There
is a real difference between the two things; the one is within

the scope of human possibilities, the other means resurrection. (Dietrich Bonhoeffer, *Letters and Papers from Prison*. The enlarged edition, ed., Eberhard Bethge (NY: Macmillan, 1972), p. 240.)

To struggle with death and dying is nothing new in human experience. That struggle has taken on a peculiar tone in our society, however. On the one hand, we seek a certain control and mastery over our fate. On the other, we are increasingly asked to find ways to accept death as no affront to our dignity and as a natural part of life. To learn to think this way is itself, of course, to exercise a certain kind of "control." Indeed, it has in some ways been the burden of a quarter century's bioethical reflection to teach us the acceptance of death free of intrusive, high-tech medicine. By contrast, Felicia Ackerman has recently suggested that the "philosophy of hospice," which affirms the importance of accepting death, is "a highly questionable ideology" that may "attempt to export religiously based attitudes . . . into a context where the religious grounding that justifies these attitudes is lacking." (Felicia Ackerman, "Goldilocks and Mrs. Ilych: A Critical Look at the 'Philosophy of Hospice,'" *Cambridge Quarterly of Healthcare Ethics*, 6 (1997), pp. 314ff.)   As the passage from Bonhoeffer used as an epigraph for this essay may indicate, we should not too readily suppose that religious belief will incline one toward acceptance of death. It is Socrates, not Jesus in Gethsemane, who more closely approximates the "ideology" that Ackerman rejects.

I want to look at some stories about dying to see what we can learn by reflection upon them, but I suspect that just looking at how people die or telling their stories will not decide for us whether death is an enemy against which we quite rightly ought to rage and struggle, or whether it is a part of life that comes naturally and ought to be accepted. What we think about such questions is likely to depend on what we think about quite a few other matters. I will, therefore, reflect upon these stories against the background of more systematic consideration of the significance of death. The stories I will draw from Ira Byock's widely read book, *Dying Well: The Prospect for Growth at the End of Life*. (NY: Riverhead Books, 1997. References will be given by page number in parentheses within the body of the text.) As a hospice doctor, Byock has cared for many suffering patients in their dying.   Moreover, he believes deeply in the importance of accepting dying and making it – as the book's subtitle indicates – a time of personal growth. But I will place these stories in the context of a pair of essays that are now more than a quarter century old: Paul Ramsey's "The Indignity of 'Death with Dignity,'" and Leon R. Kass's rejoinder, "Averting One's eyes, or Facing the Music? – On Dignity in Death." (Both were published in the *Hastings Center Studies*, 2 (May, 1974). Ramsey's essay covers pp. 47-62; Kass's, pp. 67-80. References will be given by page number in parentheses within the body of the text.) The Ramsey/Kass exchange will serve to remind us that what we make of Byock's stories depends in some considerable measure on beliefs – even metaphysical and religious beliefs – that we bring along with us when we read them. Our moral reflection on the meaning of death seems almost to require that we move back and forth between (a) particular cases, and our response to them, and (b) the larger patterns of belief that frame our response to cases and, in part, shape what we see. We cannot simply reflect on cases as if ours were a view from nowhere in particular. Neither, however, should we suppose that our beliefs about the meaning of death remain entirely unaffected by the experience of dying patients.

REVISITING AN OLD DEBATE: IS DEATH AN ENEMY?

In arguing that death itself is an affront to human dignity and that, therefore, the shibboleth of "death with dignity" can also readily become an affront, Ramsey wants to make a place for the attitude exemplified in the oft quoted passage from Dylan Thomas, which he himself also cites: "Do not go gentle into that good night . . . Rage, rage against the dying of the light." In making this claim, Ramsey does not deny that death might, sometimes, by some people, be accepted with serenity (48). He does not deny that, weighing the "comparative indignities" of different possibilities, one might sometimes conclude that continued personal deterioration was more fearful than death (51ff). His central contention is summed up in a sentence such as the following: "The more acceptable in itself death is, the less the worth or uniqueness ascribed to the dying life" (56).

Why might one hold such a view? Underlying Ramsey's position are beliefs that he draws from Christian faith but also understands to belong to any "true humanism" – as he calls it – in particular, (a) the belief that we are bodies extended in time, that human life is biological and historical in character, and (b) the belief that each person is unique and cannot be replaced by any other, because each is made for God. These are the two grounds of our individual worth.

We are finite bodies, located and connected in a particular time and place. Something of what this means is nicely expressed by C.S. Lewis in a passage discussing the way Christians tend sometimes to depict death as simply a good thing – the transition to a new and better life. Lewis does not deny that belief; he simply points to what has been lost – and seemingly lost forever – to the alien power of death. He writes,

> If a mother is mourning not for what she has lost but for what her dead child has lost, it is a comfort to believe that the child has not lost the end for which it was created . . . a comfort to the God-aimed, eternal spirit within her. But not to her motherhood. The specifically maternal happiness must be written off. Never, in any place or time, will she have her son on her knees, or bath[e] him or tell him a story, or plan for his future, or see her grandchild. (C.S. Lewis, *A Grief Observed* (London: Faber & Faber, 1961), p. 24.)

But we are not only embedded in nature and history. We are not just "a part" of it. The second ground of our uniqueness is that called into personal communion with God, we are "apart [from] and not [simply] a part" of the natural world (55). It follows, therefore, that death, in cutting off a particular "human countenance," is the enemy. My death may be part of the natural cycle of birth and death, it may seem necessary for future generations to flourish, it may bring to an end "comparative indignities" of suffering and deterioration that were themselves even more fearful, but, nonetheless, it does not bring my life to completion. It is, Ramsey says, *"finis,* not in itself *telos"* (53). It is not end as completion.

For both reasons, then, death is the enemy of our individuality and our worth. Hence, when caring for one who is dying, or when facing our own death, we need, Ramsey writes, "to acknowledge that there is grief over death which no human agency can alleviate" (62). This will be true, on Ramsey's account, not only when a child dies prematurely (as we would say) but also when someone dies "full of years." If we try to ignore or deny the loss that every death brings, we miss the dignity of the dying person. We cherish him too little if we seek "dignity" in death as a way of removing its sting – as if any "human agency," any theory of ours, any care (even the most dedicated) that we might give, could itself "alleviate" the loss of this "human countenance."

None of this means, of course, that there are not comparatively better and worse ways to die. None of this means that there might not be deaths that are comparatively more or less dignified. It means only that, even in the most dignified of deaths, we need to recognize the presence of a hostile power, the "last enemy" from which Jesus himself shrank, a power that cannot be overcome simply by mastering the art of dying. Something like that is Ramsey's understanding of "the indignity of 'death with dignity.'" (We should not overlook the fact that there may also be a kind of empirical evidence for the perception of death as hostile power. Several recent studies have concluded that seriously ill people may struggle far more to stay alive than the healthy think sensible – or than the ill themselves would have thought reasonable prior actually to facing death. See the studies cited by Ackerman in her footnotes 28, 29, and 30. Those of you who've actually read the essay will know that I've untangled a rather knotty piece of prose along the way.)

Kass's response, although largely agreeing with respect to some of the deformations brought to our experience by notions of "death with dignity," nevertheless turns in a very different direction. In part, Kass argues for an understanding of dignity as human achievement and, hence, not just a universal human possession. The dignity that we do sometimes attain is dependent not on what uniquely individuates each of us but on the way we exercise those generic qualities that distinguish the human species from others. Moreover, on his view, death is not a hostile power; it is simply the natural conclusion to the trajectory of a human life and, still more, a possibly necessary condition for the display of much that is noble in our life (68ff). It is a good, even if sometimes an "evil good."

This is, in many respects, Kass at his most Aristotelian – set over against Ramsey at his most existentialist. For Kass, our nobility lies in the exercise of the most characteristically human capacities – presumably, although he does not specify them precisely, a yearning for what is true, and good, and beautiful. For those human beings who achieve such dignity, death, simply in and of itself, cannot be an indignity – it cannot deprive them of what they have achieved. Kass offers several reasons for this judgment. He suggests, for example, that – whatever we may say of the child who dies prematurely – we do not regard death as an affront to dignity when it takes one who dies "full of days after a rich and worthy life" (74). We may pause briefly to reflect upon this claim in contrast to Ramsey's view. Certainly it is true that we react differently to the death of an old woman than to the death of a young girl. That much one must surely grant to Kass. But it is harder to know how to decide whether the death of the old woman – even if painless and at a ripe old age – should be counted an affront, a defeat by a hostile power. Simply observing such deaths will not, I suspect, make the distinction for us. Kass himself, after all, can understand a sense in which any person's death – the sheer fact of mortality – could be considered an indignity. "Only if dignity were synonymous or coextensive with life itself could we even begin to make such a case" (73). But, of course, precisely such "coextensiveness" is integral to Ramsey's case. What sets us "apart" for Ramsey is, first, the particular web of relationships and loyalties that constitutes this bodily life – to which death brings a *finis*. What also sets us "apart" for him, and makes us more than just "a part" of nature, is that each is called by God to himself. That is an alien dignity conferred or bestowed from outside; it is not human achievement. Each person has an individual dignity that is snuffed out by death. For Kass, at least the Kass of this essay, it is universal form – the generically human rather than particular matter – that really makes for human dignity (76). And death is the end point of the decay and decline built into life, not a personal force that confronts us from the outside, opposing itself to the call of God. There is no way to read the differences between Ramsey and Kass apart form these differences in worldview. Neither confronts the fact of death simply as an event to be observed. Each sees in death an event shaped by the (Aristotelian or Christian existentialist) metaphysic he brings to it.

Kass also offers a variety of angles from which we may see death as necessary to a world in which virtue and nobility are present. Heroes and martyrs demonstrate how death can provide "the occasion for the display of dignity. . . . Far from undermining their worth, their death – like the life it terminates – is a necessary condition for the display of dignity" (74). In addition, the simple fact of our mortality may be a kind of "necessary spur" to excellence, pressing us along the way by reminding us that we may not, if fact, have "world enough and time" (74). And without death, without the withering and dying of the old, there could be no place for the next generation, for the young with their vibrant sense of hope – no place for all those Ph.D. students waiting for us to step aside. In all these ways, death may serve human well being and enhance human dignity.

Finally, death is, on Kass's view, simply a natural event, a limit set within the very principle of life. "How can death be an indignity if it is the natural and necessary accompaniment of life itself?" (75). Against Ramsey's suggestion (48) that suffering, which we think it right to oppose, is also a natural part of life, Kass argues for a difference. Disease – and the suffering it brings – are "*fought* by nature working within, whereas decline is *produced* by nature working within" (75ff). Hence, "unlike all those other things which *occur* in life, decline and death are a *part* of life, an integral part which cannot be extruded without destroying the whole" (76).

There is, however, one sense in which we might wonder whether Kass is quite Aristotelian enough here. For Aristotle the "natural" is not simply what happens regularly and, even, inevitably. The "natural" is whatever is appropriate to a thing of a particular kind, whatever constitutes its flourishing. It is, then, a normative concept, and that opens up space for Ramsey's view of what is fitting and appropriate for beings of our kind, when he writes:

But the man who is dying happens not to be evolution. He is a part of evolution, no doubt: but not to the whole extent of his being or his dying. A crucial testimony to the individual's transcendence over the species is man's problem and his dis – ease in dying. Death is a natural fact of life, yet no man dies "naturally" (49).

On Ramsey's view, in other words, human self-transcendence is a sign that we are made for the living God – and that death is an affront to the "nature" of such creatures. The lesson to be drawn from this is one I need not belabor further: The different responses of Ramsey and Kass as they stand at the bedside of a dying man may not be explicable apart from the respective webs of belief which they carry along with them to that bedside. Their respective attitudes toward the man's dying will be shaped by their metaphysical accounts of human nature. That said, we are ready to consider Ira Byock's stories of the dying.

THE DYING OF THE LIGHT

Chapters ten and eleven of *Dying Well*, the last two stories narrated by Byock, form a pair – an intentional pair. The first, the story of Terry Matthews, illustrates what Byock regards as a bad death, the second, the story of Maureen Riley offers his image of perhaps the best possible death. Yet, he is willing to say that each of these women "died well," because each died in her own chosen way. In general, in fact, this seems to be the key to his evaluations. Having first, as he tells his readers, been drawn toward the concept of a "good death," he rejected it in favor of the idea of "dying well" (32). Focusing on a "good death" may not be helpful. For one thing, most people will describe it only negatively – in terms of the evils they hope to avoid in their dying. Moreover, "it tends to blur the distinction between death . . . and the preceding time of living" (32). By contrast, he writes, "Dying well expresses the sense of living, and a sense of process" (32). It invites us to think about what we may yet accomplish in our dying and sees that dying as another stage in a lifelong process of human development.

Terry Matthews was twenty-four years old and the mother of a toddler when she had a growth on her right kidney removed. To her physician's surprise the growth turned out to be a cancer of a kind very difficult to cure. She undertook a course of chemotherapy, however, went into remission for a time, conceived and gave birth to a second child, and (with her husband Paul) adopted a third. Thus, she was a mother of a son and two young daughters, and she devoted herself wholeheartedly to being that. After six years, however, she developed a persistent cough and occasionally spat up blood. Lung x-rays showed that, after years of lying dormant, the cancer "had returned with a vengeance" (195).

Over the next nine months Terry struggled with her own vengeance against her illness and in the face of, what Byock himself – although he thinks that such pain can always be relieved – calls, "unbearable pain." (The title of chapter ten is: "Facing Unbearable Pain, Unspeakable Losses: Terry Matthews." Even in this case, however, pain relief was provided – though it could be done only by means of permanent sedation. Indeed, Byock emphasizes throughout the book his conviction that "physical suffering can *always* be alleviated" – and 'always' is always italicized when he makes this point. Cf. pp. xiv, 44, 60, 215, 245.) Even in the midst of such pain, however, she hung grimly to life. Byock recounts a conversation Terry had with Vickie Kammerer, the hospice social worker assigned to help her. The issue was whether Terry should enact a directive stating that she did not want CPR if she should undergo cardiac or respiratory arrest.

> Though Vickie knew of Terry's fierce drive to stay alive, the topic required discussion. As she had with hundreds of patients with advanced cancer, Vickie gently explained to Terry, "If you had a massive heart attack in your current condition, it might be somewhat futile even if you could be briefly revived." Terry's reaction said it all: "If they could bring me back to life and if I could have one or two more days, that is what I would want" (200).

Why? Why would she rage this fiercely against the dying of the light? (Byock does, in fact, provide the obligatory citation of Dylan Thomas, Cf p. 193.) Because she loved her husband and her children. Byock says of her case: "By the end of her life, Terry's pain was as bad as it gets, as severe as I have ever witnessed" (215). She "was absorbing – and her pain all but ignoring – more than nine hundred milligrams of morphine per hour," and yet she clung to life (207). Indeed, in choosing every possible life-prolonging option she certainly brought upon herself – and willingly accepted in return for life – much greater pain than might otherwise have been hers. He says, "She clung to life far beyond the point at which most people surrender to the inevitable. Her connection to her family, being with them, was more important than the pain – and her resistance to letting go gave the disease more time to inflict its cruel torment" (214ff). Even this, however, does not tell the whole story of her suffering or the reasons for it. Byock can write that "while the physical aspects of her distress were enormous, I have no doubt that Terry's blinding grief at the thought of losing her husband and three young children contributed to her pain" (214). Clearly, hers was, in Ramsey's words, a grief that "no human agency can alleviate."

In the end, her pain could be relieved only through permanent sedation, which she finally accepted and which gave her troubled body the peace of "twilight sleep" before she died thirty hours after the barbiturate drip was begun. Even in the last hours before she was thus sedated, in the midst of almost unspeakable suffering, she spent her time making notes of her last wishes for her children, worrying about what they would wear at her funeral, and expressing to her husband her sorrow at leaving him (210). Byock writes, "Life had to be plucked from Terry; she never did let go or turn inwardly to leave the way most dying people do. This was the crux of her life: she died with arms open and outstretched toward her family. Her reluctance to leave will always be part of her legacy to them" (212).

Byock's own assessment of the death of Terry Matthews is clear . . . in a way very clear, though it's also confusing or confused. He will not deny a certain authenticity to her dying. He tells her story very powerfully. Because she died in her own chosen manner, she did, in a sense, "die well." Nevertheless, he will not call "good" a death in which one never lets go, in which life is forcibly taken by the power of death. So he says,

> Terry's was not the way I would choose for a relative or loved one to die. By my personal values, Terry did not die a "good death." Yet how Terry and her family felt, not my values, is what ultimately matters. In this respect, she died well, because she died her way – fighting for life and time with her family. In her dying, she remained true to her spirit and true to her values. It was her way, thus the only way (193).

Surely there is something to such a response; yet if this is where telling stories leads, it may have deleterious consequences for ethical reflection. One of the themes of Byock's book, *Dying Well*, for example, is that euthanasia is never necessary or choiceworthy. Physical suffering can always be relieved, and dying can become the occasion for one last stage of personal growth. Yet, if what counts most is that we each die our own way, true to our values, it is not clear how a judgment against euthanasia can be sustained. Byock does not recommend Terry Matthews's kind of death, but he is willing to stand by her throughout it and do everything he can to care for her – because it is "her way" and "thus the only way." Analogous reasoning might seem to commit him to provide assistance also to those desiring euthanasia – which would undercut one of the themes of his book and, perhaps, undercut the point of the care he has rendered to so many of the suffering dying.

If that is not where we want the argument to lead, we must step back and ask whether there is not something more positive to be said of Terry Matthews's dying. On Ramsey's terms, of course, her rage against the dying of the light, however hard it might be for many of us to emulate and however true it may be that it is not the only acceptable way to die, can be praised. In its appreciation of the moral and personal significance of her embodied life and individuality, her rage and her struggle may manifest a "true humanism." Even on Kass's terms, there is room here for praise. She neither averts her eyes nor refuses to face the music. When the time comes, when she is compelled no longer to avert her eyes, she and her husband tell their children what is soon to happen. She will not regard her death as anything other than an evil, to be sure. Not for her Kass's sense that the death of individuals may contribute to the good of the species. Yet, I think it fair to say that any reader of Byock's chapter ten will conclude that she makes of the occasion of her death an opportunity for the exercise of nobility. And finally, in saying goodbye and accepting sedation when she can bear no more, she gives nature its due. It is a more grudging acknowledgment than Kass might wish – more in the spirit of Ramsey. But it has about it an undeniable nobility that Byock's account captures quite well. As one who had won "the lottery from hell" (215), Terry Matthews seized the occasion to turn outward and die, as Byock says, "with arms open and outstretched toward her family" (212). In that sense, though she would not agree with Kass that death could be an "evil good," she made of it a "good evil."

The death of Maureen (Mo) Riley was very different indeed. For her it was a good and hardly, even, an "evil good." Of her Byock writes,

> Everything this woman did in her dying days reflected not just acceptance of her impending demise, but curiosity, anticipation, and even pleasure. She typified full, rich living through her very last breath. Mo also showed me how someone who is dying can transform herself from a vibrant, loving mother and person living in the world into an almost lofty being of beauty and spirit . . . Mo epitomized a blessedness that comes with letting go of both the burdens and the delights of daily life—ultimately letting go of life itself and willingly slipping into another realm (217).

She is, in short, the very epitome of his notion of "dying well," for hers is a death that takes seriously the possibilities for personal growth in the process of dying. If part of his problem with Terry Matthews's dying was that she focused entirely on "a deeper love for her family" rather than "experiencing a deeper love of self" (212), the same cannot be said of Mo Riley. She, by contrast, seemed "to flow smoothly out of worldly concerns and relationships and toward an ethereal, spiritual state" (218).

Sixty-five years old and retired, with six grown children and also grandchildren, Mo Riley learned that she had "a very fast-growing cancer lodged at the top of her spine and entwining the base of her brain," and was told that she probably had only weeks to live (220). She initially accepted radiation therapy to shrink the tumor and ease her pain. Her twenty-six year old daughter Emily, although seven months pregnant with her own first child, moved back in with her to provide care during her dying, and Mo accepted no further radiation therapy or chemotherapy. She seemed remarkably calm at the thought that she would die soon, showed little inclination to regret anything, and she even felt no strong urge to stay alive long enough to see Emily's child born. "'Actually,' she reflected, 'I've been ready for a while'" (224).

As it turned out, Mo lived longer than her doctors had predicted – some three months, and long enough to see the birth of her granddaughter. When she lost control of her bladder, she accepted with equanimity the fact that Emily had to "change" her as she did the baby. "Out of necessity, Mo had shed her modesty as one might set aside a favorite wool coat for the spring" (228). We could overstate the case, however. Byock does, for example, recount an occasion when she expressed concern about being a burden to her children and was overcome with tears at the thought of what they had to do for her (231). The last time he saw her, only hours before her death, he could still see, however, that "her spirit was strong and soaring" (234). He writes of her: "As much as any patient I have known, Mo personified the possibility of a joy within the process of letting go, transcending this world, and growing into an unexplored, spiritual realm" (234).

Here is one who did not rage against the dying of the light; nevertheless, her case, at least as Byock describes it, demonstrates how complex are the questions we are considering. Mo Riley did not appear to recognize death as an indignity or an enemy. Shall we, therefore, read her death as closer to the model Kass recommends? Perhaps in part, but only in part. The death that is "the natural and necessary accompaniment of life" on Kass's account is one that involves "decay and decline" (75). Consciously following Aristotle at this point, Kass sees human beings as, in this respect, like all living things: built into their life is "a principle of growth *and decay*" (75). And, although Kass would no doubt understand something of what Byock means when he speaks of continued possibilities for growth in dying – Kass himself, after all, sees death as the occasion for display of nobility – the account Byock gives of Mo Riley's death does not seem to make much place for decay and decline.

> At the edge of the transcendent – in the midst of "letting go" – a person who has completed the work of development does not disintegrate in dying. Rather, she *dissolves* out of life, becoming increasingly ephemeral – less dense or corporeal – but no less integrated, in the passage from life. Personhood becomes gauzy and translucent (238).

One begins to lose here not only Ramsey's sense that death is an enemy but also Kass's sense of our finitude and materiality. And if not everyone can or does die as Mo did, Byock is clear that becoming "increasingly ephemeral," – less body and more spirit – is, in his view, what it means really to die well.

Thus, at least at certain moments, Byock seems to see death neither (in Kass's terms) as the necessary decline of mortal beings nor (in Ramsey's terms) as the enemy that is the wages of sin. Rather, he sees it in his own particular way. One can only respect the work that Byock does, and he has surely served the well being of many suffering patients. But one would like to know more about the metaphysical underpinnings of what he thinks he sees in death; for ultimately we seek not simply comfort but the comfort of truth. (Although Byock himself is Jewish, I think that any reader of *Dying Well* would conclude that his religious views, or perhaps more accurately, his "spirituality," are decidedly eclectic.) It is not clear, to me at least, why we should be encouraged to seek continued growth – into ephemerality – in our dying. If I would not quite, with Ramsey, brand such exhortations themselves as always an additional "indignity" heaped upon the dying, I think they can be. Terry Matthews rightly recognized an enemy in death, an enemy to her continued "growth" as a human being, and she was not, I think, wrong to fight it.

Byock himself has moments when he seems compelled by the stories themselves to agree. Writing of Janelle Haldeman, a high school girl who suffered from a rare, juvenile onset form of Huntington's chorea, whose mother constantly battled the health care system and the school system on behalf of her daughter, he can say, "Janelle's battles were more directly with her illness, which was an unprincipled, vicious enemy" (120). Perhaps he needs a bit more of this language. Many of the powerful stories recounted in *Dying Well* involve severe pain or the suffering that comes with dementia, and, precisely because they are powerful, they might cause us to wonder whether Kass's vision takes full account of them. Ramsey had noted that advocates of "death with dignity" were not as inclined to speak of "suffering with dignity" or of suffering as simply a natural part of life (48). To this Kass responded, in some ways reasonably enough, that disease and injury are not "as natural, necessary, and inextricably bound up with life as are death or decay" (75). Even in the case of disease, which might seem most natural, he notes that "disease is *fought* by nature working within, whereas decline is *produced* by nature working within" (76).

The contrast between disease and decline is worth our attention. In a finely wrought essay, Lewis Thomas once developed a similar distinction, relying on a poem by Oliver Wendell Holmes. (Lewis Thomas, "The Deacon's Masterpiece," pp. 130-36 in *The Medusa and the Snail* (NY: Viking Press, 1979).) Holmes's poem is about a carriage made by a deacon, and Lewis Thomas used it to distinguish between a life that *breaks down* and a life that *wears out*. The deacon in the poem fashioned his carriage with such care that it was the "perfect organism" – each part as good as all the rest, with no weak link. Had there been a weak link, and had that link broken down, the carriage might have halted prematurely, before its time. But instead, since it never breaks down, the whole gradually wears out. As the poem puts it: "A general flavor of mild decay, / But nothing local, as one may say." Finally, one day, it simply goes to pieces: "All at once, and nothing first." That's decline. This is not Ramsey's vision of death as enemy. It is not Byock's vision of death as transition to ephemeral spirit. It is, though, quite close to Kass's vision of death as the end-point of decline. And such a vision is not without its attractions.

The problem, though, as the narratives in *Dying Well* make clear, is that many of us will not die this way: "A general flavor of mild decay, / But nothing local, as one may say." In chapter after chapter Byock tells us of patients who wrestle with dementia, ALS or MS, pancreatic, colon, or lung cancer, AIDS ... the list, of course, knows no real end. In the face of these narratives we may need to choose between death as enemy or death as transition to ephemeral spirit, between raging against the dying of the light that is death or encouraging growth and progress throughout the process of dying. Kass's vision, powerful and appealing as it may be, helpful as it is in certain instances, will not do justice to what we see in these stories. And we seem left with Ramsey or Byock.

Perhaps I need to qualify that claim. In the face of great suffering, the patients depicted in *Dying Well* do often claim for themselves a measure of nobility. To that extent Kass remains on target: dying can be the occasion for the display of much that is praiseworthy and noble. But it is an awful price some of these patients pay for that opportunity, and I am not sure many of us would wish for the chance to be quite this heroic. Moreover, the nobility displayed by these patients seems to depend in part precisely on the viciousness of the "enemy" they face. They are not just dealing with "decay and decline."

Time after time throughout his book Byock emphasizes that dying is not inherently undignified. What he means by this – namely, that it is possible to provide dying patients with the kind of support they need to retain some sense of their own worth – is generally clear. Thus, for example, he writes:

> Dignity is important to everyone, but especially to someone who is dying and has already begun losing control over much of his life. And while many people think of dignity in terms of appearance, independence, and personal embarrassment, people close to a dying patient seem to know intuitively that their loved one's dignity does not

depend on these. Dying is not inherently undignified, it is
simply part of being human. With supportive family and
friends, even needing help with basic bodily functions need
not diminish dignity (72).

In thinking of death as part of life, Byock here is like Kass. In seeing
that personal dignity should not depend on control or independence,
he is not unlike Ramsey, for whom human dignity is essentially an
alien dignity bestowed by God.

Exactly how Byock holds these several emphases together is
not always clear. In one, quite simple, sense we may say that he
always looks for goals that the dying person can meet, tasks that can
still be undertaken – if only, on occasion, the task of allowing others
the satisfaction of caring for oneself. More centrally, though I think
more problematically, he often seems to ground dignity in "the
remarkable achievements in personal growth that can occur while
someone is dying" (86). Yet, he looks for dignity even in the stories
of patients who do not really seem to achieve the kind of growth he
praises. And he is tenacious in looking for this dignity. Hence, his
narratives seem themselves to press us beyond his own conceptual
scheme – they seem to press us toward a dignity that is bestowed
rather than achieved. But the conceptual resources needed to develop
such a notion are not really on display in *Dying Well* – and one
wonders, therefore, whether the practices of care to which Byock is
committed can be sustained indefinitely without a firmer grounding.

THE ART OF DYING? OR OVERCOMING DEATH?

To recapitulate: I began with two views of death: as an enemy
to be opposed or as the end-point of natural human decline, to be
accepted with as much dignity and nobility as we can muster. I then
considered Byock's stories of dying patients within the framework of
these alternatives. His stories suggest, at least to this reader, that we
should not – and perhaps cannot – look at death with quite the
equanimity that Kass's view intimates. Dying as many people
experience it is not just the result of the decline and decay that are
natural for living organisms. What they experience in their dying is

something more like an assault upon the integrity of their person. (And in facing that assault they are, in many respects, fortunate to have Byock at their side.) This much, perhaps, we can say at a purely phenomenological level – without importing too much by way of metaphysical baggage.

But that is what they experience "in their dying." With respect to death itself, however, Byock and Kass may not be too far apart. Neither sees it as an enemy, as a loss which, in Ramsey's terms, "no human agency can alleviate." For Kass, it would be strange to talk of alleviating what is inherent in our nature and perhaps necessary for the display of our nobility. For Byock, it would be strange to speak of such grief in connection with a moment so rich in possibilities for personal growth. For Ramsey, by contrast, our ultimate problem is not dying but death. Death assaults our person, in part, precisely because we are not ephemeral beings but bodies with location and attachments. Death assaults our person, in still larger measure, because we are "apart and not [simply] a part" of the natural world. As self – transcending creatures made for God, we experience "dis-ease in dying," however commonplace and "natural" death may seem to be.

If that is true – and here we must decide what metaphysical baggage we want to carry – then we do indeed, as Ramsey put it, heap additional indignities on the dying if, in our care, we do not penetrate to a problem even deeper than dying – the indignity of death itself. Powerful as Byock's narratives are, they are told by one who is still among us, and they are therefore confined to the experience of dying. None of the subjects of these stories can come back to tell us about death itself. That is not within the scope of human possibilities, and our judgment about the meaning of death inevitably draws us beyond the limits and terrain of such stories. At least it must if we want to pay as much attention to death as to dying.

I conclude that Ramsey had his sights set on something very important: namely, that death, not just dying, is an enemy that assaults us. This, in turn, means that Terry Matthews cannot have been simply wrong to rage, as she did, against the dying of the light – and I trust that my account of Byock's stories has made clear my admiration for her "reluctance to leave." This does not mean, however, that we should simply affirm her attitude toward death. Byock says, "Life had to be plucked from Terry." But perhaps there should sometimes come a point at which – without denying that there is grief in death that "no human agency can alleviate" – we should cease to oppose our death or that of another. If the "dis-ease" that we experience in dying is rooted, finally, in the fact that we are made for God, then God must constitute the limit to our struggle against death. It must be death that we oppose – not God. "There are two attitudes towards Death," C.S. Lewis once wrote, "which the human mind naturally adopts."

> One is the lofty view, which reached its greatest intensity among the Stoics, that Death "doesn't matter," that it is "kind nature's signal for retreat," and that we ought to regard it with indifference. The other is the "natural point of view, . . . that Death is the greatest of all evils . . .. The first idea simply negates, the second simply affirms, our instinct for self-preservation; neither throws any new light on Nature, and Christianity countenances neither. Its doctrine is subtler. On the one hand Death is the triumph of Satan, the punishment of the Fall, and the last enemy . . .. On the other hand, only he who loses his life will save it. We are baptized into the *death* of Christ, and it is the remedy for the Fall. Death is . . . the thing Christ came to conquer and the means by which he conquered. (C.S. Lewis, *Miracles* (NY: Macmillan, 1947), pp. 129-30.)

Thus, death is never to be embraced – because it is an evil. But it must sometimes be acknowledged – because it is not the greatest evil.

"What madness it is," St. Augustine writes, in his famous account of the death of a friend, "not to know how to love men as they should be loved." (*Confessions*, IV, 7.) (It was Richard Miller who, in discussion of an earlier version of this paper, first pointed out to me the relevance for my analysis of Augustine's treatment of the proper way to love temporal goods, and I thank him for the insight.) Which means: as creatures – genuine goods, but not the highest good. Augustine says, "The good that you love is from Him; but its goodness and sweetness is only because you are looking toward Him;

it will rightly turn to bitterness if what is from Him is wrongly loved, He himself being left out of the account." (*Confessions*, IV, 12.) How must we think if we do not leave God "out of the account"?

We should remember that Paul Ramsey's assertion of "the indignity of 'death with dignity'" was quite self-consciously put forward not as the whole truth but as a correction. At the outset of his essay Ramsey notes that he himself, only a few years earlier in his book *The Patient as Person*, had argued that our responsibility to care for the dying should lead to "the acceptance of death, stopping our medical interventions for all sorts of good, human reasons, *only* companying with the dying in their final passage" (47). Suddenly, however, it seemed to him "that altogether too many people were agreeing with me" (47). They had grabbed hold of only one half of his view – thereby distorting it and heaping new indignities upon the dying with their talk of death as natural, or as friend, or perhaps, as the occasion for personal growth, or even as something beautiful.

In chapter three of *The Patient as Person*, a treatment that remains one of the classics of bioethics literature, Ramsey had characterized our obligation toward the dying as one of "(only) caring." That is, faithfulness to patients requires that we never cease in our efforts to care for them, while recognizing that at some point proper care means precisely ceasing from efforts any longer to cure disease or to struggle against death. And Ramsey then depicted "two opposite extremes" from which this morality of caring (but only caring) for the dying would be resisted. (Paul Ramsey, *The Patient as Person* (New Haven and London: Yale University Press, 1970), pp. 144-57.) Some would argue that if death could sometimes rightly be acknowledged, it should also sometimes be chosen and sought as a good thing. Others would argue that if death was an evil to be opposed, it should never be acknowledged or accepted. For the first, death might actually be, not an enemy, but a good. For the second, death became not just an evil, but the greatest evil, and life not just a good, but the greatest good.

Insofar, then, as Mo Riley seems (on Byock's account) to embrace, and not merely acknowledge, death, she is wrong to do so. Insofar as Terry Matthews seems (on Byock's account) to embrace temporal life not just as a creaturely good but as the greatest good, she is wrong to do so. Which mistake is the more serious? That is probably a question we cannot answer without a context. The more serious mistake is the one to which our culture is more drawn and by which we are tempted at any given moment. Judged in that light, I must say that our present temptation is to welcome and embrace death – to view it as a good to be seized and sought. We should be clear that Byock does not exactly recommend that, since, for example, he so clearly sets himself against the practice of euthanasia. Nonetheless, his stories may draw us in a direction he does not anticipate unless we are more self-conscious than he is about the background beliefs that shape our understanding of death and dying.

The question, finally, that is raised by looking at Byock's narratives in the light of the Ramsey/Kass exchange is this: Can a vision that pictures dying as "a part of full, even healthy, living" sustain over time the sense that care for the dying is "a valuable part of the life of the community" (246). If death is simply "a part" of life, and the individual who dies "a part" of the natural cycle of living and dying, it may be harder than we suppose to retain the sense that the human being who dies is "apart" from all natural cycles and quite properly experiences dis-ease when facing death. It is that dis-ease, the sense that we do stand "apart" from the natural world that best captures our individuality. It teaches us that the dying person can never be replaced and that, therefore, death blots out an utterly unique individual. If hospice were to teach us too readily to accept another's death, we might learn lessons that could not easily be unlearned. We have, therefore, good reason not simply to reflect on stories of the dying but to contemplate how the meaning of the stories may depend in good part upon the moral vision we bring to the reading of them. We have good reason not merely to try to master the art of dying, but also to reflect upon the meaning of death – even if, in such reflection, we run up against the limits of human possibilities.

Response to DEATH AND DIGNITY: "APART AND NOT A PART"

M. Cathleen Kaveny

INTRODUCTION

Toward the end of his rich and provocative essay, Gilbert Meilaender quotes a passage from C.S. Lewis that captures the common Christian understanding of the meaning of death, as it stands in counterpoint to the prevailing alternatives:

> There are two attitudes toward Death which the human mind naturally adopts. One is the lofty view, which reached its greatest intensity among the Stoics, that Death "doesn't matter," that it is "kind nature's signal for retreat," and that we ought to regard it with indifference. The other is the "natural point of view . . . that Death is the greatest of all evils . . .. The first idea simply negates, the second simply affirms, our instinct for self-preservation; neither throws any new light on Nature, and Christianity countenances neither. Its doctrine is subtler. On the one hand Death is the triumph of Satan, the punishment of the Fall, and the last enemy. . . on the other hand, only he who loses his life will save it. We are baptized into the death of Christ, and it is the remedy for the Fall. Death is . . . the thing Christ came to conquer and the means by which he conquered. (C.S. Lewis, *Miracles* (New York: Macmillan, 1947) 129-30.)

Meilaender describes the general practical implications of this common Christian meaning of death in the following way: "Death is never to be embraced – because it is an evil. But it sometimes must be acknowledged – because it is not the greatest evil". Where, however, do we move from this generalization? What, concretely, would it mean for Christians to "acknowledge" death while refusing to "embrace" it? How, exactly, should Christians situate their stance on the meaning of death with respect to the diametrically opposed views of death described by Lewis as natural for human beings to adopt? What difference does the death and resurrection of Christ make?

The answer we give to these questions is very much shaped by the particular Christian tradition to which we belong. On the one hand, we could understand the task of a Christian ethicist as insuring that the two opposing natural views of death remain in dialectical tension, not as charting a *via media* between them. Here the task of the Christian ethicist would be to intervene to support one side of the tension if it appears that the other is gaining too much power in a particular time and place. On the other hand, we could understand the task of Christian ethics as helping to reduce, if not resolve, the tension between the two natural extremes, transforming them both in light of the good news of the gospel. Rather than insuring that both poles are preserved in their oppositional purity, we might attempt to reshape the sharpest edges of each in an effort to formulate a "middle" position that is permeated by the Christian understanding of salvation history.

Meilaender's essay in this volume exemplifies the first approach, which is a characteristically Lutheran way of formulating and addressing ethical questions. In contrast, the second approach is embodied in the Roman Catholic casuistical method of medical-moral decision making, particularly its distinction between ordinary (proportionate) and extraordinary (disproportionate) means of medical treatment. The differences between the Lutheran and the Roman Catholic approaches to the theological ethics surrounding death and dying stem largely from differing theological sensibilities and the methods and rhetoric they generate; they do not necessarily reflect differences of bedrock moral or theological commitment. In my view, each demonstrates particular strength in addressing some aspects of the neuralgic contemporary discussion of end of life decision-making, while proving less helpful with respect to other aspects.   I will elaborate on these points in the remainder of the response.

LUTHERAN DIALECTICS

At risk of oversimplification, let me suggest that dialectical tension is a leitmotif of a Lutheran approach ethics.   The great twentieth century Lutheran theologian Helmut Thielicke suggests that the Christian life is encapsulated in the cry "Lord, I believe, help thou my unbelief." Christians are always *simul iustus et peccator*; at one and the same time sinners, and justified by the grace of Christ. We are driven by the law to recognize our own unworthiness, and our inability to overcome that unworthiness on our own; we are saved from utter despair by the saving word of the gospel, which assures of God's free and unconditional mercy toward us sinners. Yet justified sinners cannot do without law; its continued force insures that we do not distort the Good News, drawing from it the mistaken belief that we have improved enough to do without God's grace. (Helmut Thielicke, *Theological Ethics* (vol. 1): *Foundations*, ed. William H. Lazareth. (Philadelphia: Fortress Press, 1966), p. 95.) For Thielicke, the dialectical character of the relationship between the two cannot be overcome; it reflects the two irreducible aspects of God's relationship to humanity: God appears to us both as judge and as savior; we cannot seek to formulate a middle way without eventually falling into a monism that either denies the power of God's grace by focusing exclusively on our shortcomings, or downplays the gravity of sin by too quickly moving toward salvation as a happy ending.   Thus Christians live in the tension between law and gospel, propelled from one pole to the other and then back again.

For Lutheran theologians, the dialectical tension relationship between law and gospel is reflected in a dialectical approach to moral questions in general. It is evident in Meilaender's essay "Death and Dignity." More specifically, he develops his position with reference to the two diametrically opposed views of death that C.S. Lewis believes human beings naturally develop: 1) death as a friend, or at the very least, something to which we should be indifferent; and 2) death as the greatest enemy.   Meilaender's basic worry is that our efforts to make navigating the passage of dying easier through the hospice movement and experimentation with physician-assisted suicide, have brought contemporary Americans perilously close to the deadly cliffs of death as a friend.   He wonders, for example, whether the view of dying prominent in the hospice movement, which sees it as a part of life presenting the occasion for personal growth, might teach us to accept the death of another human being too easily.   He fears that as a result, "we might learn lessons that could not easily be unlearned."   Ironically, the result of these lessons might be the undoing of the hospice movement itself.   If dying is natural, and we do not find it within ourselves to fight it as an extinction of a unique and irreplaceable person, then why not avoid the whole process and embrace voluntary (and doubtless involuntary) euthanasia?

In order to avoid shipwreck, Meilaender makes a 180 degree turn away from the cliffs of death as a friend – and heads directly toward the land of death as the enemy.   He does not engage in the risky behavior of negotiating the rocky waters of the nearer shore in order to find and preserve its good elements; here, at least, his style is self-consciously oppositional.   In fact, in developing his position, Meilaender draws upon the most oppositional piece written by Paul Ramsey on the topic, entitled "The Indignity of Dignity."   (Paul Ramsey, "The Indignity of Death With Dignity," *Hastings Center Studies* 2 (May 1974) 47-62.)   Ramsey quotes, and Meilaender reiterates, Dylan Thomas's famous lines, "Do not go gentle into that good night. . . . Rage, rage, against the dying of the light."   He also emphasizes the fundamental reasons that Ramsey believes death – not just dying – to violate our nature as human beings in a most fundamental way.   First, because death wrenches body from soul, death undermines our nature as psychosomatic unities of body and soul.   Second, because death extinguishes the presence among us of a unique and irreplaceable human person, it contradicts our identity as children of God – as beings made for and called to communion with God in all our particularity.   Our dignity consists in these two elements, which renders us "apart" from nature, rather than making us "a part" of it.

Meilaender is quite right about the general tendency of our culture to sail far too closely to the land of "death as a friend," particularly when it appears in the form of medically managed death such as physician assisted suicide or voluntary euthanasia. As he recognizes, at the cultural level, the struggle is over the fundamental values that inform case-by-case decision making. In discussing the views of Ramsey and Leon Kass on the meaning of death, he rightly observes, "there is no way to read the differences between Ramsey and Kass apart from their differences in worldview." The priority that we Americans give to autonomous self-determination, the unwillingness we have to become dependent upon another, particularly for basic care, and the high costs we incur in caring for those who are frail, old, or ill means has meant that dying (in the right manner) looks better than living to many of us in an increasingly large number of situations. In order to address this multifaceted cultural problem effectively, we need a clear and prophetic call to reaffirm the value of human life, not the finely honed casuistical analysis characteristic of Roman Catholic medical ethics. A firm course toward the other pole of "death as the enemy," propelled by the eloquent words of Dylan Thomas, Paul Ramsey, and Gilbert Meilaender on the indignity of death, is urgently required as a cultural corrective. This is the great contribution of a Lutheran approach to ethics.

By the same token, however, this approach is less successful in dealing with particular cases in which particular individuals must make decisions about the course that their own dying will take. More specifically, I suggest that the core of human dignity that Meilaender is so rightly concerned to protect, which is bound up with the uniqueness of each person, is in fact undermined by his attempts to evaluate particular examples of end-of-life decision making in terms of the dialectic between death as a friend and death as an enemy. A closer examination of Meilaender's treatment of two cases discussed in *Dying Well: The Prospect for Growth at the End of Life*, authored by hospice physician Ira Byock, will illustrate my point.

Terry Matthews, a young mother of three small children, fought her death from cancer until the bitter end, tolerating what Dr. Boyock describes as "unbearable pain" in order to snatch more time with her family. Thirty hours before her death, when she could no longer bear it, she said good-bye to her family and agreed to terminal sedation. In contrast, Mo Riley, a sixty-five year old mother of grown children, did not rage against the dying of the light. Instead, she appeared "to flow smoothly out of worldly concerns and relationships toward an ethereal. spiritual, state." (Ira Byock, *Dying Well, The Prospect for Growth at the End of Life* (New York: Riverhead Books, 1997) 218.) Meilaender worries that Byock ultimately regards Terry's death as a "bad death," and Mo's death as a "good death," although he concedes that Byock acknowledge that each woman died well because she died in her chosen way, in a way that fit the circumstances of her life.

In contrast, Meilaender tends toward the opposite view in evaluating the deaths of the two women. He is concerned, for example, that Byock resists calling Terry's death "good," because her life was taken forcibly from her by the power of death. He is also less enthusiastic than Byock about the manner of Mo's death. According to Byock, she "epitomized a blessedness that comes with letting go of both the burdens and the delights of daily life – ultimately letting go of life itself and willingly slipping into another realm." (Byock, 217.) Meilaender fears that Mo's gentle slide from this world into the next does not take proper account of death's nature as an implacable enemy to our embodiment, to our individuality. He writes, "it is not clear, to me at least, why we should be encouraged to seek continued growth – into ephemerality – in our dying."

What ultimately drives Meilaender's judgments about these two cases? Ironically, it is not the facts and circumstances of each woman's journey through her own unique dying process, but the way in which the basic choices they make with respect to her death affect the broader and more abstract values of uniqueness and dignity. The particularities of the lives of these two women, each dying in very different circumstances, are ultimately irrelevant to him; what in the end is decisive for Meilaender is how the manner in which they die – and Byock's account of it – affects the contemporary cultural battle over the meaning of death. In the end, he asks us to interpret each dying woman as if she is exercising a fundamental option about the meaning of death. Meilaender writes, "in the face of these narratives, we may need to choose between death as enemy or death as transition to ephemeral spirit, between raging against the dying of the light that is death or encouraging growth and progress throughout the process of dying." But why do we need to choose? Each of these women knows that she is dying. Neither has any chance of living free of illness, or living very long at all. Why can't we see both women as making decisions about how long and how hard to fight the inevitable in light of their own particular circumstances, including the needs of their families?

Meilaender acknowledges that going too far in either direction is a mistake; at the end of the essay, he admits that Terry might have resisted death too fiercely, while Mo might not have fought hard enough. In a telling move, he goes to ask, "Which mistake is the more serious?" Meilaender begins his reply by acknowledging that "this is a question we cannot answer without a context." Unfortunately, however, the context he points to is not the one specific to each woman's life, but the broader social context in which they are living and dying: "The more serious mistake is the one to which our culture is more drawn and by which we are tempted at any given moment. Judged in that light, I must say that our present temptation is to welcome and embrace death – to view it as a good to be seized and sought." But why is the broader cultural situation the context for determining either the existence or the seriousness of a mistake? In making those determinations, shouldn't we take into account the particular situation of each dying woman, as well as her own unique challenges and temptations? Despite his emphasis on the importance of individuality and dignity, I fear that in the end, Meilaender reduces the particular deaths of Terry Matthews and Mo Riley to their symbolic value in the contemporary culture wars.

ROMAN CATHOLIC CASUISTRY

Is there another way to address end-of-life decision making in particular cases that also "acknowledges" death without "embracing" it? In my view, this is the sphere in which the Roman Catholic tradition of moral analysis can offer the most help. In contrast to Lutheranism, which moves dialectically between the two poles of death as friend and death as enemy, the Catholic traditions tries to formulate an integrated approach that incorporates the (partial) truths found at both poles, while avoiding the falsehoods and exaggerations of each. It offers a more promising way to honor the uniqueness of each dying person, precisely it directs us to apply general norms to concrete situations in a fashion that takes account of individual differences.

The Catholic casuistical tradition pays attention both to what human beings have in common and to what distinguishes us from one another. Certain courses of action, such as physician-assisted suicide and euthanasia, are ruled out from the start, because they are inconsistent with respect for human dignity. The focus here is on the agent's intention in acting, not the full range of consequences that she foresees her action will bring about. There is no way that anyone can act with the intention of bringing about the death of a dying person without denigrating the value of her earthly life (which encompasses the course of her dying) and undermining her dignity. This negative prohibition insures that no one sets a course too close to the shores of death as a friend. More importantly, it reminds believers that their decision-making is best construed as discernment of God's will, rather than completely autonomous self-determination. It both expresses and anchors the idea that human beings do not exercise complete dominion over their lives, but are stewards whose scope of decision-making is real, but limited.

Precisely because it has so firmly ruled out intentional killing of the dying, the Catholic tradition can give a wide scope to individual discernment regarding the means used to preserve life in particular cases, without fear of eroding the dignity of each person. Accordingly, it does not require patients to avail themselves of each measure designed to preserve their lives; they are required to use ordinary (proportionate) means, but can omit extraordinary (disproportionate) ones. On a general level, this distinction is designed to guide individual patients in determining what counts as "acknowledging" death while refusing to "embrace" it in their own situations. For example, the *Ethical and Religious Directives for Catholic Health Care Services* define ordinary (proportionate) means are "those that in the judgment of the patient offer a reasonable hope of benefit and do not entail an excessive burden, or impose excessive expense on the family or the community." Conversely, extraordinary (disproportionate) means as "those that in the patient's judgment do not offer a reasonable hope of benefit or entail an excessive burden, or impose excessive expense on the family or the community." (National Conference of Catholic Bishops, *Ethical and Religious Directives for Catholic Health Care Services* (Washington, D.C.: United States Catholic Conference, 1995) §§ 55-56.)

The tradition has been extremely sensitive to the fact that individuals face death in very different circumstances, with very different strengths and weaknesses. Not everyone can bear the same level of physical pain. Not everyone is as able to tolerate the same level of risk of success or failure. Not everyone is at the same stage of life, with the same set of practical familial and social responsibilities to be fulfilled before death. Nor do we all have the same amount of spiritual work to do before dying; the tasks of reflecting on our lives, repairing strained bonds with one and other, and deepening our relationship with God may loom larger in some cases than others. What is a disproportionate means for a person who has met all of these responsibilities may, all other things being equal, be a proportionate means for one who has not yet done so.

It is also true that the Catholic view of death is in some sense more hopeful than that advocated by Meilaender in this essay. Acknowledging death is not simply a matter of acknowledging defeat. This not because the Catholic view falls closer to the "death as friend" pole of the dichotomy than it does to the "death as enemy" pole, but because it transforms the whole relationship between the two in light of salvation history. In essence, it adds an entirely new dimension to the question. The Catechism of the Catholic Church observes that:

> [B]ecause of Christ, Christian death has a positive meaning:
> "For to me to live is Christ, and to die is gain." "The saying
> is sure: if we have died with him, we will also live with
> him." What is essentially new about Christian death is this:
> through Baptism, the Christian has already "died with
> Christ"sacramentally, in order to live a new life; and if we
> die in Christ's grace, physical death completes this "dying
> with Christ" and so completes our incorporation into him in
> his redeeming act." (*Catechism of the Catholic Church*
> (New York: Doubleday (An Image Book), 1995 § 1010.)

The positive meaning of death that the Catechism speaks of is not detached from death's darker aspects. In fact, it is inseparable from it, and in some sense grounded in it, because it is realized by those who unite themselves to Christ's suffering and death – and through them, to his resurrection. The last words in Meilaender's quotation from C.S. Lewis, with which I began this essay, point to the same insight. Lewis writes: "We are baptized into the *death* of Christ, and it is the remedy for the Fall. Death is . . . the thing Christ came to conquer and the means by which he conquered." Ultimately, the casuistry is integrated by this theological vision, enabling it to exert its power in the messy details of concrete cases.

The Catholic casuistical approach, I think, allows us to honor the uniqueness of Terry and Mo, by taking account of the very different circumstances under which they confronted their respective deaths. Terry seems to have discerned that her vocation as a mother called her to bear the unbearable pain in order to impress upon her children her unconditional love for them; the cancer forced her to compress a lifetime of maternal love into a cruelly short period of time. In contrast, Mo had already raised her children; there was no danger that they would experience her death as abandonment. She discerned that her work in this life was essentially done. In religious terms, she might have described her situation not by saying that she saw nothing of value in this life, but that she perceived that God was now calling her to friendship with him in the next.

For Meilaender, the imperative of affirming the indignity of death in a culture that is far too taken with its countenance presses him to downplay the significant differences between the deaths of Terry and Mo. In contrast, at the bedside, the Catholic casuistical tradition gives priority to the recognition that God calls every person by name to die and rise again in Christ, each in our own particular way. It understands its task as formulating an approach to end-of-life decision-making that acknowledges what is true from each pole of the death as friend / death as enemy dichotomy, while situating everything within the context of God's loving and saving will. Within this integrated framework, it can find more room to acknowledge these differences in particular cases without fear of tipping the overall balance in either direction.

CONCLUSION

On October 31, 1999, the Lutheran and Roman Catholic Churches took an important step toward unity by signing a *Joint Declaration on the Doctrine of Justification*, (available on the Vatican's website at http://www.vatican.va/ roman_curia/p...cath-luth-joint-declaration_en.html) in which each church withdrew its sixteenth century condemnations of the other with respect to the doctrine of justification. In so doing, the Joint Declaration both reflected and gave new impetus to ecumenism, encouraging Lutherans and Catholics to continue to learn from each other's traditions. In my view, Pope John Paul II's encyclical *Evangelium Vitae* incorporates with great effectiveness the dialectical style of Lutheran moral reflection. In a striking step outside traditional Catholic discourse on medical-moral matters, the encyclical functions as an exercise in cultural criticism; it does not offer a close analysis of particular cases. The Pope writes to challenge a social context in which "we are facing an enormous and dramatic clash between good and evil, death and life, the 'culture of death' and the 'culture of life.'" (Pope John Paull II, *Evangelium Vitae* (Boston: Pauline Books and Meida, 1995) ¶ 28.) In its effort to expose and counteract the distortions in the broad social value system, the encyclical resonates strongly with the themes of Meilaender's essay, as well as those found in Paul Ramsey's "The Indignity of Death with Dignity."

By the same token, Protestant theologians have incorporated aspects of Roman Catholic thought into their work. In both *The Patient as Person* (New Haven: Yale University Press, 1970) and *Ethics at the Edges of Life* (New Haven: Yale University Press, 1978), Paul Ramsey draws upon the Catholic casuistical tradition to explore the meaning of covenant fidelity with respect to dying patients. As Meilaender himself describes it in another essay, Ramsey here develops and applies "love's casuistry." ("Love's Casuistry: Paul Ramsey on Caring for the Terminally Ill," *The Journal of Religious Ethics* 19:2 (Fall 1991): 1330-56.) No doubt Ramsey's Protestant theological sensibilities, lead him to use that casuistry in ways that differs from the Catholics engaged in the same project. One can argue, as Meilaender has done, about the degree to which the changing cultural context affected the content of Ramsey's casuistry from one book to the next. The key point, however, is that in making decisions about what life-prolonging treatment to provide to particular patients, he never wavered from his call for attention to concrete circumstances of individual patients. By its very nature, "love's casuistry" cannot subordinate the call to care for a human being in the unique course of her dying into an abstract and symbolic defense of a principle – even the principle of love itself.